Pediatric Oncology

Editors

JENNIFER H. ALDRINK
ROSHNI DASGUPTA

SURGICAL ONCOLOGY CLINICS OF NORTH AMERICA

www.surgonc.theclinics.com

Consulting Editor
TIMOTHY M. PAWLIK

October 2026 • Volume 35 • Number 4

ELSEVIER

1818 Market Street • Suite 3323 • Philadelphia, Pennsylvania, 19103-2899

http://www.theclinics.com

SURGICAL ONCOLOGY CLINICS OF NORTH AMERICA Volume 35, Number 4
October 2026 ISSN 1055-3207, ISBN-13: 978-0-443-43228-6

Editor: Megan Ashdown (m.ashdown@elsevier.com)
Developmental Editor: Malvika Shah

Publishing Office: *Surgical Oncology Clinics of North America* (ISSN 1055-3207) is published quarterly by Elsevier Inc., 1818 Market Street, Philadelphia, PA 19103, United States. Periodicals postage paid at New York, NY and additional mailing offices. USA POSTMASTER: Send address changes to *Surgical Oncology Clinics of North America*, Elsevier Customer Service Department, 3251 Riverport Lane, Maryland Heights, MO 63043, USA Months of publication are January, April, July, and October. Subscription prices are $351.00 per year (US individuals), $100.00 (US student/resident), $393.00 (Canadian individuals), $100.00 (Canadian student/resident), $509.00 (foreign individuals), and $205.00 (foreign student/resident). For institutional access pricing please contact Customer Service via the contact information below. Foreign air speed delivery is included in all *Clinics* subscription prices. All prices are subject to change without notice. Orders, claims, and journal inquiries: Please visit our Support Hub page https://service.elsevier.com for assistance.

Reprints. For copies of 100 or more, of articles in this publication, please contact the Commercial Reprints Department, Elsevier Inc., 360 Park Avenue South, New York, New York 10010-1710. Tel. 212-633-3874; Fax: 212-633-3820; E-mail: reprints@elsevier.com.

Surgical Oncology Clinics of North America is covered in *MEDLINE/PubMed (Index Medicus) and EMBASE/Excerpta Medica, Current Contents/Clinical Medicine, and ISI/BIOMED.*

Contributors

CONSULTING EDITOR

TIMOTHY M. PAWLIK, MD, PhD, MPH, MTS, MBA, FACS, FSSO, FRACS (Hon)
Professor and Chair, Department of Surgery; The Urban Meyer III and Shelley Meyer Chair for Cancer Research; Professor of Surgery, Oncology, and Health Services Management and Policy; Surgeon in Chief; The Ohio State University, Wexner Medical Center, Columbus, Ohio

EDITORS

JENNIFER H. ALDRINK, MD
Professor of Clinical Surgery and Pediatrics, Division of Pediatric Surgery, Department of Surgery, Director of Surgical Oncology, Nationwide Children's Hospital, The Ohio State University College of Medicine, Columbus, Ohio, USA

ROSHNI DASGUPTA, MD, MPH
Professor of Surgery, University of Cincinnati College of Medicine, Pediatric Surgeon, Division of General and Thoracic Surgery, Directory of Surgical Oncology, Cincinnati Children's Hospital Medical Center, University of Cincinnati, Cincinnati, Ohio, USA

AUTHORS

JENNIFER H. ALDRINK, MD
Professor of Clinical Surgery and Pediatrics, Division of Pediatric Surgery, Department of Surgery, Director of Surgical Oncology, Nationwide Children's Hospital, The Ohio State University College of Medicine, Columbus, Ohio, USA

ERICA C. ARNOLD, MD
Pediatric Surgical Oncology Research Fellow, Center for Surgical Outcomes Research, Nationwide Children's Hospital, Columbus, Ohio, USA

STEFANO AVANZINI, MD
Consultant Pediatric Surgeon, Pediatric Surgery Department, IRCCS Istituto Giannina Gaslini, Genova, Italy

ODION BINITIE, MD
Assistant Member, Department of Sarcoma, Moffitt Cancer Center, Tampa, Florida, USA

THOMAS BLANC, MD, PhD, FEAPU
Professor of Pediatric Surgery, Department of Paediatric Urology, Paediatric Surgery and Transplantation, Hôpital Necker-Enfants Malades, Assistance Publique-Hôpitaux de Paris, Université Paris Cité, Paris, France

ERIN G. BROWN, MD
Associate Professor, Division of Pediatric Surgery, UC Davis Medical Center, Sacramento, California, USA

AMANDA BUCHANAN, MD
Associate Professor of Urology, Chief of Pediatric Urology, Golisano Children's Hospital, University of Kentucky, Lexington, Kentucky, USA

DANIELLE B. CAMERON, MD, MPH
Assistant Professor, Department of Surgery, Harvard Medical School, Director of Pediatric Surgical Oncology, Division of Pediatric Surgery, Massachusetts General Brigham, Boston, Massachusetts, USA

EMILY CHRISTISON-LAGAY, MD
Associate Professor of Surgery (Pediatrics), Surgical Director, Pediatric Thyroid Center, Division of Pediatric Surgery, Yale School of Medicine, New Haven, Connecticut, USA

NICHOLAS G. COST, MD
Associate Professor, Department of Surgery, Division of Urology, University of Colorado School of Medicine, Co-Director, Surgical Oncology Program, Children's Hospital Colorado, Aurora, Colorado, USA

KRISTINE S. CORKUM, MD
Assistant Professor, Department of Surgery, University of Colorado Anschutz Medical Campus, Director, Fertility Preservation and Reproductive Late Effects Program, Children's Hospital Colorado, Aurora, Colorado, USA

ROSHNI DASGUPTA, MD, MPH
Professor of Surgery, University of Cincinnati College of Medicine, Director of Surgical Oncology, Division of General and Thoracic Surgery, Cincinnati Children's Hospital Medical Center, University of Cincinnati, Cincinnati, Ohio, USA

ANDREW DAVIDOFF, MD, FACS
Chair, Department of Surgery, St. Jude Children's Research Hospital, Memphis, Tennessee, USA

BRYAN J. DICKEN, MD, MSc
Associate Professor, Division of Pediatric Surgery, Stollery Children's Hospital, University of Alberta, Edmonton, Alberta, Canada

BRIAN R. ENGLUM, MD, MHS
Assistant Professor, Division of Pediatric Surgery, Department of Surgery, University of Maryland School of Medicine, Baltimore, Maryland, USA

JOSEPH C. FUSCO, MD, MPH
Assistant Professor, Department of Pediatric Surgery, Monroe Carrel Jr Children's Hospital at Vanderbilt, Nashville, Tennessee, USA

CHRISTA N. GRANT, MD
Associate Professor, Department of Pediatric Surgery, New York Medical College, Maria Fareri Children's Hospital, Westchester Medical Center, Valhalla, New York, USA

RAJUL GUPTA, MD
Fellow, Division of Musculoskeletal Oncology, Nationwide Children's Hospital, Columbus, Ohio, USA

KATE HARRISON, MD
Fellow, Department of Sarcoma, Moffitt Cancer Center, Tampa, Florida, USA

MEERA KOTAGAL, MD, MPH
Associate Professor, Division of Pediatric General and Thoracic Surgery, Department of Surgery, Cincinnati Children's Hospital, University of Cincinnati College of Medicine, Cincinnati, Ohio, USA

LUCAS KRAUEL, MD, PhD, FACS, FEBPS
Associate Professor of Surgery, Pediatric Surgery Department, SJD Barcelona Children's Hospital, Universitat de Barcelona, Barcelona, Spain

DAVE R. LAL, MD, MPH
Professor of Surgery, Chief, Division of Pediatric Surgery, Children's Wisconsin, Medical College of Wisconsin, Milwaukee, Wisconsin, USA

TIMOTHY B. LAUTZ, MD
Assistant Professor, Department of Surgery, Ann & Robert H Lurie Children's Hospital of Chicago, Northwestern University, Chicago, Illinois, USA

HAU D. LE, MD
Associate Professor, Division of Pediatric Surgery, American Family Children's Hospital, University of Wisconsin School of Medicine and Public Health, Madison, Wisconsin, USA

MARCUS M. MALEK, MD
Associate Professor of Surgery, Clinical Director, Division of Pediatric General and Thoracic Surgery, UPMC Children's Hospital of Pittsburgh, Pittsburgh, Pennsylvania, USA

SARA A. MANSFIELD, MD, MS
Assistant Professor, Department of Surgery, Division of Pediatric Surgery, Nationwide Children's Hospital, The Ohio State University College of Medicine, Columbus, Ohio, USA

ANDREW JACKSON MURPHY, MD
Assistant Professor, Division of Pediatric Surgery, Department of Surgery, University of Tennessee Health Science Center, Associate Member, Department of Surgery, St. Jude Children's Research Hospital, Memphis, Tennessee, USA

ERIKA A. NEWMAN, MD, MBA
Chief, Division of Pediatric Surgery, University of Michigan, Ann Arbor, Michigan, USA

NELSON PICHÉ, MD, MSc
Professor, Division of Pediatric Surgery, Centre Hospitalier Universitaire Sainte-Justine, Université de Montréal, Montréal, Québec, Canada

STEPHANIE F. POLITES, MD, MPH
Pediatric Surgeon and Chair, Department of Surgery, Mayo Clinic, Rochester, Minnesota, USA

DANIEL S. RHEE, MD, MPH
Associate Professor, Division of Pediatric Surgery, Department of Surgery, Memorial Sloan Kettering Cancer Center, Baltimore, Maryland, USA

BARRIE S. RICH, MD
Associate Professor, Division of Pediatric Surgery, Cohen Children's Medical Center, Zucker School of Medicine, Northwell/Hofstra, New York, USA

DAVID A. RODEBERG, MD
Professor, Department of Surgery, Chief, Division of Pediatric Surgery, Kentucky Children's Hospital, Lexington, Kentucky, USA

JOSÉLIO RODRIGUES DE OLIVEIRA FILHO, MD
Postdoctoral Research Fellow, Division of Pediatric Surgery, Department of Surgery, Harvard Medical School, Massachusetts General Brigham, Boston, Massachusetts, USA

JOHN C. ROUTH, MD, MPH
Associate Professor of Surgery, Pediatrics and Population Health Sciences, Pediatric Urologist, Chief of Children's Surgery, Duke University School of Medicine, Durham, North Carolina, USA

ERIN E. ROWELL, MD
Professor, Department of Surgery, Northwestern Feinberg School of Medicine, Director, Fertility and Hormone Preservation and Restoration Program, Ann & Robert H. Lurie Children's Hospital of Chicago, Chicago, Illinois, USA

TERESA SANTIAGO, MD
Associate Member, Department of Pathology, St. Jude Children's Research Hospital, Memphis, Tennessee, USA

THOMAS J. SCHARSCHMIDT, MD
Professor, Division of Musculoskeletal Oncology, Nationwide Children's Hospital, The Ohio State University, Columbus, Ohio, USA

SOPHIA M.V. SCHERMERHORN, MD, MPH
Research Fellow, Department of Pediatric General and Thoracic Surgery, Cincinnati Children's Hospital Medical Center, University of Cincinnati College of Medicine, Cincinnati, Ohio, USA

SHAHAB SHAFFIEY, MD, MSc
Pediatric Surgeon, Department of Pediatric and Thoracic Surgery, Director of Surgical Oncology, Nicklaus Children's Hospital, Miami, Florida, USA

HATIM THAKER, MD
Pediatric Urologist, Department of Urology, Boston Children's Hospital, Boston, Massachusetts, USA

ALIDA F.W. VAN DER STEEG, MD, PhD, MBA
Surgeon, Princess Máxima Center for Pediatric Oncology, Heidelberglaan, Utrecht, Netherlands

BRENT R. WEIL, MD, MPH
Associate Professor, Department of Pediatric Surgery, Boston Children's Hospital, Boston, Massachusetts, USA

Contents

Foreword: Pediatric Oncology xiii

Timothy M. Pawlik

Preface: Pediatric Surgical Oncology xv

Jennifer H. Aldrink and Roshni Dasgupta

Wilms Tumor 695

Andrew Jackson Murphy, Teresa Santiago, and Nicholas G. Cost

Wilms tumor (WT) is the most common pediatric renal malignancy, characterized by triphasic histology and strong links to disrupted kidney development. Advances in molecular profiling and international collaboration have refined risk stratification using histology, stage, and biomarkers. Treatment combines surgery, chemotherapy, and radiation, with protocol differences between Children's Oncology Group (upfront nephrectomy) and International Society of Pediatric Oncology (preoperative chemotherapy). Nephron-sparing surgery is prioritized for bilateral disease to preserve renal function. Despite excellent survival for favorable histology WT, diffuse anaplasia and adverse molecular features require intensified therapy. Emerging trials aim to reduce toxicity while maintaining cure rates.

Neuroblastoma 715

Meera Kotagal, Christa N. Grant, Erin G. Brown, Dave R. Lal, and Erika A. Newman

Neuroblastoma (NB) is the most common extracranial pediatric solid tumor. The most common location for development of NB is in the adrenal glands, but primary tumors may develop along the developmental pathway of neural crest progenitor cells. NB may vary in severity and prognosis from low-risk congenital neuroblastic lesions to aggressive high-risk neuroblastoma. Therapy is risk-based with intensification of therapy for those at greater risk and de-escalation for patients with lower risk tumors. Surgical resection has a critical role in local control of NB for the most optimal outcome.

Management of Rhabdomyosarcoma in Pediatric Patients 731

Sophia M.V. Schermerhorn, John C. Routh, Stephanie F. Polites, and Roshni Dasgupta

Treatment of rhabdomyosarcoma (RMS) involves a multimodality approach, including chemotherapy, surgery, and radiotherapy, while minimizing the long-term treatment-related morbidities. This article outlines the key points related to the diagnosis and management of RMS with a focus on current surgical management of RMS at specific tumor sites. There is a need for improved local control approaches and systemic therapy in RMS to reduce locoregional and metastatic relapse, reduce late sequelae of treatment, and improve functional outcomes. Better understanding of the biology of the RMS subtypes found in adult patients, with increased enrollment into cooperative group studies, is required.

Non-rhabdomyosarcoma Soft Tissue Sarcoma **749**

Daniel S. Rhee and David A. Rodeberg

Non-rhabdomyosarcoma soft tissue sarcomas (NRSTS) is a diverse group of soft tissue sarcomas with a wide range of behavior, presentation, and response to treatment. As most NRSTS are not responsive to chemotherapy, surgery remains the cornerstone of treatment and excellent outcomes for low-risk tumors can be achieved with surgery alone. The prognosis for high-risk, metastatic, or advanced tumors remains poor despite aggressive multi-modal treatment and new treatment modalities are needed. Studying NRSTS as a combined classification in cooperative group trials has been successful in identifying prognostic factors and optimizing treatment strategies for this diverse group of tumors.

Primary Bone Tumors: Osteosarcoma and Ewing Sarcoma **765**

Thomas J. Scharschmidt, Rajul Gupta, Kate Harrison, and Odion Binitie

Substantial recent progress has been made in the management of osteosarcoma and Ewing sarcoma, the most common childhood bone sarcomas. Surgical treatment continues to evolve through navigation, 3D printing, biomaterials, and custom-growing implants. New targeted therapies on the horizon have the potential to achieve a breakthrough improvement in survivorship. Newer radiation modalities, such as proton and carbon-ion radiotherapy, have greater therapeutic potential than conventional photon-beam radiotherapy. This article provides a comprehensive review of common childhood sarcomas and highlights recent advances.

Management of Extracranial Germ Cell Tumors in Pediatric Patients **785**

Brent R. Weil, Hatim Thaker, Bryan J. Dicken, and Barrie S. Rich

This article aims to summarize the fundamentals of pediatric and adolescent extracranial germ cell tumors (GCTs) and to review current best practices regarding surgical and overall management. An understanding of the principles of surgical management of GCTs is critical to ensure optimal outcomes for patients. Details of surgical management vary based on tumor site of origin, but the role of surgery is central to ensuring adequate treatment and staging for tumors of all locations. For pediatric patients, the role of surgery is to maximize chances for disease cure while also maintaining organ function, including future fertility.

Rare Tumors: Part One **801**

Erica C. Arnold, Brian R. Englum, Emily Christison-Lagay, and Jennifer H. Aldrink

Differentiated thyroid carcinoma (DTC) and melanoma are 2 rare cancers seen in pediatric patients. Both pediatric DTC and melanoma present with more advanced disease than their adult counterparts but also have improved long-term outcomes compared to adults. The primary treatment for DTC is surgery with compartment-based lymph node dissection in patients with clinically involved nodes. Wide local excision is the foundation of melanoma treatment, with sentinel lymph node biopsy and completion lymph node dissection based on disease characteristics. For both pediatric melanoma and thyroid carcinoma, molecular testing is an important component for diagnosis, risk stratification, and targeted therapies.

Rare Tumors: Part Two 817

Erica C. Arnold, Josélio Rodrigues de Oliveira Filho, Danielle B. Cameron, and Sara A. Mansfield

Adrenocortical carcinoma (ACC) and colorectal cancer (CRC) are rare tumors that can be seen in pediatric and adolescent patients. Both are associated with underlying cancer predisposition syndromes, most commonly Li-Fraumeni syndrome for ACC and familial adenomatous polyposis and Lynch syndrome for CRC. The mainstay of treatment for these diseases is surgical resection, with chemotherapy and other targeted therapies being used for advanced disease. Pediatric CRC and ACC have distinct molecular characteristics from those of their adult counterparts, and should be managed at specialized centers with a multidisciplinary approach to optimize outcomes.

Surgical Management of Metastatic Pediatric Solid Tumors: Histology-specific Strategies and Multidisciplinary Approaches 831

Shahab Shaffiey and Timothy B. Lautz

Metastatic pediatric solid tumors require tailored surgical approaches guided by tumor histology, treatment response, and multidisciplinary collaboration. This article reviews current strategies for surgical management of metastases across common pediatric cancers, including osteosarcoma, Ewing sarcoma, Wilms tumor, rhabdomyosarcoma, hepatoblastoma, and nonrhabdomyosarcoma soft tissue sarcomas. Emphasis is placed on indications for metastasectomy and the integration of surgery with systemic therapies. Special considerations for extrapulmonary metastases including liver, lymph node, bone, and brain involvement are also addressed. The article underscores the importance of multidisciplinary care to balance aggressive tumor control with preservation of long-term function and reduction of late treatment-related morbidity.

Minimally Invasive Surgery and New Technologies in Pediatric Oncology 847

Lucas Krauel, Stefano Avanzini, Thomas Blanc, and Andrew Davidoff

Minimally invasive surgery (MIS) has become a cornerstone in many areas of pediatric surgery, with proven benefits including reduced postoperative pain, shorter hospitalization, faster return to normal activity, and improved cosmesis. In pediatric surgical oncology, however, the application of MIS has historically been limited by concerns about compromising oncologic principles, the technical challenges posed by small anatomy, and the lack of robust data compared to adult series. Over the past 2 decades, advances in technology, perioperative care, and collaborative research have led to a gradual expansion of indications for MIS in children with solid tumors.

Image-Guided and Fluorescence-Guided Surgery in Pediatric Oncology: Current State of the Art 867

Alida F.W. van der Steeg, Marcus M. Malek, and Joseph C. Fusco

This article reviews the evolving role of image-guided surgery (IGS) and fluorescence-guided surgery (FGS) in pediatric solid tumor surgery. Owing to tumor biology, small anatomy, and the need for organ preservation, pediatric surgical oncology demands exceptional precision. IGS enhances spatial orientation through 3-dimensional modeling, navigation, and augmented reality, while FGS provides real-time functional and molecular visualization of tumors, lymph nodes, and critical structures. The integration of these complementary technologies enables more accurate resections, improved margin control, and reduced morbidity. Emerging advances in artificial intelligence, targeted fluorescent tracers, and multimodal data fusion signal a shift toward personalized, data-driven pediatric surgical oncology.

Fertility Preservation for Children and Adolescents with Cancer **885**

Kristine S. Corkum, Amanda Buchanan, and Erin E. Rowell

Survivors of pediatric cancer are at an increased risk for infertility and premature hormonal failure. Surgeons caring for children with cancer are important advocates for infertility risk assessment and can perform appropriate fertility preservation (FP) procedures. FP options in male individuals and female individuals vary by pubertal status and include nonexperimental (oocyte harvest, ovarian tissue cryopreservation, and sperm cryopreservation) and experimental (testicular tissue cryopreservation) options. This review summarizes infertility risk assessment and FP options, explores important factors in access to pediatric FP, and highlights the current status of FP research.

Pediatric Palliative Surgical Oncology: Principles, Practice, and Evolving Roles **899**

Nelson Piché and Hau D. Le

Pediatric cancer care has changed dramatically over the past several decades, with survival rates increasing to nearly 85% across many childhood malignancies. Yet, despite these advances, children with cancer and their families continue to confront significant physical, emotional, and psychosocial burdens. The expanding role of surgery in both curative and noncurative contexts demands proficiency in operative skill and also in communication, shared decision-making, prognostication, and the delivery of primary palliative care. This article presents a comprehensive, evidence-informed framework for pediatric palliative surgical oncology. We discuss the current literature, guiding principles, and communication models, and ethical complexities unique to pediatric patients.

SURGICAL ONCOLOGY CLINICS OF NORTH AMERICA

FORTHCOMING ISSUES

January 2027
Sarcoma
Ricardo J. Gonzalez, *Editor*

April 2027
Updates in Colorectal Cancer
Gregory D. Kennedy, *Editor*

July 2027
Contemporary Advances in Breast Cancer Management: From Precision Diagnosis to Personalized Treatment
Doreen M. Agnese and Erin E. Burke, *Editors*

RECENT ISSUES

July 2026
Minimally Invasive and Robotic Surgery for Cancer
Melissa E Hogg, *Editor*

April 2026
Immunotherapy for Solid Tumors
Jashodeep Datta, *Editor*

January 2026
Pancreatic Cancer
Kimberly Washington, *Editor*

Foreword

Pediatric Oncology

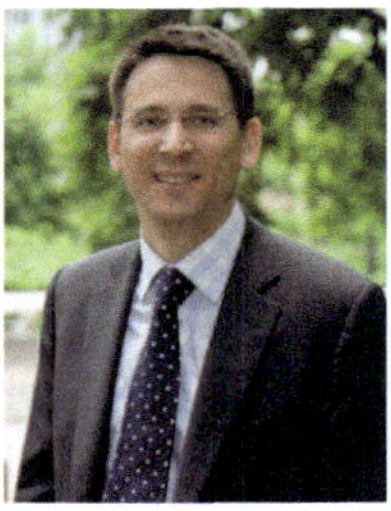

Timothy M. Pawlik, MD, PhD, MPH, MTS, MBA, FACS, FSSO, FRACS (Hon.)
Consulting Editor

This issue of the *Surgical Oncology Clinics of North America* focuses on updates in the surgical management of pediatric malignancies. Pediatric Oncology has evolved over the last century from primarily radical, often palliative operations to a nuanced, multidisciplinary specialty that now can provide oncologic control with preserved organ function and quality of life. Beginning in the early twentieth century and led by William E. Ladd and others, surgical care of children advanced to a more systematic operative approach that paralleled advances in pediatric anesthesia, intensive care, and chemotherapy. More recently, cooperative clinical trials and study groups have increasingly standardized the staging and treatment of cancer in children—significantly improving the outcomes for kids with Wilms tumors, sarcomas, neuroblastoma, and other childhood cancers. Currently, pediatric oncology increasingly focuses on the integration of molecular diagnostics to tailor surgical and medical interventions, and there has been a dramatically greater use of minimally invasive techniques to extirpate malignant lesions while enhancing survivorship and quality of life. In the current issue of *Surgical Oncology Clinics of North America*, our two guest editors, Dr Roshni Dasgupta and Dr Jennifer Aldrink, have put together an amazing collection of expert authors to provide a definitive source of information on pediatric surgical oncology for providers.

Roshni Dasgupta, MD, MPH is a professor with the University of Cincinnati College of Medicine. Dr Dasgupta obtained her medical degree at the University of Toronto. She finished her residency at Massachusetts General Hospital at Harvard Medical School. She completed a Rhodes scholarship at the University of Oxford in Oxford, England, followed by a Pediatric Surgery Fellowship at the Hospital for Sick Children in Toronto, Canada. She also completed her Master of Public Health at the Harvard School of Public Health. Her clinical interests are in surgical oncology and vascular anomalies. Jennifer Aldrink, MD is a graduate of the Brody School of Medicine at East Carolina University, She is the Director of Surgical Oncology and the Surgical Discipline Chair of the Childrens Oncology Group (COG) and completed her general surgery residency at Duke University Medical Center. Dr Aldrink completed a

Surg Oncol Clin N Am 35 (2026) xiii–xiv
https://doi.org/10.1016/j.soc.2026.05.006
1055-3207/26/© 2026 Published by Elsevier Inc.
surgonc.theclinics.com

fellowship in pediatric surgery at Nationwide Children's Hospital. Dr Aldrink's surgical interests focus on pediatric and adolescent surgical oncology and endocrine surgery, including chest and abdominal solid tumors, such as neuroblastoma, Wilms tumor, ovarian tumors, sarcoma, melanoma, thyroid cancer, and metastatic disease. She is the director of Surgical Oncology at Nationwide Children's Hospital, a member of the Thyroid Disease team, Pigmented Skin Lesion team, and vascular malformations team at Nationwide Children's Hospital.

This issue of *Surgical Oncology Clinics of North America* covers a wide array of pediatric oncology topics. An expert team of physicians review various diseases, including Wilms tumor, neuroblastoma, osteosarcomas, and germ cell tumors. In addition, several articles are devoted to rare tumors, as well as surgical management of metastatic pediatric solid tumors. In addition, attention is given to minimally invasive and image-guided surgical techniques, as well as important topics such as fertility preservation and palliative oncology.

I express my sincere thanks to Dr Dasgupta and Dr Aldrink for inviting a fantastic group of pediatric oncology experts to contribute to this issue of *Surgical Oncology Clinics of North America*. The issue will be an important contribution to assist providers and trainees caring for children with pediatric cancers. Thanks again to our guest editors and all the expert authors who contributed to this issue of the *Surgical Oncology Clinics of North America*.

Timothy M. Pawlik, MD, PhD, MPH, MTS, MBA, FACS, FSSO, FRACS (Hon.)
Department of Surgery
The Urban Meyer III and Shelley Meyer Chair for Cancer Research
The Ohio State University
Wexner Medical Center
395 W. 12th Avenue, Suite 670
Columbus, OH 43210, USA

E-mail address:
Tim.Pawlik@osumc.edu

Preface

Pediatric Surgical Oncology

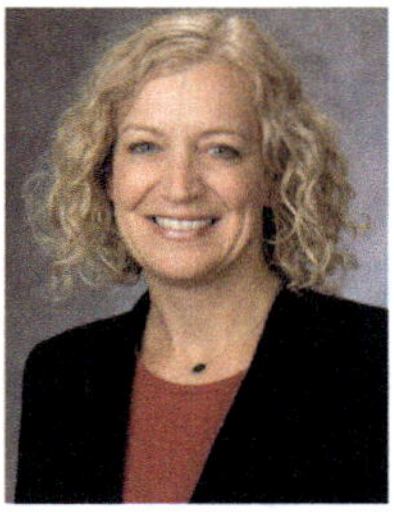

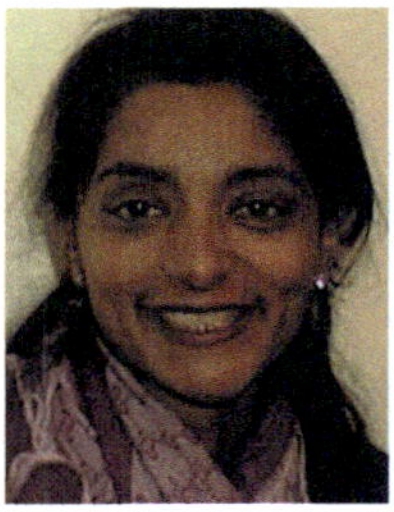

Jennifer H. Aldrink, MD Roshni Dasgupta, MD, MPH
Editors

Cancer remains the leading disease-related cause of death among children and adolescents. In response to the increasing complexity of pediatric cancer care, pediatric surgical oncology has emerged as a distinct and evolving subspecialty within pediatric surgery. Advances in precision medicine, paralleling transformative developments in adult oncology, have significantly reshaped the management of pediatric malignancies. Improved molecular and genetic characterization of tumors has enhanced risk stratification, refined prognostication, and enabled more individualized treatment strategies.

Multimodal therapy remains the cornerstone of treatment for most pediatric solid tumors; however, increasingly precise risk stratification now allows select patients to be managed with reduced-intensity therapy, including observation or surgery alone, with the goal of minimizing long-term treatment-related morbidity. As pediatric oncologic care continues to advance, specialized surgical expertise is essential to address the unique technical and multidisciplinary challenges inherent to the management of pediatric solid tumors.

The guest editors and contributing authors of this issue are internationally recognized leaders in their respective fields. Given the rarity and biologic diversity of pediatric tumors, collaborative research efforts and multi-institutional data sharing remain critical to the development of standardized treatment protocols and adequately powered clinical trials aimed at improving outcomes for children with cancer.

This issue provides a comprehensive overview of the most common solid tumors encountered in pediatric oncology, including Wilms tumor, neuroblastoma, rhabdomyosarcoma, non-rhabdomyosarcoma soft tissue sarcomas, hepatoblastoma, primary bone tumors, germ cell tumors, and select rare malignancies. It also addresses key multidisciplinary topics relevant to contemporary pediatric oncologic care, including oncofertility, minimally invasive surgery, advanced localization techniques, and palliative care.

Surg Oncol Clin N Am 35 (2026) xv–xvi
https://doi.org/10.1016/j.soc.2026.05.004
1055-3207/26/© 2026 Published by Elsevier Inc.
surgonc.theclinics.com

The unique biology of pediatric cancers, coupled with the distinct physiologic considerations of children, necessitates specialized expertise to achieve optimal surgical outcomes while minimizing long-term treatment-related morbidity. Effective care of children with cancer requires close multidisciplinary collaboration among pediatric surgeons, medical oncologists, radiation oncologists, radiologists, and pathologists to ensure the highest-quality, patient-centered outcomes.

Jennifer H. Aldrink, MD
Division of Pediatric Surgery
Department of Surgery
Nationwide Children's Hospital
The Ohio State University
College of Medicine
Columbus, OH, USA

Roshni Dasgupta, MD, MPH
Division of General and
Thoracic Surgery
Cincinnati Children's Hospital Medical Center
University of Cincinnati
Cincinnati, OH, USA

E-mail addresses:
jennifer.aldrink@nationwidechildrens.org (J.H. Aldrink)
roshni.dasgupta@cchmc.org (R. Dasgupta)

Wilms Tumor

Andrew Jackson Murphy, MD[a,b,*], Teresa Santiago, MD[c],
Nicholas G. Cost, MD[d,e]

KEYWORDS

- Wilms tumor • Favorable histology • Diffuse anaplasia • Surgery • Staging
- Risk-stratification

KEY POINTS

- *Wilms tumor (WT)* is the most common pediatric kidney cancer (~85%), peaks at ages 2–4, and is usually sporadic, though several syndromes increase risk.
- *Histology and molecular features* guide risk stratification: favorable-histology WT has ~90% survival, whereas diffuse anaplasia (often *TP53*-mutant) predicts poor outcomes and requires intensified therapy.
- *International protocols differ*: COG favors upfront nephrectomy for unilateral WT, while SIOP uses preoperative chemotherapy; both achieve high survival but differ in sequencing and staging.
- *Prognosis* depends on stage, histology, molecular biomarkers (1q gain, LOH 1p/16q), and pulmonary metastatic response; these guide therapy intensity and eligibility for treatment reduction.
- *Surgical principles* emphasize complete tumor removal, lymph node sampling, and minimizing intraoperative spill; nephron-sparing surgery is prioritized for bilateral WT to preserve renal function.

INTRODUCTION

Epidemiology and Presentation

Wilms tumor (WT) is the most common pediatric kidney cancer and the second most frequent pediatric extracranial solid tumor after neuroblastoma.[1] It occurs at a rate of 8.2 per million children aged under 15 years, with peak incidence between ages 2 and 4 years.[2] WT comprises approximately 85% of renal tumors and 6% to 7% of all pediatric cancers in this age group.[1] About 85% to 90% of cases lack an identifiable

[a] Division of Pediatric Surgery, Department of Surgery, University of Tennessee Health Science Center, Memphis, TN, USA; [b] Department of Surgery, St. Jude Children's Research Hospital, Memphis, TN, USA; [c] Department of Pathology, St. Jude Children's Research Hospital, Memphis, TN, USA; [d] Department of Surgery, Division of Urology, University of Colorado School of Medicine; [e] Surgical Oncology Program, Children's Hospital Colorado, Aurora, CO, USA
* Corresponding author. Department of Surgery, St. Jude Children's Research Hospital, 262 Danny Thomas Place, Memphis, TN 38105.
E-mail address: Andrew.murphy@stjude.org

Surg Oncol Clin N Am 35 (2026) 695–714
https://doi.org/10.1016/j.soc.2026.03.002 surgonc.theclinics.com
1055-3207/26/

Abbreviations	
COG	Children's Oncology Group
CT	computed tomography
DHPLN	diffuse hyperplastic perilobar nephroblastomatosis
FH	favorable histology
IVC	inferior vena cava
LOH	loss of heterozygosity
NSS	nephron-sparing surgery
RCC	renal cell carcinoma
SIOP	International Society of Pediatric Oncology
VAD	vincristine, actinomycin-D, and doxorubicin
WT	Wilms tumor

genetic predisposition, though 10% to 15% are linked to congenital anomalies or syndromes.[3] Improved molecular diagnostics suggest predisposition may be underrecognized, especially in bilateral cases, which occur in 5% to 8% of patients.[4–6]

High-risk WT predisposition syndromes (>20% WT incidence) include Wilms tumor, Aniridia, Genitourinary anomalies, intellectual disability syndrome (WAGR) (11p13 deletion), *WT1* disorder, Perlman (*DIS3L2*), Fanconi anemia (*BRCA2/PALB2*), and mosaic variegated aneuploidy (*BUB1B/TRIP13*). Moderate-risk syndromes (5%–20% WT incidence) include Beckwith-Wiedemann (11p15.5 imprinting defects) and Simpson-Golabi-Behmel (*GPC3*).[3] Other rare predisposition mechanisms have been reported, including Phosphatidylinositol-4,5-bisphosphate 3-kinase catalytic subunit alpha (PIK3CA)-related overgrowth disorders such as Congenital Lipomatous Overgrowth, Vascular malformations, Epidermal nevi, Skeletal anomalies (CLOVES) syndrome, and germline alterations in *RE1-silencing transcription factor (REST), Tripartite motif–containing protein 28 (TRIM28), Dicer 1, ribonuclease III (DICER1),* and *Phosphatase and tensin homolog (PTEN).*[7,8]

Children typically present with large, asymptomatic abdominal masses. Screening programs for children with predisposition syndromes may detect smaller tumors in patients at an increased risk. Unlike neuroblastoma, systemic symptoms are rare (<10%). Abdominal pain occurs in 15% to 40% and may signal rupture, anaplasia, or advanced disease.[9] Hypertension (up to 25%) results from renin-angiotensin activation. Hematuria may occur due to collecting system involvement.[10]

Pathophysiology

WT was first described by Max Wilms in 1899 as a "mixed tumor" due to its characteristic triphasic histology (blastemal, stromal, and epithelial elements) resembling the fetal kidney (**Fig. 1**A–J).[11] Beyond this histologic similarity, multiple lines of evidence support WT as an embryonal tumor arising from disrupted fetal kidney development. Pathogenic variants and/or copy number changes in key developmental genes (*Wilms tumor 1 [WT1], Sine oculis homeobox homolog 2 [SIX2], MYCN proto-oncogene [MYCN], Catenin beta 1 [CTNNB1], Insulin-like growth factor 2 [IGF2], and microRNA processing genes like DiGeorge syndrome critical region gene 8 [DGCR8], Drosha ribonuclease III [DROSHA] ,and Lin-28 homolog B [LIN28B]*) are strongly linked to WT pathogenesis.[12,13] Bulk and single-cell RNA sequencing studies show that WT expresses gene profiles and contains cell types similar to those in the fetal kidney, in contrast to renal cancers found in adolescents and adults, like renal cell carcinoma (RCC), which more closely resemble mature tubular epithelium.[12,14] Furthermore, nephrogenic rests (undifferentiated metanephric blastema) are nonobligate precursor lesions often found with WT.[15]

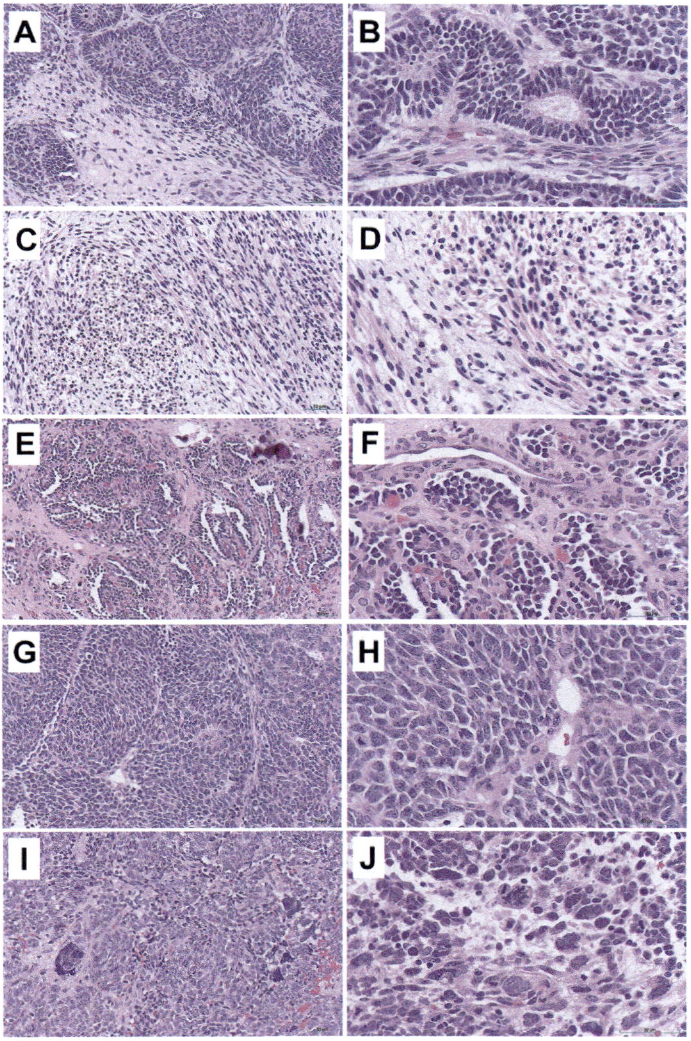

Fig. 1. Histologic features of Wilms tumor (WT). (*A, B*) WT with a classic triphasic morphology composed of clusters of blastema (undifferentiated round cells), stromal elements (spindle cells), and epithelial tubules; no anaplasia is identified (favorable histology—FH). (*C, D*) FH stromal predominant WT is mainly composed of spindle cells with occasional skeletal muscle (rhabdomyomatous/rhabdomyoblastic) differentiation. (*E, F*) FH epithelial predominant WT composed of epithelial tubes and glomeruli-like structures. (*G, H*) Postchemotherapy blastemal predominant WT with greater than 33% residual viable tumor and greater than 66% blastemal elements (high-risk). (*I, J*) Anaplastic WT displaying enlarged and hyperchromatic tumor cells and atypical multipolar mitoses (high-risk). Hematoxylin-eosin: A, C, E, G, and I, 200×; B, D, F, H, and J, 400×.

Perilobar nephrogenic rests (linked to 11p15.5/*IGF2* imprinting defects) form peripherally (subcapsular); intralobar rests (associated with 11p13/*WT1* pathogenic variants) are centrally located. These rests may be incidental or expansile, detectable on imaging. Multiple or diffuse rests are termed nephroblastomatosis. Diffuse hyperplastic perilobar nephroblastomatosis (DHPLN) presents as bilateral, rind-like peripheral kidney expansion, preserving architecture, and resembling a "giant kidney."[15] Distinguishing DHPLN from bilateral WT is critical, as DHPLN is managed nonoperatively unless WT is suspected to be present.[16] Radiographic features favoring WT over nephrogenic rests include exophytic growth, size greater than 1.75 cm, spherical shape, and invasion into noncortical tissue.[17] Biopsy differentiation is challenging without sampling the lesion–nonneoplastic kidney parenchyma interface; WT typically has a pseudocapsule, which is mostly absent in nephrogenic rests, making core needle biopsy unreliable.

Diagnosis

Evaluation begins with a thorough history and physical examination focused on syndromic features associated with WT predisposition, including hemihypertrophy, somatic overgrowth, developmental delay, aniridia, disorders of sexual development, hypospadias, cryptorchidism, and other genitourinary anomalies. Signs of Beckwith–Wiedemann syndrome (macroglossia, abdominal wall defects, and hemihypertrophy) can be subtle.[18] A family history of WT may also indicate genetic susceptibility.

Initial laboratories should include complete blood count (CBC), basic metabolic panel, and coagulation studies. Renal dysfunction is rare at presentation, but up to 5% of patients may have paraneoplastic coagulopathy due to acquired von Willebrand disease, warranting coagulation screening.[19] Imaging begins with abdominal ultrasound to confirm renal origin, assess solid versus cystic components, and evaluate for tumor thrombus in the renal vein or inferior vena cava (IVC). Contrast-enhanced dual-phase computed tomography (CT) or MRI provides superior characterization, including the "claw sign," where normal renal parenchyma is compressed around the tumor (**Fig. 2**A–K). WT typically displaces rather than encases vessels, rarely crosses the midline, and infrequently contains calcifications, features that help distinguish it from neuroblastoma.[20]

Cross-sectional imaging may also aid in a suspicion of preoperative tumor rupture, indicated by free fluid outside the cul-de-sac, capsular disruption, retroperitoneal fat stranding, or peritumoral collections (see **Fig. 2**).[21] Final determination of rupture requires intraoperative confirmation. "Rupture" refers to preoperative tumor disruption confirmed during surgery; "intraoperative spill" describes tumor capsular breach occurring during resection or biopsy. CT is considered more sensitive than ultrasound for detecting retroperitoneal and para-aortic lymphadenopathy. However, CT can both overestimate and underestimate nodal disease: enlarged nodes may be reactive, while microscopic metastases can occur in normal-sized nodes. For this reason, surgical lymph node sampling remains essential for accurate staging.[22–25]

Chest CT is essential for staging, as the lungs are the most common site of metastasis, occurring in up to 10% to 15%. Chest radiography may miss small pulmonary lesions, increasing relapse risk; therefore, noncontrast chest CT is preferred to guide appropriate therapy .[26]

Staging, Risk Stratification, and Sequencing of Multimodal Therapy

From the late nineteenth to mid-twentieth century, treatment of patients with WT evolved through the integration of nephrectomy, radiotherapy, and systemic chemotherapy. WT was the first human solid tumor shown to respond to systemic chemotherapy, demonstrated by Dr Sidney Farber's use of actinomycin-D in 1955.[27] Since then, large-scale observational studies—initially through the National Wilms Tumor Study 1 to 5, and later via the Children's Oncology Group (COG) in North America and the International Society of Pediatric Oncology (SIOP) in Europe—have led to excellent survival rates for patients with favorable histology WT using a multimodal

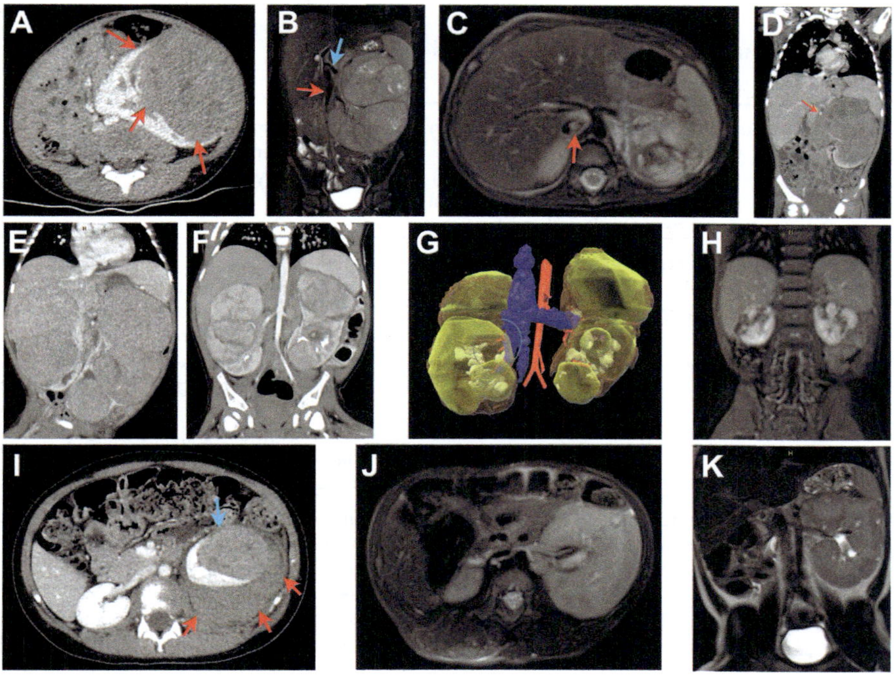

Fig. 2. Radiographic features of Wilms tumor. (*A*) Left WT with interface of normal renal parenchyma and tumor demonstrating the claw sign (*red arrows*). (*B*) Same left WT demonstrating rightward displacement of the celiac axis (*blue arrow*) and superior mesenteric artery (*red arrow*) rather than encasement. (*C*) Left WT with retrohepatic intracaval tumor thrombus extension (*red arrow*). (*D*) Left-sided WT with medial nodal conglomerate abutting the superior mesenteric artery (SMA). (*E*) Extensive bilateral WT at diagnosis. (*F*) Bilateral WT in the same patient demonstrating response to 12 weeks of vincristine, actinomycin-D, and doxorubicin. (*G*) Preoperative 3 dimensional model demonstrates extensive bilateral WT (yellow). (*H*) Despite the extensive appearance, bilateral nephron-sparing surgery was performed using a staged approach. Long-term follow-up MRI demonstrates bilateral kidneys with postoperative changes. (*I*) Left WT (*blue arrow*) with surrounding retroperitoneal fluid consistent with preoperative rupture. (*J*) Diffuse hyperplastic perilobar nephroblastomatosis (DHPLN) on the left side with a peripheral cortical rim and maintenance of the reniform appearance. (*K*) Same left DHPLN demonstrating coronal perspective of maintained reniform appearance.

approach.[28] Despite similarly good outcomes, COG and SIOP differ in how they sequence surgery, chemotherapy, and radiation within treatment protocols.

COG protocols advocate for up-front radical nephroureterectomy for the treatment of most unilateral WT in patients without genetic predisposition.[28] Advantages of this approach include avoiding inappropriate treatment of rare histologies, earlier identification and intensification of therapy for unfavorable histology disease (anaplasia) or high-risk molecular features (1q gain, 1p/16q loss of heterozygosity [LOH]), and the ability to identify groups of patients with very-low-risk disease who can be successfully treated with nephrectomy alone.[29–34] On COG protocols, WT is a surgically staged disease (**Table 1**). In cases of metastatic disease (stage IV) or bilateral WT (stage V), each involved kidney is assigned a local stage (stage I–III), which can then guide the radiotherapy plan.

Table 1
Wilms tumor staging according to the Children's Oncology Group

Stage	Criteria	Notes
Stage I	Tumor completely contained within the kidney capsule; negative resection margins; no more than minimal involvement of the renal sinus; negative lymph nodes	Adequate sampling of resection margins, renal sinus, and lymph nodes is key
Stage II	Tumor extends beyond renal capsule; negative resection margins; negative lymph nodes	Examples: • Viable tumor penetration through renal capsule, perirenal soft tissue, but confined to Gerota's fascia • Viable tumor infiltration into the renal vein (with negative margins) • More than minimal involvement of the renal sinus by viable tumor • Viable tumor infiltrates the wall of the pelvis or the ureter
Stage III	Residual tumor after surgery confined to the abdomen	Examples: • Surgical margins involved by viable or nonviable tumor (positive margins) • Preoperative tumor rupture • Intraoperative tumor spill • Positive lymph nodes • Peritoneal implant of viable or nonviable tumor • Presurgical biopsy
Stage IV[a]	Metastatic disease	Examples: • Lung • Liver • Bone
Stage V[a]	Bilateral tumors	—

[a] Stages IV and V are overall disease stages; each involved kidney will also be assigned a local stage I–III that can affect the radiotherapy plan.

COG guidelines generally recommend upfront radical nephroureterectomy for WT, but exceptions exist. These include cases with intracaval tumor thrombus extending above the hepatic veins, extensive local invasion requiring en bloc resection of organs beyond the diaphragm or adrenal gland, significant pulmonary compromise due to tumor burden or metastases, a solitary kidney, or when the surgeon determines that upfront resection would risk major morbidity, incomplete removal, or tumor spill. In such scenarios, neoadjuvant chemotherapy may be indicated.[35] For patients receiving preoperative therapy under COG protocols, a percutaneous, retroperitoneal image-guided core needle biopsy should be performed to confirm histology before treatment begins. However, this method may not reliably detect anaplasia due to its potential patchy distribution within the tumor. Patients with bilateral WT or known predisposition syndromes also receive neoadjuvant chemotherapy under COG protocols.[36,37] In these cases, biopsy at diagnosis is typically omitted, as non-Wilms bilateral renal tumors in children are exceedingly rare. Following surgical resection, histology, stage, molecular genetic biomarkers, patient demographic features, and response characteristics of pulmonary nodules (for patients with metastatic disease) are combined to assign a risk group and select an adjuvant therapy regimen (**Table 2**).

Table 2
Children's Oncology Group favorable histology Wilms tumor treatment stratification

COG Stage	Age	Molecular	Lymph Node Positive	Lung Nodule Response	Extrapulmonary Metastases	Postchemotherapy Histology	Other	AREN2231 Stratum Assignment
I	Any	Normal	NA	NA	NA	NA	Epithelial histology and no WT predisposition	Nephrectomy only
I	<4y	Normal	NA	NA	NA	NA	No WT predisposition	Nephrectomy only
I	Any	Combined 1p/16q LOH, 1q gain, OR 11p15 LOH	NA	NA	NA	NA	NA	EE-4A
I	>4y	Any	NA	NA	NA	NA	NA	EE-4A
II	Any	Normal	NA	NA	NA	NA	NA	EE-4A
II	Any	1p OR 16q isolated LOH	NA	NA	NA	NA	NA	EE-4A
III	Any	Normal	Any	NA	NA	NA or low-risk or intermediate-risk	NA	EE-4A ± XRT
III	Any	1p OR 16q isolated LOH	No	NA	NA	NA or low-risk or intermediate-risk	NA	EE-4A ± XRT
II	Any	Combined 1p/16q LOH or 1q gain	NA	NA	NA	NA	NA	DD-4A vs VIVA
IV	Any	Normal	Any	Rapid complete	No	NA or low-risk or intermediate-risk	NA	DD-4A ± XRT
IV	Any	1p or 16q isolated LOH	Any	Rapid complete	No	NA or low-risk or intermediate-risk	NA	DD-4A ± XRT

(continued on next page)

Table 2
(continued)

COG Stage	Age	Molecular	Lymph Node Positive	Lung Nodule Response	Extrapulmonary Metastases	Postchemotherapy Histology	Other	AREN2231 Stratum Assignment
III	Any	Combined 1p/16q LOH	Any	NA	NA	NA or low-risk or intermediate-risk	NA	Regimen M vs MVI ± XRT
III	Any	1p or 16q isolated LOH	Yes	NA	NA	NA or low-risk or intermediate-risk	NA	Regimen M vs MVI + XRT
IV	Any	Combined 1p/16q LOH or 1q gain	Any	Any	No	NA or low-risk or intermediate-risk	NA	Regimen M vs MVI + XRT
IV	Any	1p or 16q isolated LOH	Yes	Any	No	NA or low-risk or intermediate-risk	NA	Regimen M vs MVI + XRT
IV	Any	Any	Any	Slow incomplete	No	NA or low-risk or intermediate-risk	NA	Regimen M vs MVI + XRT
IV	Any	Any	Any	Any	Yes	NA or low-risk or intermediate-risk	NA	Regimen M vs MVI + XRT
III	Any	Any	Any	NA	NA	High-risk	NA	Regimen UH-3 + XRT
IV	Any	Any	Any	Any	Any	High-risk	NA	Regimen UH-3 + XRT

Adapted from Benedetti DJ, Varela CR, Renfro LA, et al. Treatment of children with favorable histology Wilms tumor with extrapulmonary metastases: A report from the COG studies AREN0533 and AREN03B2 and NWTSG study NWTS-5. Cancer. Mar 15 2024;130(6):947–961. https://doi.org/10.1002/cncr.35099

In contrast, SIOP protocols follow an alternate sequencing of multimodality therapy, with neoadjuvant chemotherapy preceding surgical resection.[28] Neoadjuvant chemotherapy with vincristine and actinomycin-D is administered to patients with localized WT for 4 weeks, and vincristine, actinomycin-D, and doxorubicin (VAD) are given for 6 weeks in patients with metastatic disease.[28,38] The underlying rationale for this sequence is that up-front nephroureterectomy was associated with a higher rate of intraoperative tumor spill, positive margins, and postoperative complications in previous SIOP studies.[38–40] Furthermore, when compared to prior SIOP studies, the utilization of doxorubicin or radiotherapy decreased by 20% when preoperative chemotherapy was used.[39] Exceptions to this sequence are made for patients less than 6 months of age, when alternate histologies such as congenital mesoblastic nephroma or malignant rhabdoid tumor of the kidney are more common and for patients who have tumors with atypical radiographic findings (no visible normal renal parenchyma, extrarenal tumor, very large lymph nodes, intratumoral calcifications, pulmonary metastases in patients aged <2 years). Patients aged older than 10 years should also be carefully evaluated for non-WTs, as the incidence of RCC increases, and upfront resection or biopsy is more appropriate.[38] Posttreatment histology then guides risk stratification and further adjuvant therapy selection (**Table 3**).[38,41]

Prognostic Features that Guide Risk Stratification and Treatment

Histology

Histologic classification remains the most critical determinant of prognosis in children with WT. Within the COG framework, tumors are broadly categorized as having either favorable or unfavorable histology. Most WT cases fall into the favorable category, respond well to current multimodal therapies, and achieve approximately 90% 5 year overall survival. In contrast, about 5% to 10% of WTs exhibit diffuse anaplasia, a histologic subtype marked by enlarged, hyperchromatic nuclei and atypical multipolar mitoses.[42] This form is notably resistant to standard treatment and is implicated in roughly half of all WT-related mortalities. Anaplastic WT is further subdivided into focal (1 to 2–3 small anaplastic foci within the primary tumor) and diffuse (when diffusely present within the primary tumor or identified in any extrarenal site, such as vessels, lymph nodes, or metastatic sites). Stage I and II focal anaplastic WT have 100% 4 year event-free and overall survival when treated with DD-4A and

Table 3
Postchemotherapy Wilms tumor histology risk-group assignment

Posttreatment Histology Risk Group	Histologic Features	Notes
Low	Completely necrotic	No residual viable tumor is identified except for scattered small tubules
Intermediate	Regressive Mixed (Triphasic) Epithelial predominant Stromal predominant Focal anaplasia	<33% residual viable tumor, regardless of the tumor composition; or, >33% residual viable tumor, but <66% residual blastemal component
High	Blastemal predominant Diffuse anaplasia	Must be >33% viable and have >66% blastemal component Presence of diffuse anaplasia, regardless of the amount of residual viable tumor

radiation. Stage III and IV focal anaplastic WT receive intensified regimens but continue to exhibit poor outcomes.[43]

Diffuse anaplasia is strongly correlated with pathogenic variants in *TP53* and/or loss of chromosomal material at 17p13.1, suggesting a clonal evolution from initially favorable histology.[44] This is further supported by the tendency for unfavorable histology WT to present at older ages. Historically, diffuse anaplastic WT has shown poor responsiveness to VAD, the cornerstone agents for favorable histology WT. Nevertheless, stage I anaplastic tumors have demonstrated successful outcomes with the same agents when combined with flank irradiation, although recent data indicate that radiation may be unnecessary in select cases.[45] For patients with stage II to IV diffuse anaplastic WT, intensified chemotherapy regimens incorporating vincristine, doxorubicin, cyclophosphamide, and etoposide (often preceded by a vincristine/irinotecan window) have led to improved survival rates.[46] However, these aggressive protocols are associated with significant treatment-related toxicity. The ongoing study COG AREN1921 (ClinicalTrials.gov ID NCT04322318) is assessing whether intensified chemotherapy, improved surgical timing, and enhanced metastatic control can meaningfully improve survival for children with stage 2 to 4 diffuse anaplastic WT.

The SIOP classification system also stratifies WT risk based on histologic features. However, unlike the COG approach, SIOP evaluates histology after neoadjuvant chemotherapy (see **Table 3**).[47] Tumors showing complete necrosis are considered low-risk, while those with diffuse anaplasia, or blastemal predominance (defined as >33% residual viable tumor and >66% blastema), are classified as high-risk. An important concept is that blastemal predominance is only associated with a higher risk of relapse when present after neoadjuvant chemotherapy treatment. All other postchemotherapy histologic patterns (<33% residual viable tumor of any histology, >33% residual viable tumor with blastemal component <66%, and focal anaplasia) fall into the intermediate-risk category.[41,47] Notably, the SIOP posttreatment histology criteria are applied in the COG system for bilateral WT and are also being used in the ongoing COG AREN2231 trial (ClinicalTrials.gov ID NCT06501330) for patients undergoing delayed nephrectomy.[48,49]

Epithelial-predominant histology, particularly in stage I tumors, is associated with excellent outcomes. This subtype has been linked to germline mutations in genes such as *TRIM28*, which may confer a predisposition to WT. The COG AREN2231 (ClinicalTrials.gov ID NCT06401330) protocol is currently investigating whether patients of any age with stage I prechemotherapy epithelial-predominant tumors and favorable molecular features can be safely managed with nephrectomy followed by observation alone, potentially sparing them from adjuvant chemotherapy.[48]

Stage

Stage is the cornerstone of risk stratification for favorable histology WT in the COG system (see **Table 1**). Among patients with stage III disease (residual tumor is known, suspected, nodal involvement, or capsular breach has occurred), the reason for the tumor being designated stage III confers additional prognostic significance. For example, among patients with stage III disease, patients with positive lymph nodes have an inferior prognosis when compared to those with stage III tumors due to positive surgical margins or intraoperative spill.[50] Similarly, among patients with stage IV (metastatic) disease, extrapulmonary metastases confer an inferior prognosis when compared to pulmonary metastases.[51]

Patient age and tumor weight

In favorable histology WT, younger age has traditionally been linked to improved outcomes.[52] The COG AREN0532 study highlighted that children aged under 2 years without known genetic predisposition and with stage I favorable histology WT weighing less than 550 g achieved excellent survival with nephrectomy alone (very-low risk cohort). Importantly, those who relapsed after surgery-only treatment responded well to salvage chemotherapy, underscoring the effectiveness of rescue chemotherapy with EE-4A (vincristine, actinomycin-D) in this setting. Molecular profiling of very-low risk tumors that went on to relapse revealed associations with adverse genetic features such as combined LOH at 1p/16q, gain of 1q, and LOH at 11p15.5. Accordingly, the identification of these adverse biomarkers renders patients ineligible for a nephrectomy-only approach on the currently enrolling COG AREN2231 trial (ClinicalTrials.gov ID NCT06401330).[31,48]

However, a more recent pooled analysis of over 1700 children with stage I and II favorable histology WT found that age alone was not independently predictive of event-free or overall survival once adverse tumor biology (more common in older children) was accounted for. In this cohort, larger tumor weight correlated with higher relapse risk in stage I and increased mortality in stage II, though these associations did not hold in children aged younger than 4 years.[53] Building on these insights, the ongoing COG AREN2231 trial (ClinicalTrials.gov ID NCT06401330) is investigating the safety and efficacy of nephrectomy-only management in nonsyndromic children aged under 4 years with stage I favorable histology WT, regardless of tumor weight, provided lymph nodes are sampled and negative for tumor, and no adverse molecular features are present.[48]

Molecular genetic biomarkers

Several genetic alterations have been linked to increased relapse risk in WT, including mutations in *TP53* and *SIX1/2* when accompanied by defects in microRNA-processing genes.[13,44,54] Additionally, chromosomal copy number changes such as gain of 1q and LOH at 1p and 16q are associated with poor outcomes and warrant intensification of therapy.[29,30,32,34] Concomitant studies published by the COG and SIOP demonstrated that 1q gain has prognostic significance when found in the context of upfront nephrectomy or after neoadjuvant chemotherapy.[29,30] While mutations in *TP53*, *SIX1/2*, and microRNA-processing genes are biologically significant, they are not yet clinically actionable.[13,44,54]

In contrast, the actively enrolling COG AREN2231 protocol incorporates several molecular biomarkers into risk stratification and treatment planning.[48] These include 1q gain and combined LOH of 1p and 16q across all patient groups. For patients with stage III to IV disease, LOH of either 1p or 16q in combination with lymph node positivity is also considered actionable.[33,48] Furthermore, LOH at 11p15 is recognized as an adverse prognostic marker in children who would otherwise qualify for very-low-risk therapy, specifically those aged under 4 years with stage I favorable histology WT and no known predisposition, regardless of tumor weight.[48]

Metastatic disease—extrapulmonary metastases and response of pulmonary nodules

Stage IV disease is characterized by metastasis, with the lungs being the most common site.[1] Children with extrapulmonary metastases, liver being the most common site, experience inferior event-free and overall survival when compared to children with pulmonary metastases, and are not eligible for therapy reduction based on response characteristics.[51] Historically, all children with WT and pulmonary metastases received whole-lung radiotherapy. The COG AREN0533 study demonstrated that up to 40% of patients with pulmonary metastases exhibit a rapid complete response (total disappearance of all pulmonary nodules) after 2 cycles/6 wk of chemotherapy and can be spared pulmonary irradiation and continued on DD-4A chemotherapy while maintaining excellent 5 year overall survival (96.1%). In contrast, for slow incomplete responders in whom the pulmonary nodules do not resolve after 6 weeks of induction DD-4A (vincristine, actinomycin-D, doxorubicin) pulmonary irradiation is administered, and systemic chemotherapy is intensified to regimen M (vincristine, actinomycin-D, doxorubicin, cyclophosphamide, and etoposide). Patients with combined 1p/16q LOH were not eligible for sparing of pulmonary irradiation on AREN0533, regardless of the response to initial therapy.[55]

Surgical resection

Radical nephroureterectomy The goals of WT surgery include local control of the primary tumor mass (clearance of all local disease), accurate staging of lymph nodes, and obtaining tissue for complete pathologic evaluation. Radical nephroureterectomy with lymph node sampling remains the standard approach for unilateral WT.[56] The procedure is typically performed via a transperitoneal route with the patient supine, using a transverse or chevron incision tailored to tumor size and location. A thoracoabdominal incision is rarely needed for extremely large tumors that exhibit significant superior mass effect on the diaphragm.

Intra-abdominal entry should be cautious, especially when the colon is displaced anteriorly. If the tumor is found to invade adjacent organs such as the spleen, pancreas, or colon, upfront resection is deferred in favor of biopsy and neoadjuvant chemotherapy, given the tumor's chemosensitivity and the morbidity of extensive en bloc resections. However, in rare circumstances in which such local invasion persists after completion of neoadjuvant chemotherapy, en bloc resections may be required in favor of obtaining complete tumor resection.

Exposure techniques vary by tumor location. Both sides require colonic mobilization and varying degrees of medial visceral rotation. Right-sided tumors may require duodenal kocherization and hepatic mobilization; left-sided tumors may necessitate medial rotation of the spleen and pancreas. Adrenal preservation is recommended when invasion is absent, but en bloc resection is warranted if oncologic margins are at risk.[57] Diaphragmatic involvement is managed with limited resection and primary repair, though synthetic patches can be needed if significant diaphragmatic resection is required, and chest tubes may be needed for larger defects or pleural entry. Contralateral renal exploration is generally only of historical significance and typically not indicated, as preoperative imaging is extremely sensitive for the detection of contralateral renal lesions.[58]

To minimize intraoperative tumor spill, a key determinant of staging and adjuvant therapy, gentle, broad-handed retraction is essential. Intraoperative spill mandates stage III classification and may require flank or whole-abdominal radiotherapy depending on the extent of the spill.[59] If an intraoperative tumor spill occurs, whether it is confined to the ipsilateral flank or more broadly throughout the abdomen, it should be carefully documented in the operative report. Spill confined to the flank is treated with flank irradiation, while a broader distribution of spill requires whole abdominal radiotherapy.[59] Intraoperative spill should be distinguished from preoperative tumor rupture. All intraoperative findings, including spill or rupture, must be documented in the operative report and communicated to the oncology team for coordinated postoperative care. Synoptic operative reports for renal tumors facilitate appropriate documentation of such details and are being adopted.[60]

Optimal vascular control during WT resection begins with near-complete mobilization of the mass by dividing its lateral, posterior, superior, and inferior attachments. This allows for safer and clearer access to the renal hilum. If exposure is limited, extending the incision is often effective. The ureter is divided distally near the bladder, and the gonadal vein is typically sacrificed.[56] Preoperative imaging should be reviewed carefully to anticipate variations in renal vascular anatomy, including multiple vessels or anomalous courses such as retroaortic renal veins. Ureteral involvement is present in approximately 2% of WT and may be suggested by hematuria, hydronephrosis, or rarely passage of tissue per urethra.[61] If ureteral involvement is suspected, cystoscopy with retrograde urethrogram can aid in the preoperative evaluation. When encountered intraoperatively, the entire course of the ureter and any component of the mass within the bladder should be resected with clear margins if possible.

During hilar dissection, the renal vein is usually encountered as the most anterior vascular structure, followed by the renal artery posteriorly. Although traditional practice favors ligating the artery before the vein to reduce tumor engorgement, this sequence is less critical if the tumor is already mobilized. For large left-sided tumors, particularly with adjacent nodal masses, distorted anatomy may bring the superior mesenteric artery into the field early; tracing the aorta from its bifurcation upward or dividing the left diaphragmatic crus to access the supraceliac aorta can aid in safe vessel identification. Vascular structures should never be ligated until their identity is confirmed to avoid catastrophic errors.

Lymph node sampling is essential for accurate staging and treatment planning. Failure to sample nodes can result in understaging and inadequate therapy. Current protocols require sampling of at least 1 lymph node, with 5 nodes encouraged for optimal sensitivity.[22,23,48] Renal hilar, paraaortic, aortocaval, and paracaval nodes should be sampled, while radical lymphadenectomy and sampling of parailiac, mesenteric, or periportal nodes are not indicated.[25] Lymphatic tributaries should be securely ligated to prevent chyle leaks. Fluorescence-guided lymphatic mapping of WT is achievable with either intrarenal (normal kidney) or perihilar indocyanine green injection, but its impact on improving lymph node sampling remains unknown and requires prospective investigation.[62–64]

Bowel obstruction is a known postoperative risk, with adhesions and intussusception being the primary causes. Intussusception should be suspected in patients who initially recover bowel function but then develop sudden distension and vomiting. Ultrasound is diagnostic, and surgical intervention is typically required.[65] Adhesive obstruction may occur within weeks postop, but can also present later in life and is potentiated by radiation therapy.[66,67]

Intravascular extension WT may extend into the renal vein (11%) or further into the IVC and right atrium (4%). For thrombus at or above the hepatic veins, neoadjuvant chemotherapy is recommended to reduce thrombus burden and avoid cardiopulmonary bypass, which is often unnecessary after regression. Chemotherapy also has the potential to lower surgical risk and improve resectability.[68]

Intravascular tumors confined below the hepatic veins can be approached abdominally. Right liver mobilization and circumferential IVC dissection are required for retrohepatic caval thrombus, including ligation of the right posterior section hepatic and lumbar vein branches. Vascular control is achieved with clamps or vessel loops, and a cavotomy is performed to extract the thrombus, often en bloc with the kidney and tumor. Closure is typically done with a running nonabsorbable suture, and vein patches may be necessary after resection of thrombus that has invaded the vascular wall.

If the IVC is chronically occluded, collateral venous pathways (especially via gonadal and periureteral vessels) may complicate resection. Restoration of IVC flow is unlikely, and partial cavectomy may be necessary, with care to preserve contralateral renal and hepatic venous drainage.[69] In select cases, ligation of the contralateral renal vein is safe due to compensatory flow through the azygos system.

For thrombus reaching or entering the right atrium, cardiac surgical collaboration is essential. Median sternotomy with bypass is standard, though limited approaches, including partial sternotomy or balloon occlusion, may be considered in experienced centers.[70] Lymph node sampling and tailored radiation remain critical for staging and treatment, especially when margins are positive due to intravascular involvement.

Nephron-sparing surgery Bilateral WTs are managed with neoadjuvant chemotherapy (VAD) to reduce tumor volume and enable nephron-sparing surgery (NSS), which is feasible in up to 90% of cases at experienced centers.[36,71] Unlike unilateral disease, where radical nephroureterectomy is preferred due to low risk of long-term renal failure, bilateral cases carry a higher risk (~14%) of end-stage renal disease, making renal preservation critical.[72]

Surgical access is typically via a bilateral subcostal or transverse incision. Tumors are fully mobilized before parenchymal dissection. Renal vessels are isolated with loops, and bleeding is controlled with manual pressure or selective ligation. Temporary vascular clamping may be performed, but is typically avoidable in most cases, especially when tumors are exophytic, well-encapsulated, or have responded well to preoperative chemotherapy. Conversely, more infiltrative or central tumors may benefit from temporary vascular occlusion to ensure margin control. When clamping is performed, techniques such as selective arterial branch clamping, segmental clamping, renal cooling, or early unclamping can reduce warm ischemia time while still enabling adequate visualization of the tumor plane. In some cases, NSS may require enucleation over partial nephrectomy to enable renal parenchyma preservation. Intraoperative ultrasound aids in identifying multifocal lesions, especially in the setting of concomitant nephroblastomatosis. Tumors are resected individually, and adjacent nephrogenic rests may be biopsied. Lesions with complete chemotherapy response and residual scar are biopsied if identifiable.[73] Collecting system involvement is not a contraindication to NSS and collecting system defects can typically be repaired primarily. Intraoperative urine leaks from the collecting system can be visualized using methylene blue. Because leaks are uncommon, drains and ureteral stents are not routinely needed and may be used selectively when a leak is detected.

Hemostasis is achieved using sutures, pressure, and topical agents. Entry into the collecting system is repaired with absorbable suture. Postoperative complications (such as urine leak) are more common with NSS than with radical nephroureterectomy but are usually manageable with drainage and stenting. Alternative NSS techniques, including longitudinal partial nephrectomy, have been described. Renal cooling and vascular clamping are not routinely used but may reduce blood loss and preserve visualization during resection of complex tumors with hilar involvement. Lymph node sampling (paraaortic, aortocaval, paracaval, and parailiac) is performed for staging. NSS is also indicated in unilateral WT with solitary kidneys or syndromic predisposition.[37,73] While initial experiences suggested that completion nephrectomy was indicated for diffuse anaplasia, the COG AREN0534 BWT study demonstrated no difference in outcomes according to margin status, even for patients with anaplastic disease.[74]

Standardized reporting of NSS, as developed by the SIOP Renal Tumors Study Group, is now incorporated into prospective protocols to correlate surgical technique with outcomes.[75]

Wilms tumor in adults Adult WT is an exceptionally rare entity, accounting for less than 1% of all renal malignancies. In most cases, it is an unexpected histopathological diagnosis following nephrectomy performed for a presumed RCC. There are no distinguishing radiographic or histologic features that differentiate adult WT from its pediatric counterpart. Despite histologic similarities, clinical outcomes in adults are significantly worse. The 5 year overall survival rate in adults is approximately 70%, compared to over 90% in children.[76,77]

This disparity is likely multifactorial. Adults more frequently present with advanced-stage disease—stage III or IV in nearly 50% of cases, versus 30% in children. Additionally, adult oncologists may lack familiarity with WT and often do not follow pediatric-derived, risk-adapted treatment protocols, leading to delays in diagnosis and suboptimal therapy. Treatment-related decisions may also be influenced by comorbidities and concerns about toxicity, resulting in lower relative chemotherapy dosing in adults.[76,77]

Emerging molecular data suggest that adult WT may harbor distinct genetic alterations compared to pediatric cases. While some adult tumors exhibit mutations seen in children (eg, *WT1*, *ASXL1*, and *TERT* promoter), others show unique profiles, including *BRAF* V600E mutations in subsets with metanephric adenoma-like features (although debate exists about whether these are a unique histology and not truly WT).[78] These findings raise the possibility of divergent tumorigenic pathways and underscore the need for further genomic characterization to inform tailored therapeutic strategies.

Extrarenal Wilms tumor Rarely, a WT may occur in an extrarenal location, defined as being completely outside the kidney capsule. The most common location is in the retroperitoneum. Additional reported sites include the inguinal regions, female genital organs (ovary and uterus), mediastinum, adrenal glands, pelvis, bladder, colon, prostate, or scrotum. Because these tumors arise completely outside the kidney capsule, they are given a minimum designation of stage II. Treatment protocols are similar to renal WT, but diagnosis and sequencing of multimodality therapies may be altered, given the unexpected histology in many cases.[79]

CLINICS CARE POINTS

- Obtain noncontrast chest CT at diagnosis; chest radiography alone may miss pulmonary metastases and lead to undertreatment.
- Avoid percutaneous biopsy when Wilms tumor is resectable, as biopsy upstages disease according to some management guidelines and increases need for radiotherapy.
- Perform systematic lymph node sampling during nephrectomy; inadequate sampling risks understaging and insufficient adjuvant therapy.
- Distinguish nephrogenic rests from Wilms tumor, as diffuse hyperplastic perilobar nephroblastomatosis is managed nonoperatively unless malignant transformation occurs.
- Prioritize nephron-sparing surgery in bilateral Wilms tumor after neoadjuvant chemotherapy to reduce long-term risk of end-stage renal disease.

DECLARATION OF ARTIFICIAL INTELLIGENCE AND ARTIFICIAL INTELLIGENCE-ASSISTED TECHNOLOGIES IN THE WRITING PROCESS

During the preparation of this article, the authors used GEN AI. After using this tool/service, the authors reviewed and edited the content as needed and take full responsibility for the content of the publication.

DISCLOSURE

The authors have no relevant commercial, financial, or other conflicts of interest to disclose.

REFERENCES

1. Davidoff AM. Wilms tumor. Adv Pediatr 2012;59(1):247–67.
2. Howlader N, Noone AM, Krapcho M, et al. SEER cancer statistics review, 1975-2016. Bethesda (MD): National Cancer Institute; 2019.
3. Turner JT, Brzezinski J, Dome JS. Wilms tumor predisposition. In: Adam MP, Feldman J, Mirzaa GM, editors. GeneReviews. University of Washington, Seattle; 2003. Available at: https://www.ncbi.nlm.nih.gov/books/NBK1294/.
4. Charlton J, Irtan S, Bergeron C, et al. Bilateral wilms tumour: a review of clinical and molecular features. Expert Rev Mol Med 2017;19:e8.
5. Murphy AJ, Cheng C, Williams J, et al. Genetic and epigenetic features of bilateral Wilms tumor predisposition in patients from the Children's Oncology Group AREN18B5-Q. Nat Commun 2023;14(1):8006.
6. Hol JA, Kuiper RP, van Dijk F, et al. Prevalence of (epi)genetic predisposing factors in a 5-Year unselected National Wilms Tumor cohort: a comprehensive clinical and genomic characterization. J Clin Oncol 2022;40(17):1892–902.
7. Kim JK, Hansen A, Peard L, et al. Bilateral Wilms Tumor in CLOVES syndrome. Urology 2023;177:178–80.
8. Maciaszek JL, Oak N, Nichols KE. Recent advances in Wilms' tumor predisposition. Hum Mol Genet 2020;29(R2):R138–49.
9. Davidoff AM, Soutter AD, Shochat SJ. Wilms tumor presenting with abdominal pain: a special subgroup of patients. Ann Surg Oncol 1998;5(3):213–5.
10. Green DM. Wilms' tumor. In: Green DM, editor. Diagnosis and management of malignant solid tumors in infants. Boston (MA): Martinus Nijhoff Publishing; 1985. p. 129–86.
11. Raffensperger J. Max Wilms and his tumor. J Pediatr Surg 2015;50(2):356–9.
12. Gadd S, Huff V, Walz AL, et al. A Children's Oncology Group and TARGET initiative exploring the genetic landscape of Wilms tumor. Nat Genet 2017;49(10):1487–94.
13. Walz AL, Ooms A, Gadd S, et al. Recurrent DGCR8, DROSHA, and SIX homeodomain mutations in favorable histology wilms tumors. Cancer Cell 2015;27(2):286–97.
14. Young MD, Mitchell TJ, Vieira Braga FA, et al. Single-cell transcriptomes from human kidneys reveal the cellular identity of renal tumors. Science 2018;361(6402):594–9.
15. Beckwith JB, Kiviat NB, Bonadio JF. Nephrogenic rests, nephroblastomatosis, and the pathogenesis of Wilms' tumor. Pediatr Pathol 1990;10(1–2):1–36.
16. Ehrlich PF, Tornwall B, Chintagumpala MM, et al. Kidney preservation and Wilms tumor development in children with diffuse hyperplastic perilobar nephroblastomatosis: a report from the Children's Oncology Group Study AREN0534. Ann Surg Oncol 2022;29(5):3252–61.
17. Sandberg JK, Chi YY, Smith EA, et al. Imaging characteristics of nephrogenic rests versus small wilms tumors: a report from the Children's Oncology Group Study AREN03B2. AJR Am J Roentgenol 2020;214(5):987–94.
18. Duffy KA, Cielo CM, Cohen JL, et al. Characterization of the beckwith-Wiedemann spectrum: diagnosis and management. Am J Med Genet C Semin Med Genet 2019;181(4):693–708.

19. Coppes MJ, Zandvoort SW, Sparling CR, et al. Acquired von Willebrand disease in Wilms' tumor patients. J Clin Oncol 1992;10(3):422–7.
20. Dumba M, Jawad N, McHugh K. Neuroblastoma and nephroblastoma: a radiological review. Cancer Imaging 2015;15(1):5.
21. Khanna G, Naranjo A, Hoffer F, et al. Detection of preoperative Wilms tumor rupture with CT: a report from the Children's Oncology Group. Radiology 2013; 266(2):610–7.
22. Zhuge Y, Cheung MC, Yang R, et al. Improved survival with lymph node sampling in Wilms tumor. J Surg Res 2011;167(2):e199–203.
23. Kieran K, Anderson JR, Dome JS, et al. Lymph node involvement in Wilms tumor: results from National Wilms Tumor Studies 4 and 5. J Pediatr Surg 2012;47(4): 700–6.
24. Ehrlich PF, Hamilton TE, Gow K, et al. Surgical protocol violations in children with renal tumors provides an opportunity to improve pediatric cancer care: a report from the Children's Oncology Group. Pediatr Blood Cancer 2016;63(11):1905–10.
25. Qureshi SS, Bhagat M, Kazi M, et al. Standardizing lymph nodal sampling for Wilms tumor: a feasibility study with outcomes. J Pediatr Surg 2020;55(12):2668–75.
26. Owens CM, Veys PA, Pritchard J, et al. Role of chest computed tomography at diagnosis in the management of Wilms' tumor: a study by the United Kingdom Children's Cancer Study Group. J Clin Oncol 2002;20(12):2768–73.
27. Nakayama DK, Bonasso PC. The history of multimodal treatment of wilms' tumor. Am Surg 2016;82(6):487–92.
28. Dome JS, Graf N, Geller JI, et al. Advances in Wilms Tumor treatment and biology: progress through international collaboration. J Clin Oncol 2015;33(27): 2999–3007.
29. Chagtai T, Zill C, Dainese L, et al. Gain of 1q as a prognostic biomarker in wilms tumors (WTs) treated with preoperative chemotherapy in the international Society of Paediatric Oncology (SIOP) WT 2001 trial: a SIOP renal tumours Biology consortium study. J Clin Oncol 2016;34(26):3195–203.
30. Gratias EJ, Dome JS, Jennings LJ, et al. Association of chromosome 1q gain with inferior survival in favorable-histology Wilms tumor: a report from the Children's Oncology Group. J Clin Oncol 2016;34(26):3189–94.
31. Fernandez CV, Perlman EJ, Mullen EA, et al. Clinical outcome and biological predictors of relapse after nephrectomy only for very low-risk Wilms tumor: a report from Children's Oncology Group AREN0532. Ann Surg 2017;265(4):835–40.
32. Grundy PE, Breslow NE, Li S, et al. Loss of heterozygosity for chromosomes 1p and 16q is an adverse prognostic factor in favorable-histology Wilms tumor: a report from the National Wilms Tumor Study Group. J Clin Oncol 2005;23(29): 7312–21.
33. Evageliou N, Renfro LA, Geller J, et al. Prognostic impact of lymph node involvement and loss of heterozygosity of 1p or 16q in stage III favorable histology Wilms tumor: a report from Children's Oncology Group Studies AREN03B2 and AREN0532. Cancer 2024;130(5):792–802.
34. Dix DB, Fernandez CV, Chi YY, et al. Augmentation of therapy for combined loss of heterozygosity 1p and 16q in favorable histology Wilms tumor: a Children's Oncology Group AREN0532 and AREN0533 study report. J Clin Oncol 2019;37-(30):2769–77.
35. Aldrink JH, Heaton TE, Dasgupta R, et al. Update on Wilms tumor. J Pediatr Surg 2019;54(3):390–7.

36. Ehrlich P, Chi YY, Chintagumpala MM, et al. Results of the first prospective multi-institutional treatment study in children with bilateral Wilms tumor (AREN0534): a report from the Children's Oncology Group. Ann Surg 2017;266(3):470–8.
37. Ehrlich PF, Chi YY, Chintagumpala MM, et al. Results of treatment for patients with multicentric or bilaterally predisposed unilateral Wilms tumor (AREN0534): a report from the Children's Oncology Group. Cancer 2020;126(15):3516–25.
38. van den Heuvel-Eibrink MM, Hol JA, Pritchard-Jones K, et al. Position paper: rationale for the treatment of Wilms tumour in the UMBRELLA SIOP-RTSG 2016 protocol. Nat Rev Urol 2017;14(12):743–52.
39. Mitchell C, Pritchard-Jones K, Shannon R, et al. Immediate nephrectomy versus preoperative chemotherapy in the management of non-metastatic Wilms' tumour: results of a randomised trial (UKW3) by the UK Children's Cancer Study Group. Eur J Cancer 2006;42(15):2554–62.
40. Fuchs J, Kienecker K, Furtwangler R, et al. Surgical aspects in the treatment of patients with unilateral Wilms tumor: a report from the SIOP 93-01/German society of pediatric oncology and hematology. Ann Surg 2009;249(4):666–71.
41. Vujanic GM, Gessler M, Ooms A, et al. The UMBRELLA SIOP-RTSG 2016 wilms tumour pathology and molecular biology protocol. Nat Rev Urol 2018;15(11): 693–701.
42. Faria P, Beckwith JB, Mishra K, et al. Focal versus diffuse anaplasia in Wilms tumor–new definitions with prognostic significance: a report from the National Wilms Tumor Study Group. Am J Surg Pathol 1996;20(8):909–20.
43. Armstrong AE, Daw NC, Renfro LA, et al. Treatment of focal anaplastic Wilms tumor: a report from the Children's Oncology Group AREN0321 and AREN03B2 studies. Cancer 2025;131(2):e35713.
44. Ooms AH, Gadd S, Gerhard DS, et al. Significance of TP53 mutation in wilms tumors with diffuse anaplasia: a report from the Children's Oncology Group. Clin Cancer Res 2016;22(22):5582–91.
45. Daw NC, Chi YY, Kim Y, et al. Treatment of stage I anaplastic Wilms' tumour: a report from the Children's Oncology Group AREN0321 study. Eur J Cancer 2019;118: 58–66.
46. Daw NC, Chi YY, Kalapurakal JA, et al. Activity of vincristine and Irinotecan in diffuse anaplastic Wilms tumor and therapy outcomes of stage II to IV disease: results of the Children's Oncology Group AREN0321 study. J Clin Oncol 2020;38-(14):1558–68.
47. Vujanic GM, D'Hooghe E, Vokuhl C, et al. Dataset for the reporting of nephrectomy specimens for Wilms' tumour treated with preoperative chemotherapy: recommendations from the International Society of Paediatric Oncology Renal Tumour Study group. Histopathology 2021;79(5):678–86.
48. Benedetti DJ, Cost NG, Ehrlich PF, et al. Updated favourable-histology Wilms tumour risk stratification: rationale for future Children's Oncology Group clinical trials. Nat Rev Urol 2025;22(11):775–88.
49. Chintagumpala MM, Perlman EJ, Tornwall B, et al. Outcomes based on histopathologic response to preoperative chemotherapy in children with bilateral Wilms tumor: a prospective study (COG AREN0534). Cancer 2022;128(13):2493–503.
50. Fernandez CV, Mullen EA, Chi YY, et al. Outcome and prognostic factors in stage III favorable-histology Wilms Tumor: a report from the Children's Oncology Group Study AREN0532. J Clin Oncol 2018;36(3):254–61.
51. Benedetti DJ, Varela CR, Renfro LA, et al. Treatment of children with favorable histology Wilms tumor with extrapulmonary metastases: a report from the COG

studies AREN0533 and AREN03B2 and NWTSG study NWTS-5. Cancer 2024; 130(6):947–61.

52. Hol JA, Lopez-Yurda MI, Van Tinteren H, et al. Prognostic significance of age in 5631 patients with Wilms tumour prospectively registered in International Society of Paediatric Oncology (SIOP) 93-01 and 2001. PLoS One 2019;14(8):e0221373.
53. Renfro LA, Vallance KL, Tfirn IC, et al. Associations of patient age, tumor nephrectomy weight, and tumor diameter with event-free and overall survival in stage I or II favorable histology Wilms tumor: a pooled analysis of Children's Oncology Group studies AREN0532 and AREN03B2. Ann Surg 2025. https://doi.org/10.1097/SLA.0000000000006726.
54. Wegert J, Ishaque N, Vardapour R, et al. Mutations in the SIX1/2 pathway and the DROSHA/DGCR8 miRNA microprocessor complex underlie high-risk blastemal type wilms tumors. Cancer Cell 2015;27(2):298–311.
55. Dix DB, Seibel NL, Chi YY, et al. Treatment of stage IV favorable histology Wilms tumor with lung metastases: a report from the Children's Oncology Group AREN0533 study. J Clin Oncol 2018;36(16):1564–70.
56. de Campos Vieira Abib S, Chui CH, Cox S, et al. International society of Paediatric Surgical Oncology (IPSO) Surgical Practice Guidelines. ecancermedicalscience 2022;16:1356.
57. Kieran K, Anderson JR, Dome JS, et al. Is adrenalectomy necessary during unilateral nephrectomy for Wilms tumor? A report from the Children's Oncology Group. J Pediatr Surg 2013;48(7):1598–603.
58. Kessler O, Franco I, Jayabose S, et al. Is contralateral exploration of the kidney necessary in patients with Wilms tumor? J Urol 1996;156(2 Pt 2):693–5.
59. Green DM, Breslow NE, D'Angio GJ, et al. Outcome of patients with stage II/favorable histology Wilms tumor with and without local tumor spill: a report from the National Wilms Tumor Study Group. Pediatr Blood Cancer 2014;61(1):134–9.
60. Petrushkevich A, Livingston E, Davidson J, et al. Dictation precision: evaluating paediatric oncology operative reports as an impetus for synoptic reports. J Pediatr Surg 2025;60(4):162186.
61. Ritchey M, Daley S, Shamberger RC, et al. Ureteral extension in Wilms' tumor: a report from the National Wilms' Tumor Study Group (NWTSG). J Pediatr Surg 2008;43(9):1625–9.
62. Abdelhafeez AH, Davidoff AM, Murphy AJ, et al. Fluorescence-guided lymph node sampling is feasible during up-front or delayed nephrectomy for Wilms tumor. J Pediatr Surg 2022. https://doi.org/10.1016/j.jpedsurg.2022.06.002.
63. Roberts R, Pachl M. Intraparenchymal indocyanine green use improves nodal yield during minimally invasive tumor nephrectomy in children. J Laparoendosc Adv Surg Tech 2024;34(11):1039–43.
64. Pachl MJ. Fluorescent guided lymph node harvest in laparoscopic wilms nephroureterectomy. Urology 2021;158:189–92.
65. VanHouwelingen LT, Seims AD, Ortega-Laureano L, et al. Use of ultrasound in diagnosing postoperative small-bowel intussusception in pediatric surgical oncology patients: a single-center retrospective review. Pediatr Radiol 2018;48(2):204–9.
66. Ritchey ML, Kelalis PP, Etzioni R, et al. Small bowel obstruction after nephrectomy for Wilms' tumor. A report of the National Wilms' tumor Study-3. Ann Surg 1993; 218(5):654–9.
67. Weil BR, Murphy AJ, Liu Q, et al. Late health outcomes among survivors of Wilms tumor diagnosed over three decades: a report from the childhood cancer survivor study. J Clin Oncol 2023;41(14):2638–50.

68. Shamberger RC, Ritchey ML, Haase GM, et al. Intravascular extension of Wilms tumor. Ann Surg 2001;234(1):116–21.
69. Ribeiro RC, Schettini ST, Abib Sde C, et al. Cavectomy for the treatment of Wilms tumor with vascular extension. J Urol 2006;176(1):279–83 [discussion: 283–4].
70. Cox SG, Davidson A, Thomas J, et al. Surgical management and outcomes of 12 cases of Wilms tumour with intracardiac extension from a single centre. Pediatr Surg Int 2018;34(2):227–35.
71. Davidoff AM, Interiano RB, Wynn L, et al. Overall survival and renal function of patients with synchronous bilateral Wilms tumor undergoing surgery at a single institution. Ann Surg 2015;262(4):570–6.
72. Breslow NE, Collins AJ, Ritchey ML, et al. End stage renal disease in patients with Wilms tumor: results from the National Wilms Tumor Study Group and the United States Renal Data System. J Urol 2005;174(5):1972–5.
73. Murphy AJ, Davidoff AM. Nephron-sparing surgery for Wilms tumor. Front Pediatr 2023;11:1122390.
74. Romao RLP, Aldrink JH, Renfro LA, et al. Bilateral Wilms tumor with anaplasia: a report from the Children's Oncology Group Study AREN0534. Pediatr Blood Cancer 2024;71(7):e30981.
75. Mrad C, Coulomb-Lhermine A, Tabone MD, et al. Evaluation of the nephron-sparing surgery formula in Wilms tumors. Pediatr Blood Cancer 2020;67(12):e28661.
76. Spreafico F, Ferrari A, Mascarin M, et al. Wilms tumor, medulloblastoma, and rhabdomyosarcoma in adult patients: lessons learned from the pediatric experience. Cancer Metastasis Rev 2019;38(4):683–94.
77. Segers H, van den Heuvel-Eibrink MM, Pritchard-Jones K, et al. Management of adults with Wilms' tumor: recommendations based on international consensus. Expert Rev Anticancer Ther 2011;11(7):1105–13.
78. Argani P, Tickoo SK, Matoso A, et al. Adult Wilms tumor: genetic evidence of origin of a subset of cases from metanephric adenoma. Am J Surg Pathol 2022;46(7):988–99.
79. Karim A, Shaikhyzada K, Abulkhanova N, et al. Pediatric extra-renal nephroblastoma (Wilms' tumor): a systematic case-based review. Cancers (Basel) 2023;15(9). https://doi.org/10.3390/cancers15092563.

Neuroblastoma

Meera Kotagal, MD, MPH[a,*], Christa N. Grant, MD[b],
Erin G. Brown, MD[c], Dave R. Lal, MD, MPH[d,1],
Erika A. Newman, MD, MBA[e,1]

KEYWORDS

• Neuroblastoma • Pediatric oncology • Surgical oncology • Childhood cancer

KEY POINTS

- Neuroblastoma (NB) is the most common extracranial pediatric solid tumor, accounting for 8% of childhood cancer and 15% of cancer-related mortality in children.
- NB may vary in severity and prognosis from low-risk congenital neuroblastic masses to aggressive high-risk NB.
- A revised risk stratification system from the Children's Oncology Group stratifies patients as low, intermediate, and high risk.
- Therapy is risk-directed with intensification of therapy for those at greater risk and de-escalation for patients with lower risk tumors.

INTRODUCTION

Neuroblastoma (NB) is the most common extracranial pediatric solid tumor, accounting for 8% of childhood cancers and 15% of cancer-related mortality in children.[1–3] First described in 1864 by the German physician Rudolf Virchow, NB is a small, round, and blue cell tumor. The most common location for development of NB is the adrenal glands, but primary tumors may develop along the developmental pathway of neural crest progenitor cells.[4] NB may vary in severity and prognosis from low-risk congenital neuroblastic tumors to aggressive high-risk neuroblastoma. The former often spontaneously regress; while the latter requires high intensity multi-modal therapy. Surgical resection has a critical role in local control of NB for the most optimal outcome.

[a] Division of Pediatric General and Thoracic Surgery, Department of Surgery, Cincinnati Children's Hospital, University of Cincinnati College of Medicine, Cincinnati, OH, USA; [b] Department of Pediatric Surgery, New York Medical College/Maria Fareri Children's Hospital, Westchester Medical Center, Valhalla, NY, USA; [c] Division of Pediatric Surgery, UC Davis Medical Center, Sacramento, CA, USA; [d] Division of Pediatric Surgery, Children's Wisconsin/Medical College of Wisconsin, Milwaukee, WI, USA; [e] Division of Pediatric Surgery, University of Michigan, Ann Arbor, MI, USA
[1] These authors contributed equally and are co-senior authors of this work.
* Corresponding author. Division of Pediatric General and Thoracic Surgery, Cincinnati Children's Hospital, 3333 Burnet Avenue, Cincinnati, OH 45229.
E-mail address: meera.kotagal@cchmc.org

Surg Oncol Clin N Am 35 (2026) 715–729
https://doi.org/10.1016/j.soc.2026.04.012 surgonc.theclinics.com

Abbreviations	
ALK	anaplastic lymphoma kinase
CBC	complete blood count
COG	Children's Oncology Group
EFS	event-free survival
ERAS	enhanced recovery after surgery
IDRF	image-defined risk factors
MIBG	metaiodobenzylguanidine
MKI	mitotic karyorrhexis index
NB	neuroblastoma
SBO	small bowel obstruction
SCA	segmental chromosome aberrations

EPIDEMIOLOGY

The median age at diagnosis of NB is 17 to 19 months, with 90% of cases diagnosed before 10 years of age. While NB may be diagnosed in older children or adults, it is uncommon over the age of 10 years.

There are approximately 650 new diagnoses of NB in the United States annually, and the prevalence is approximately 1 in 7000 live births.[5] Overall, the incidence of NB has slightly increased globally over the last 30 years.[5] NB is more prevalent in high-income countries. NB is slightly more common in males than females with the most noticeable difference in children ages 2 to 4 years in whom the incidence ratio of boys to girls is 2:1. In the United States, the incidence of NB is highest in non-Hispanic White children than any other race and ethnicity group; survival is higher for non-Hispanic White and Hispanic patients than non-Hispanic Black patients.[6]

To date, no environmental factors have been associated with the development of neuroblastoma. The majority of NB cases are spontaneous, with only 2% of cases arising from familial causes.[7] Patients with familial NB present at a younger age and are more likely to present with multifocal tumors, particularly bilateral adrenal masses. The most common germline mutations associated with familial NB are the PHOX2B gene, anaplastic lymphoma kinase (*ALK*) oncogene, KIF1Bβ tumor suppressor gene, RAS pathway mutations, and deletions at the 1p36 or 11q14 to 23 locus. Children with cancer predisposition syndromes such as Beckwith-Wiedemann, Costello, Noonan, Li-Fraumeni, ROHHAD, and hereditary pheochromocytoma also have an increased risk of developing NB.

HISTOLOGY

Tumors along the neuroblastic spectrum originate from neural crest cells, allowing for the development along the sympathetic axis from the neck to the pelvis. The tumors can span the spectrum of differentiation from undifferentiated small blue cells (neuroblastoma) to intermediate differentiation (ganglioneuroblastoma) to highly differentiated (ganglioneuroma; **Fig. 1**A–C).[8] Tumor histology is divided into favorable and unfavorable. Favorable histology tumors are stroma-rich with Schwannian stroma and have evidence of differentiation of cells, as well as low mitotic karyorrhexis index (MKI).[9]

Histologic analysis of neuroblastic tumors, requires this assessment of the differentiation, as well as cytogenics for evaluation of segmental chromosome aberrations (SCA). Loss of heterozygosity of 1p, 11q, and 14q are present in 50% of neuroblastomas.[10] These chromosomal changes, as well as gain of 17p are most commonly associated with poor outcomes. In particular, deletion of 11q is associated with

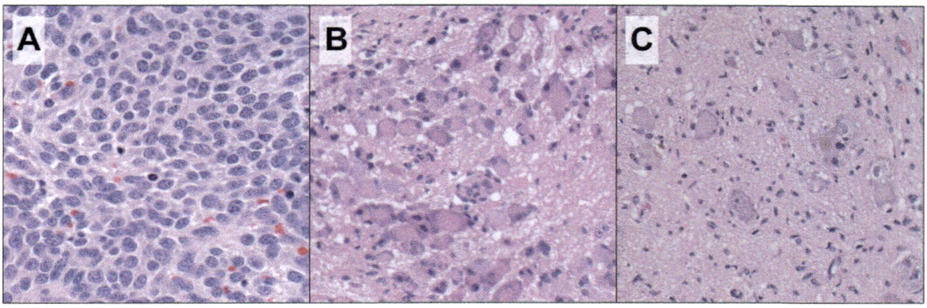

Fig. 1. Histologic spectrum of neuroblastic tumors. NB (*A*) composed of poorly differentiated neuroblasts embedded within neuropil and lacking accompanying Schwannian stroma. Ganglioneuroblastoma, intermixed (*B*), with a range of poorly differentiated neuroblasts to maturing ganglion cells and patchy neuropil set in an overall background of at least 50% Schwannian stroma. Ganglioneuroma (*C*) with only mature/maturing ganglion cells within Schwannian stroma, and lacking immature neuroblasts and neuropil. (*Figure courtesy of* Jason Jarzembowski, MD, PhD.)

high risk of recurrence and worse outcomes overall.[11] Tumors may also be hyperdiploid, or have gene amplifications.[12] Hyperdiploid status is associated with improved overall survival—long-term disease free survival in more than 90%—compared to diploid tumors, which may be associated with early treatment failure.[12] The MYCN oncogene is amplified in approximately 30%, and this amplification is associated with poorer prognosis.[13] Amplification of this gene implies greater than 10 copies, and presence of this amplification remains one of the most powerful prognostic indicators for tumor behavior and survival, with resistance to therapy more frequently observed among this subset of children with neuroblastoma.[14] There is some overlap between these factors, with MYCN amplification more frequent among patients with diploid tumors.[12]

Additionally, ALK mutations causing proto-oncogene activation are associated with hereditary neuroblastoma.[15] These mutations, as well as amplification of the gene, can be somatically acquired, and may be targets for ALK inhibitors such as crizotinib and loratinib.[16] Mutations in ATRX, a transcriptional regulator that plays a role in telomere maintenance to prevent shortening and chromosomal instability, have been found in older patients with advanced stage NB.[17]

Often histologic analysis of tumors is performed at diagnosis through percutaneous core needle biopsy, and patients are stratified based on their histologic, imaging, and genetic features to determine treatment approach.

STAGING

Staging for patients with NB is performed using a pretreatment risk stratification system. This system considers pretreatment image-defined risk factors (IDRFs), as well as evidence of metastasis, to determine the therapeutic strategy.

IDRFs were established by the International Neuroblastoma Risk Group (INRG) to allow for standardized interpretation of risk. A list of IDRFs is included in **Box 1**. Based upon the presence of IDRFs and metastatic disease, a tumor is staged as L1, L2, M, or MS. L1 disease is localized without IDRFs; L2 disease indicates the presence of at least one IDRF and may include ipsilateral contiguous body compartments (eg, right thorax and abdomen). Stage M disease includes distant metastases, including contralateral body compartments, and infiltration of the bone marrow over 10%. MS disease

Box 1
Image-define risk factors by anatomic compartment

Neck:
- Tumor encasing carotid and/or vertebral artery and/or internal jugular vein
- Tumor extending to base of skull
- Tumor compressing the trachea

Cervico-thoracic junction:
- Tumor encasing brachial plexus roots
- Tumor encasing subclavian vessels and/or vertebral and/or carotid artery
- Tumor compressing the trachea

Thorax:
- Tumor encasing the aorta and/or major branches
- Tumor compressing the trachea or principal bronchi
- Lower left mediastinal tumor, infiltrating the costovertebral junction between T9-12

Thoraco-abdominal:
- Tumor encasing the aorta and/or vena cava

Abdomen:
- Tumor infiltrating the porta hepatic and/or the hepatoduodenal ligament
- Tumor encasing branches of the superior mesenteric artery at the mesenteric root
- Tumor encasing the origin of the celiac axis, and/or of the superior mesenteric artery
- Tumor invading one or both renal pedicles[a]
- Tumor encasing the aorta and/or vena cava
- Tumor encasing the iliac vessels
- Pelvic tumor crossing the sciatic notch

Dumbbell tumors with signs of spinal cord compression (any compartment)

Infiltration of adjacent organs/structures:
- Pericardium, diaphragm, kidney, liver, duodenopancreatic block, or mesentery

[a]Updated guideline in 2011 that any contact with the renal pedicle was to be considered an IDRF [Ref].[18]

can only be established in patients less than 18 months of age with metastases confined to the skin, liver, and/or less than 10% of bone marrow.

Using INRG Stage (**Table 1**) as well as age, tumor histologic and genetic characteristics, and extent of resection for L1 tumors, the Children's Oncology Group created a revised risk classification system, which is now the standard of care for risk

Table 1
International neuroblastoma risk group stage

Stage	Definition
L1	localized tumor contained within one body compartment without IDRF, including intraspinal tumors not meeting IDRF definition
L2	local-regional tumor with one or more IDRF, ipsilateral contiguous body compartments
M	distant metastases excluding MS disease (see later), contralateral contiguous body compartments
MS	L1 or L2 primary, less than 18 months of age with metastases confined to skin, liver, and/or bone marrow (<10% of nucleated cells) and negative MIBG for bone/bone marrow

classification and treatment in Children's Oncology Group (COG) NB trials (**Fig. 2**A, B)[14] This system classifies children as low-risk, intermediate-risk, or high-risk. Ongoing determination of risk stratification balances the need for treatment intensification in those with greatest risk, while minimizing treatment intensity in children with lower risk to mitigate late effects and toxicity.

MULTIDISCIPLINARY MANAGEMENT: LOW-RISK, INTERMEDIATE-RISK, HIGH-RISK

The heterogeneity of neuroblastic tumors results in highly variable prognosis and outcomes. In the current COG V2 stratification system, low risk patients have a 5-year EFS of 91%, while intermediate risk patients have an EFS of 85% and high risk patients with EFS of 51%.[14] These differential outcomes have led to heterogeneity of treatment approaches as well. Therapy is risk-directed with intensification of therapy for those at greater risk and de-escalation for patients with lower risk tumors. Determination of necessary therapy centers on risk stratification – which includes both INRG staging, as well as tumor biology including histology, diploid status, and presence or absence of segmental chromosomal abnormalities (SCA).[14] With the exception of low risk tumors, much of the management of NB requires a multi-modal approach.

Low Risk Disease

Patients in the low-risk stratum include those with L1 tumors without MYCN amplification, as well as a small subset of L2 and MS patients. Patients less than 6 months of age with tumors limited to the adrenal gland can be observed and their tumors will frequently regress spontaneously. COG ANBL00P2 found that these patients have a 100% survival rate, and fewer than 20% ever required a surgical intervention.[19] COG ANBL1232 is evaluating an expansion of this observation cohort, to include

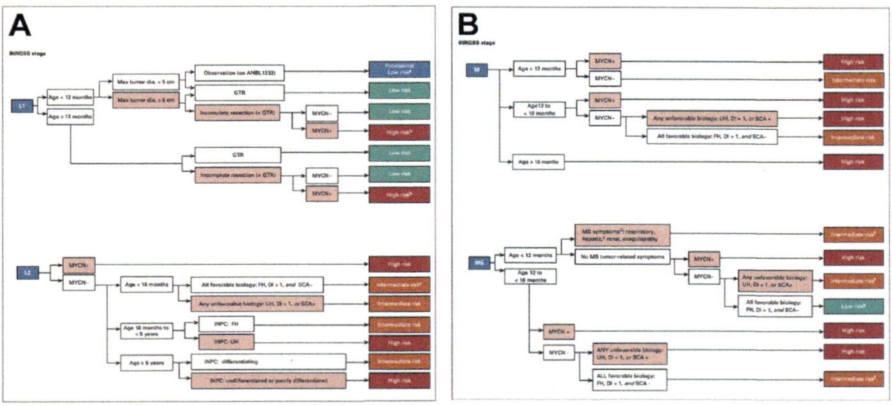

Fig. 2. Revised COG Risk Classification System for (*A*) L1 and L2 patients and (*B*) M and MS patients. [a]If tumor progresses during observation, biopsy or resect and reclassify with biomarkers (as in COGANBL1232); [b]Consider complete resection if feasible; [c]If no tumor burden symptoms, consider observation (as in COG ANBL1232); [d]Biopsy contraindicated, defer biopsy until stable (note: biomarker results may modify Risk Class); [e]Hepatomegaly alone is an MS symptom in patients age , 3 months of age (see COG ANBL1232); [f]Response-based therapy (as in COG ANBL1232); [g]MS score–based therapy (as in COG ANBL1232). (*From* Irwin MS, Naranjo A, Zhang FF, et al. Revised Neuroblastoma Risk Classification System: A Report From the Children's Oncology Group. J Clin Oncol 2021;39(29):3229–3241. https://doi.org/10.1200/JCO.21.00278. Epub 2021 Jul 28. PMID: 34319759; PMCID: PMC8500606.)

patients less than 12 months of age with either an adrenal or nonadrenal primary. In addition, patients less than 18 months of age with L2 tumors and favorable biology (favorable histology, hyperdiploid, and no SCAs) can also be observed on study. Lastly, patients with MS stage disease (metastasis to the skin, liver, and/or 10% bone marrow) who are less than 12 months with favorable biology (favorable histology, hyperdiploid, and no SCAs) and MYCN nonamplified can be observed. For others with L1 tumors, which are non MYCN-amplified, surgical resection is usually the only therapy required. Chemotherapy and radiation are generally not required for this patient population, with excellent event-free and long-term survival outcomes.

Intermediate Risk Disease

Overall, using the COG V2 risk group stratification, patients with intermediate risk disease have a 5-year event-free survival (EFS) of 85%.[14] As such, the primary goal is to balance improved survival with minimization of late effects. The majority of patients with intermediate risk disease are stage L2. As such, most will have neoadjuvant chemotherapy before surgical resection. Patients who have greater than 50% reduction in tumor burden with neoadjuvant chemotherapy can safely be observed without surgical resection. A small subset, deemed resectable at diagnosis with minimal risk, can undergo upfront resection. For all others requiring surgery as part of their multimodal disease control, the goal is to resect as much as possible while ensuring there is no disability, injury to adjacent organs, or compromised neurologic function. This may result in residual tumor left alongside critical structures (eg, renal pedicle); this is acceptable as long as a greater than 50% reduction in tumor burden is achieved.

In addition to L2 patients, a subset of M and MS patients are also intermediate risk. These include patients without MYCN amplification less than 1 year of age, and those without MYCN amplification and overall favorable biology (favorable histology, hyperdiploid, and no SCAs) between 12 and 18 months of age.

High-Risk Disease

While patients with low-risk and intermediate-risk have largely excellent outcomes—and have been able to have reductions in therapy–high risk patients have continued to have suboptimal 5-year EFS of only 50%. This has resulted in on-going intensification of therapy to provide the best possible long-term outcomes. This multimodal approach includes induction chemotherapy, surgical resection, myeloablative consolidation with stem cell rescue, radiation, isotretinoin, and chemoimmunotherapy. High risk disease includes nearly all patients with MYCN amplification (except for L1 patients who undergo upfront gross total resection), as well L2 patients with MYCN nonamplification and unfavorable histology, patients with metastatic disease greater than 18 months (regardless of MYCN amplification status), and M and MS patients 12 to 18 months of age with MYCN nonamplification and unfavorable biology. Surgical resection usually occurs after 4 cycles of neoadjuvant chemotherapy to maximize tumor response and reduce fibrotic changes.[20]

In addition to neoadjuvant chemotherapy and surgical resection, additional therapies have been added to the treatment regimen for high-risk disease to improve outcomes. Myeloablative consolidation therapy with stem cell rescue was found initially not to increase overall survival.[21] However, addition of a second tandem transplant on ANBL0532 improved 3-year EFS from 48% to 62%.[22] Furthermore, 13-cis retinoic acid (isotretinoin) has been included in the treatment of high-risk neuroblastoma as part of maintenance therapy after tandem transplant for improved EFS.[23] Lastly, immunotherapy—in the form of anti-GD2 antibodies—have also demonstrated improved EFS for patients with high-risk disease.[24] GD2 is a glycolipid expressed on the surface of neuroblastoma cells, and use of anti-GD2 antibodies results in both antibody-dependent and complement-dependent cytotoxicity.

INDICATIONS FOR SURGERY

Surgery is a cornerstone of treatment of NB, with treatment largely based on risk stratification and stage as described. When considering surgical resection, local stage of the primary tumor is a significant factor. Resectable L1 tumors in low-risk patients should be removed entirely unless they meet specific criterion for observation, as discussed earlier. Additionally, stage MS patients usually receive supportive care without surgery due to high rates of spontaneous tumor regression. Complete resection of intermediate-risk tumors has not been shown to improve survival, and current guidance recommends greater than 50% resection.[25] In contrast, gross total resection of all macroscopic disease is the recommendation for high-risk neuroblastoma, with greater than 90% resection being shown to improve outcomes in several large cooperative group trials, although ongoing debate exists regarding the impact of complete resection on long-term outcomes.[26–28] Complete resection with microscopically negative margins is not indicated and is often not achievable due to the nature of NB encasing vital organs and vessels. Preoperative risk stratification, including tumor stage and risk group, should be considered when determining how aggressive surgical intervention should be. Importantly, vital structures should not be resected to achieve an R0 resection.

PREOPERATIVE PREPARATION/RISK/IMAGE-DEFINED RISK FACTORS

Preoperative preparation for children with NB begins with a complete history and physical examination. Laboratory studies should include serum chemistries, complete blood count (CBC), coagulation studies and tumor markers including urine vanillylmandelic acic (VMA) and homovanillic acid (HVA). A complete nutritional assessment should be performed at diagnosis and preoperatively to optimize surgical outcomes.

Radiographic studies at diagnosis include ultrasound of palpable abdominal lesion if present, followed by cross-sectional imaging of the relevant body compartments with either computed tomography (CT) or magnetic resonance imaging (MRI). A metaiodobenzylguanidine (MIBG) scan along with chest imaging if not already performed, completes the staging imaging. If neoadjuvant chemotherapy is administered, cross-sectional imaging should be repeated before surgery for preoperative planning. Imaging should be carefully reviewed with a pediatric radiologist to assess for the presence of IDRFs, radiographic features of vascular encasement and invasion of critical structures. This list of locally aggressive radiographic features is defined for each body compartment and was established by the International Neuroblastoma Risk Group in 2005 as a means to preoperatively assess the risk of surgical resection (see **Table 1**).[29] The presence of any IDRF strongly correlates with increased risk of surgical complications and lesser extent of tumor resection, and IDRF assessment is a critical component of preoperative staging and risk stratification for patients with neuroblastoma.[30–33] Given the complexity of these tumors, emerging evidence supports the role of 3-dimension imaging technology as a tool for preoperative planning for neuroblastoma resection, but additional research is to better assess the implementation and benefits of this resource (**Fig. 3**A–D).[34]

Preparation for the operating room (OR) should consider the unique anatomic considerations based on location of the tumor. Tracheal compression may be present in cervical and thoracic tumors and airway precautions should be considered when

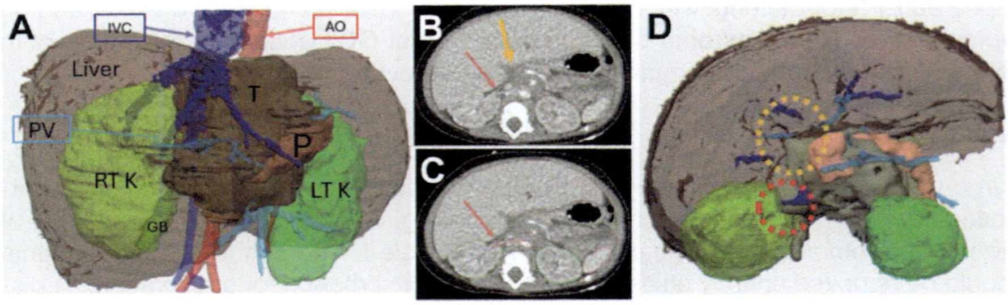

Fig. 3. (*A*) 3D digital model of a neuroblastoma tumor (T, *dark brown*) encasing the aorta (AO, *red*), inferior vena cava (IVC, *blue*), portal vein (PV, *cyan*), and invading the porta hepatis and pancreas (P). (*B*) Axial postcontrast image of the abdomen clearly demonstrates the tumor infiltrating the porta hepatis (*orange arrow*); however, invasion of the right renal pedicle remains unclear (*red arrow*). (*C*) Postsegmentation MRR images, obliqued to clarify the right renal pedicle infiltration, confirm involvement of the right renal pedicle (*red arrow*). (*D*) Top view of the 3D digital model in slice mode, intuitively demonstrating porta hepatis infiltration (*orange circle*) and infiltration of the right renal pedicle (*red circle*).

present. Peripheral nerve monitoring should be used in high-risk paraspinal tumor excisions and tumors with extensive nerve involvement.[35] When feasible, consideration should be given to enhanced recovery after surgery (ERAS) protocols, which have demonstrated improved outcomes, including reduced length of stay and decreased complications, for patients with NB.[36] Key components of these protocols include early postoperative enteral nutrition, reduced intraoperative and postoperative crystalloid fluid use, multimodal pain control to minimize opioid use including regional anesthesia, and minimization of lines and tubes such as Foley catheters, nasogastric tubes, and drains.

For L1 tumors, complete resection of the tumor, is often safe and feasible up front. For patients with favorable biology, a complete tumor resection may be the only treatment needed, and overall outcomes are excellent. For localized tumors without evidence of metastatic disease, tumor biopsy before surgical resection is typically unnecessary. Patients up to 6 months of were observed without biopsy, surgery, or chemotherapy on COG study ANBL00P2. Most of these tumors will spontaneously regress, but a greater than 50% increase in tumor volume was the threshold at which to offer resection. Three-year EFS was 100% and 81% of patients on the observation-only arm were spared surgery. ANBL1232.[19] Expansion of the age criteria up to 12 months with L1 tumors was explored on COG study ANBL1232. Trial results for these expanded criteria are pending.

L2 tumors, by definition, have IDRF present. Given this, surgical resection at the time of diagnosis may not be safe or feasible. Therefore, surgical indications at time of diagnosis are typically related to biopsy and placement of a vascular access device for therapy. Neoadjuvant chemotherapy followed by delayed tumor resection is recommended to reduce the risk of surgical complications and therapy delays.[37,38] COG guidelines recommend resection after 4 cycles of neoadjuvant chemotherapy for patients with high-risk disease, but resection after 2 cycles can be considered[39] in patients who achieve a good response to initial chemotherapy (resolution of the IDRF) and in whom resection is deemed safe. Finally, children younger than 18 months of age with L2 tumors and favorable histology and genomics (as defined by biopsy) were also observed on COG study ANBL1232 without surgery or chemotherapy due to their overall excellent prognosis and tendency to spontaneously regress.

For patients with metastatic disease, the diagnosis of neuroblastoma is most commonly confirmed by bone marrow aspirate and/or elevated catecholamines in the urine. Therefore, tumor biopsy is indicated only if tumor histopathology is required for risk classification such as when the bone marrow is negative or there is insufficient tissue for complete molecular characterization. Molecular characterization cannot be done without biopsy and BM is often not helpful. While definitive resection for local control remains important, this should be performed after neoadjuvant chemotherapy.[38]

Lastly, patients with MS disease typically demonstrate a high incidence of spontaneous regression, and their overall outcomes are quite favorable.[40] Therefore, supportive therapy is recommended and surgery is not typically indicated. The exception to this rule is infants presenting with prominent liver metastases and severe hepatomegaly who develop abdominal compartment syndrome. In these cases, decompressive laparotomy and temporary abdominal closure or use of a mesh for abdominal coverage has been recommended to reduce the intra-abdominal pressure.[39]

INTRAOPERATIVE MANAGEMENT/DECISION-MAKING

The goal of NB tumor resection varies by risk group and tumor stage; therefore, it is imperative that the surgeon understands the anatomy and presence/absence of IDRFs before tumor resection.

The operative approach to NB is influenced primarily by tumor location and the extent of involvement of surrounding structures. The key principles of vascular dissection during resection include (i) obtaining proximal and distal control of all named vessels abutted, encased or displaced by the tumor (ii) bivalving the tumor over encased vessels and nerves, (iii) piecemeal tumor excision as needed to maintain the integrity of vital structures and organs, and (iv) avoiding dissection deep to the adventitial layer of vessels during dissection. En bloc resection of adjacent organs should not be performed and is associated with increased morbidity. In addition to these key tenets, the following considerations are specific to each primary tumor site.

Cervical Tumors

Cervical tumors can be approached via a lateral neck dissection or cervicothoracic incision based on the inferior extent of the tumor. The vagus and phrenic nerves should be identified and preserved along their course. Use of intraoperative nerve monitoring is recommended for cervical tumors abutting or encasing the brachial plexus.

Thoracic Tumors

Small L1 thoracic tumors can be safely approached by thoracoscopy.[41] Thoracotomy is the incision of choice for larger tumors or those with IDRFs. Sternotomy may be required to gain proximal and distal control of encased central vessels and their primary branches. Except in cases of concomitant laminotomy/laminectomy and tumor resection by neurosurgery, dissection should not be continued into the vertebral foraminae, rather transected at the edge of the vertebral column. Minimal residual disease at this location has not been shown to affect outcome.[42,43]

Abdominal and Adrenal Tumors

L1 abdominal and pelvic tumors may be approached by laparoscopy. Minimally invasive techniques have been associated with decreased need for analgesics, faster return of bowel function, and shorter hospital stay.[44] Larger abdominal tumors and those with IDRFs are approached by transverse or vertical laparotomy. After initial exploration of the peritoneum, the tumor is exposed widely using fixed retractors, proximal and distal control of named vessels abutted or encased by the tumor is obtained, and initial findings are correlated with preoperative cross-sectional imaging to confirm resectability. Dissection proceeds following the key tenets described earlier, taking care to avoid injuring or removing adjacent organs such as the kidney or spleen. Use of ultrasonic sealers, ligation, or clips is encouraged for control of retroperitoneal lacteals to minimize the risk of chyle leak. Stimulation of chyle production by enteral introduction of lipid emulsion has been described to visualize the thoracic duct or cisterna chyli and to aid in identifying and sealing lymphatic leaks before closure.[45]

Pelvic Tumors

While small L1 pelvic tumors may be approached minimally invasively, larger pelvic tumors and L2 tumors are approached by lower midline laparotomy for best exposure. Pelvic paraspinal NB extending into the spinal canal (dumbbell tumors) may require laminotomy or laminectomy if symptomatic. Use of intraoperative nerve monitoring should be considered for tumors involving lumbosacral nerves.

COMPLICATIONS

Neuroblastoma complications can be caused by the tumor itself; patients may present with Horner's syndrome, pleural effusions, compartment syndrome, or paralysis at diagnosis.

Intraoperative complications such as hemorrhage, injury to major vessels or nerves, and chyle leak are more common in tumors with IDRFs and those requiring complex resection. Tumor adherence or encasement of named blood vessels or vital organs increases the risk of ischemia and unplanned resections including splenectomy, colectomy, bowel resection, and nephrectomy. There is a risk of nerve or spinal cord injury, cerebrospinal fluid leakage, and uncontrollable intraspinal bleeding during resection of dumbbell tumors, with laminectomy having a higher risk of morbidity than laminotomy.

Postoperative complications after neuroblastoma resection range from 5% to 25% and can impact the course and efficacy of neuroblastoma treatment.[46] The expected complications vary by primary site. Paralytic ileus is common following laparotomy, and usually resolves within 2 to 3 days. Persistent distension, vomiting, and lack of bowel function should raise suspicion for small bowel obstruction (SBO). The risk of SBO is higher in patients who undergo extensive retroperitoneal dissection. Adhesion of the serosa to the tumor bed can lead to adhesive SBO or intussusception requiring reoperation. Other complications of abdominal neuroblastoma resection include hypertension and diarrhea. Horner's syndrome may develop postoperatively following resection of low cervical and apical thoracic tumors, and presents with ptosis, miosis of the ipsilateral pupil, and/or anhidrosis. Pneumothorax and hemothorax may develop following resection of thoracic tumors. Chyle leaks may develop after left neck or right chest tumor resection and are particularly common following extensive retroperitoneal dissection of central abdominal neuroblastomas; typical treatment involves parenteral nutrition or a medium-chain triglyceride formula. Chyle leaks that persist despite nonoperative measures may require return to the operating room for identification and ligation, and may be diagnosed and treated by interventional radiology techniques such as lymphatic embolization and lipiodol injection where available.[47,48] Paralysis may develop if there is injury to the artery of Adamkewiecz during resection of thoracic or thoracoabdominal tumors. Ureteral injury may be diagnosed intraoperatively or postoperatively after resection of pelvic tumors. Most acute postoperative complications are resolved with early identification and diligent postoperative management. Long term surgical complications include incisional hernias, diaphragmatic hernias when diaphragm resections are performed as part of tumor excision. Adhesions increase the risk of intestinal obstruction, with one report citing 8.15% incidence of bowel obstruction at a median of 12 years after the initial surgery.[49,50] A larger study of 12,316 survivors of childhood cancer reported an intestinal obstruction rate of 5.8% among survivors, with the higher risk being abdominopelvic tumors and abdominal/pelvic radiotherapy.[49]

In addition to surgical complications, short-term and long-term complications can be attributed to adjuvant therapies. Chemotherapeutic agents and radiation increase the risks of secondary malignancies and other long-term toxicities, growth stunting, cardiopulmonary toxicities (anthracyclines), renal failure (ifosfamide and cisplatin), and infertility and impotency (alkylating agents and radiation therapy). Sensorineural hearing loss is multifactorial, caused primarily by platinum chemotherapy; other ototoxic components of NB treatments include loop diuretics, aminoglycoside antibiotics, and radiation. Neuroblastoma treatment also has long-term effects on the cardiovascular, renal, pulmonary, endocrine, musculoskeletal, and nervous systems.[51]

OUTCOMES

Neuroblastoma outcomes vary widely by risk group. Older children with unfavorable biological factors are at high risk and have the poorest outcomes. The COG P9641 study of children with low-risk NB evaluated outcomes after surgery alone. Chemotherapy was reserved for patients with, or at risk for, symptomatic disease, with less than 50% tumor resection at diagnosis, or with unresectable progressive disease after surgery alone. Excellent outcomes were achieved with surgery alone: for all 915 eligible patients, 5-year (EFS) and OS were 89% and 97% respectively.[52] Another low-risk group, Stage MS patients with favorable biology have excellent 5-year survival outcomes regardless of surgical extent. Given the overall good outcomes for patients with intermediate-risk neuroblastoma, treatment protocols have gradually de-escalated chemotherapy and radiation intensity with the goal of minimizing toxic side effects. COG A3961 addressed treatment toxicity by substituting carboplatin for cisplatin and decreasing total cumulative doses of chemotherapy while maintaining dose intensity and eliminating radiation therapy in all patients except those with unresectable primary tumors and unfavorable biologic features at the end of chemotherapy. Three-year EFS and OS was 88% and 96% respectively,[53] setting the stage for the current treatment strategy of surgery and risk-adjusted doses of chemotherapy for intermediate-risk patients. Current high-risk treatment protocols involve induction chemotherapy, surgery, consolidation chemotherapy, radiation, autologous stem cell transplant, immunotherapy, and MIBG therapy where applicable. Despite this, high-risk neuroblastoma carries the worst survival outcomes with 5-year EFS around 50%, thus the treatment strategy is accordingly aggressive. A 2021 report from Children's Oncology Group conducted retrospective analysis of patient outcome on 4832 patients enrolled on the COG neuroblastoma biology study ANBL00B1 to validate a revised INRG stage risk classification system. This study is the largest contemporary neuroblastoma study to report on prognosis; they reported 5-year event-free survival and overall survival as low-risk: 90.7% $\pm$ 1.1% and 97.9% $\pm$ 0.5%; intermediate-risk: 85.1% $\pm$ 1.4% and 95.8% $\pm$ 0.8%; high-risk: 51.2% $\pm$ 1.4% and 62.5% $\pm$ 1.3%.[14]

In addition to risk group, primary tumor site also affects neuroblastoma outcomes. Adrenal tumors have less favorable clinical and pathologic features and, therefore, the worst prognosis, while patients with thoracic and cervical neuroblastomas have better outcomes. A longitudinal analysis of the INRG database including 8800 patients with neuroblastoma between 1900 and 2002 evaluated relative risk based on the primary tumor site. The unadjusted 5-year EFS and OS rates according to the 6 primary tumor sites were as follows: adrenal, 56% and 62%; abdominal/retroperitoneal, 64% and 72%; neck, 79% and 90%; thoracic, 80% and 88% and pelvic, 81% and 91%, respectively.[54]

CLINICS CARE POINTS

- Surgical resection has a critical role in local control of neuroblastoma for the most optimal outcome.
- Staging for patients with neuroblastoma is performed using the International Neuroblastoma Risk Group (INRG) staging system.
- The Children's Oncology Group revised risk classification system should be used to stratify children as low-risk, intermediate-risk, or high-risk. This risk group classification should be used to balance the need for treatment intensification with mitigating late effects.

ACKNOWLEDGMENTS

The authors gratefully acknowledge Jason Jarzembowski, MD, PhD (Children's Wisconsin) for generously providing **Fig. 1**.

DISCLOSURE

The authors have nothing to disclose.

REFERENCES

1. Smith V, Foster J. High-risk neuroblastoma treatment review. Children (Basel) 2018;5(9).
2. Nong J, Su C, Li C, et al. Corrigendum to "Global, regional, and national epidemiology of childhood neuroblastoma (1990-2021): a statistical analysis of incidence, mortality, and DALYs". EClinicalMedicine 2025;88:103466.
3. Yan P, Qi F, Bian L, et al. Comparison of incidence and outcomes of neuroblastoma in children, adolescents, and adults in the United States: a surveillance, epidemiology, and end results (SEER) Program population Study. Med Sci Monit 2020;26:e927218.
4. Maris JM. Recent advances in neuroblastoma. N Engl J Med 2010;362(23): 2202–11.
5. Neuroblastoma treatment (PDQ). National Cancer Institute; 2025.
6. Campbell K, Siegel DA, Umaretiya PJ, et al. A comprehensive analysis of neuroblastoma incidence, survival, and racial and ethnic disparities from 2001 to 2019. Pediatr Blood Cancer 2024;71(1):e30732.
7. Barr EK, Applebaum MA. Genetic predisposition to neuroblastoma. Children (Basel) 2018;5(9).
8. Shimada H, Ambros IM, Dehner LP, et al. The international neuroblastoma pathology classification (the Shimada system). Cancer 1999;86(2):364–72.
9. Shimada H, Stram DO, Chatten J, et al. Identification of subsets of neuroblastomas by combined histopathologic and N-myc analysis. J Natl Cancer Inst 1995;87(19):1470–6.

10. Lavarino C, Cheung NK, Garcia I, et al. Specific gene expression profiles and chromosomal abnormalities are associated with infant disseminated neuroblastoma. BMC Cancer 2009;9:44.
11. Attiyeh EF, London WB, Mosse YP, et al, Children's Oncology Group. Chromosome 1p and 11q deletions and outcome in neuroblastoma. N Engl J Med 2005;353(21):2243–53.
12. Look AT, Hayes FA, Shuster JJ, et al. Clinical relevance of tumor cell ploidy and N-myc gene amplification in childhood neuroblastoma: a Pediatric Oncology Group study. J Clin Oncol 1991;9(4):581–91.
13. Bordow SB, Norris MD, Haber PS, et al. Prognostic significance of MYCN oncogene expression in childhood neuroblastoma. J Clin Oncol 1998;16(10):3286–94.
14. Irwin MS, Naranjo A, Zhang FF, et al. Revised neuroblastoma risk classification system: a report from the children's oncology group. J Clin Oncol 2021;39(29): 3229–41.
15. Mosse YP, Laudenslager M, Longo L, et al. Identification of ALK as a major familial neuroblastoma predisposition gene. Nature 2008;455(7215):930–5.
16. Carpenter EL, Mosse YP. Targeting ALK in neuroblastoma–preclinical and clinical advancements. Nat Rev Clin Oncol 2012;9(7):391–9.
17. Cheung NK, Zhang J, Lu C, et al, St Jude Children's Research Hospital–Washington University Pediatric Cancer Genome Project. Association of age at diagnosis and genetic mutations in patients with neuroblastoma. JAMA 2012; 307(10):1062–71.
18. Brisse HJ, McCarville MB, Granata C, et al, International Neuroblastoma Risk Group Project. Guidelines for imaging and staging of neuroblastic tumors: consensus report from the International neuroblastoma risk group project. Radiology 2011;261(1):243–57.
19. Nuchtern JG, London WB, Barnewolt CE, et al. A prospective study of expectant observation as primary therapy for neuroblastoma in young infants: a Children's Oncology Group study. Ann Surg 2012;256(4):573–80.
20. Rojas Y, Jaramillo S, Lyons K, et al. The optimal timing of surgical resection in high-risk neuroblastoma. J Pediatr Surg 2016;51(10):1665–9.
21. Yalcin B, Kremer LC, Caron HN, et al. High-dose chemotherapy and autologous haematopoietic stem cell rescue for children with high-risk neuroblastoma. Cochrane Database Syst Rev 2013;(8):CD006301.
22. Park JR, Kreissman SG, London WB, et al. Effect of tandem autologous stem cell transplant vs single transplant on event-free survival in patients with high-risk neuroblastoma: a randomized clinical trial. JAMA 2019;322(8):746–55.
23. Matthay KK, Villablanca JG, Seeger RC, et al. Treatment of high-risk neuroblastoma with intensive chemotherapy, radiotherapy, autologous bone marrow transplantation, and 13-cis-retinoic acid. Children's cancer group. N Engl J Med 1999; 341(16):1165–73.
24. Yu AL, Gilman AL, Ozkaynak MF, et al, Children's Oncology Group. Anti-GD2 antibody with GM-CSF, interleukin-2, and isotretinoin for neuroblastoma. N Engl J Med 2010;363(14):1324–34.
25. Twist CJ, Schmidt ML, Naranjo A, et al. Maintaining outstanding outcomes using Response- and biology-based therapy for intermediate-risk neuroblastoma: a report from the Children's Oncology Group Study ANBL0531. J Clin Oncol 2019;37(34):3243–55.
26. Holmes K, Potschger U, Pearson ADJ, et al, International Society of Paediatric Oncology Europe Neuroblastoma Group SIOPEN. Influence of surgical excision

on the survival of patients with stage 4 high-risk neuroblastoma: a report from the HR-NBL1/SIOPEN study. J Clin Oncol 2020;38(25):2902–15.
27. Cecchetto G, Mosseri V, De Bernardi B, et al. Surgical risk factors in primary surgery for localized neuroblastoma: the LNESG1 study of the European International Society of Pediatric Oncology Neuroblastoma Group. J Clin Oncol 2005;23(33):8483–9.
28. Yoneda A, Nishikawa M, Uehara S, et al. Can neoadjuvant chemotherapy reduce the surgical risks for localized neuroblastoma patients with image-defined risk factors at the time of diagnosis? Pediatr Surg Int 2016;32(3):209–14.
29. Monclair T, Mosseri V, Cecchetto G, et al. Influence of image-defined risk factors on the outcome of patients with localised neuroblastoma. A report from the LNESG1 study of the European International Society of Paediatric Oncology Neuroblastoma Group. Pediatr Blood Cancer 2015;62(9):1536–42.
30. Avanzini S, Pio L, Erminio G, et al. Image-defined risk factors in unresectable neuroblastoma: SIOPEN study on incidence, chemotherapy-induced variation, and impact on surgical outcomes. Pediatr Blood Cancer 2017;64(11).
31. Phelps HM, Ndolo JM, Van Arendonk KJ, et al. Association between image-defined risk factors and neuroblastoma outcomes. J Pediatr Surg 2019;54(6): 1184–91.
32. Saksiri P, Sripornsawan P, Kritsaneepaiboon S, et al. Correlation between image-defined risk factors and surgical complications in patients with neuroblastoma: a retrospective study. Pediatr Surg Int 2023;39(1):70.
33. Pohl A, Erichsen M, Stehr M, et al. Image-defined risk factors correlate with surgical radicality and local recurrence in patients with neuroblastoma. Klin Pädiatr 2016;228(3):118–23.
34. Pereira HR, Barzegar M, Hamadelseed O, et al. 3D surgical planning of pediatric tumors: a review. Int J Comput Assist Radiol Surg 2022;17(4):805–16.
35. Rich BS, Brown EG, Rothstein DH, et al, American Pediatric Surgical Association APSA Cancer Committee. The utility of intraoperative neuromonitoring in pediatric surgical oncology. J Pediatr Surg 2023;58(9):1708–14.
36. Mansfield SA, Kotagal M, Hartman SJ, et al. Enhanced Recovery After Surgery (ERAS) improves length of stay and decreases complications after resection of abdominal neuroblastoma. Pediatr Blood Cancer 2025;72(11):e31971.
37. La Quaglia MP, Kushner BH, Su W, et al. The impact of gross total resection on local control and survival in high-risk neuroblastoma. J Pediatr Surg 2004; 39(3):412–7 [discussion: 7].
38. Adkins ES, Sawin R, Gerbing RB, et al. Efficacy of complete resection for high-risk neuroblastoma: a Children's Cancer Group study. J Pediatr Surg 2004; 39(6):931–6.
39. Harper L, Perel Y, Lavrand F, et al. Surgical management of neuroblastoma-related hepatomegaly: do material and method really count? Pediatr Hematol Oncol 2008;25(4):313–7.
40. Nickerson HJ, Matthay KK, Seeger RC, et al. Favorable biology and outcome of stage IV-S neuroblastoma with supportive care or minimal therapy: a Children's Cancer Group study. J Clin Oncol 2000;18(3):477–86.
41. Malek MM, Mollen KP, Kane TD, et al. Thoracic neuroblastoma: a retrospective review of our institutional experience with comparison of the thoracoscopic and open approaches to resection. J Pediatr Surg 2010;45(8):1622–6.
42. Horiuchi A, Muraji T, Tsugawa C, et al. Thoracic neuroblastoma: outcome of incomplete resection. Pediatr Surg Int 2004;20(9):714–8.
43. Adams GA, Shochat SJ, Smith EI, et al. Thoracic neuroblastoma: a Pediatric Oncology Group study. J Pediatr Surg 1993;28(3):372–7 [discussion: 7–8].

44. Kelleher CM, Smithson L, Nguyen LL, et al. Clinical outcomes in children with adrenal neuroblastoma undergoing open versus laparoscopic adrenalectomy. J Pediatr Surg 2013;48(8):1727–32.
45. Hemyari ADA, Evans MA. Enteral administration of a methylene blue and 20% lipid emulsion slurry to aid in diagnosis of intraoperative thoracic duct injury. Ann Thorac Surg 2025;1–3.
46. Canete A, Jovani C, Lopez A, et al. Surgical treatment for neuroblastoma: complications during 15 years' experience. J Pediatr Surg 1998;33(10):1526–30.
47. Gupta A, Naranje P, Vora Z, et al. Intranodal lipiodol injection for the treatment of chyle leak in children - a preliminary experience. Br J Radiol 2022;95(1137): 20211270.
48. Koester TM, Chewning RH, Weldon CB, et al. Lymphatic embolization for the management of post-operative chyle leaks following solid tumor resection in pediatric patients. J Pediatr Surg 2023;58(11):2141–8.
49. Madenci AL, Fisher S, Diller LR, et al. Intestinal obstruction in survivors of childhood cancer: a report from the childhood cancer survivor Study. J Clin Oncol 2015;33(26):2893–900.
50. Cooke-Barber J, Scorletti F, Rymeski B, et al. Long-term follow-up of surgical outcomes for patients with Wilms tumor and neuroblastoma. Cancer 2021;127(17): 3232–8.
51. Landier W, Armenian S, Bhatia S. Late effects of childhood cancer and its treatment. Pediatr Clin North Am 2015;62(1):275–300.
52. Strother DR, London WB, Schmidt ML, et al. Outcome after surgery alone or with restricted use of chemotherapy for patients with low-risk neuroblastoma: results of children's oncology group study P9641. J Clin Oncol 2012;30(15):1842–8.
53. Baker DL, Schmidt ML, Cohn SL, et al, Children's Oncology Group. Outcome after reduced chemotherapy for intermediate-risk neuroblastoma. N Engl J Med 2010;363(14):1313–23.
54. Vo KT, Matthay KK, Neuhaus J, et al. Clinical, biologic, and prognostic differences on the basis of primary tumor site in neuroblastoma: a report from the international neuroblastoma risk group project. J Clin Oncol 2014;32(28):3169–76.

Management of Rhabdomyosarcoma in Pediatric Patients

Sophia M.V. Schermerhorn, MD, MPH[a], John C. Routh, MD, MPH[b], Stephanie F. Polites, MD, MPH[c], Roshni Dasgupta, MD, MPH[a,*]

KEYWORDS

- Rhabdomyosarcoma • Pediatric soft tissue sarcoma • Surgical management
- Local control • Multidisciplinary treatment

KEY POINTS

- Rhabdomyosarcoma (RMS) may occur at a myriad of sites with varied symptoms, requiring a high index of suspicion to avoid delays in diagnosis and treatment.
- Surgical lymph node assessment should be performed for certain named primary tumor sites with significant risk of lymph node metastases and relapse.
- Definitive locoregional control is integral, and the optimal approach for each patient should be determined by experienced multidisciplinary teams, including surgeons, radiation oncologists, and oncologists.
- Surgical resection is most often indicated following neoadjuvant chemotherapy and should be performed when feasible within site-specific principles, given improved outcomes compared to radiation alone.

BACKGROUND

Rhabdomyosarcoma (RMS) is the most common soft tissue sarcoma in children, accounting for 4.5% of all childhood cancers. It follows neuroblastoma and nephroblastoma as the third most common extracranial solid tumor of childhood.[1] The incidence is 4.6 cases per million children/adolescents per year.[2] It is rare in adults, where soft tissue sarcomas constitute less than 1% of all malignancies, and RMS comprises only 3% of all soft tissue sarcomas with an incidence of 0.9 cases per million per year.[3]

[a] Department of Pediatric General and Thoracic Surgery, Cincinnati Children's Hospital Medical Center, University of Cincinnati College of Medicine, Cincinnati, OH, USA; [b] Department of Urology, Duke University School of Medicine, Durham, NC, USA; [c] Department of Surgery, Mayo Clinic, Rochester, MN, USA

* Corresponding author. Department of Pediatric General and Thoracic Surgery, Cincinnati Children's Hospital Medical Center, 3333 Burnet Avenue, Cincinnati, OH 45229.
E-mail address: Roshni.Dasgupta@cchmc.org

Surg Oncol Clin N Am 35 (2026) 731–748
https://doi.org/10.1016/j.soc.2026.02.009 **surgonc.theclinics.com**

Abbreviations	
COG	Children's Oncology Group
CT	computed tomography
DPE	delayed primary excision
EFS	event-free survival
EOT	end-of-therapy
EpSSG	European Paediatric Soft Tissue Sarcoma Study Group
FDG	fluorodeoxyglucose
ICG	indocyanine green
IMRT	intensity-modulated radiotherapy
IRS	Intergroup Rhabdomyosarcoma
INSTRuCT	International Soft Tissue Sarcoma Consortium
OS	overall survival
PT-RMS	paratesticular rhabdomyosarcoma
PRE	pretreatment reexcision
RMS	rhabdomyosarcoma
RT	radiotherapy
SNLB	sentinel lymph node biopsy

RMS is a malignant tumor of mesenchymal origin that can occur at any anatomic site, often showing cellular differentiation toward muscle tissue. RMS is characterized by small round blue cells that usually express (and immunohistochemically stain for) the proteins desmin, vimentin, myoglobin, actin, and myoD.[4]

There are 2 primary peaks of incidence: in children 2 to 6 years of age, with tumors generally within the head and neck and genitourinary tract; and in adolescents, who present with extremity, truncal, or paratesticular tumors.[1,5]

Outcomes in localized RMS have improved substantially owing to multimodal therapy; contemporary risk-adapted regimens achieve long-term survival rates of ~90% for very-low-risk/low-risk disease and 50% to 70% for intermediate-risk disease, but remain poor (<30%) for high-risk or relapsed disease, prompting the need for novel treatment approaches.[6] Adult patients with RMS have a poorer overall survival (OS) than pediatric patients: 43% for localized RMS and 5% for metastatic RMS.[3,7–9]

Molecular Classification of Rhabdomyosarcoma

Modern RMS classification has moved away from relying on embryonal versus alveolar histology, instead focusing on molecular features that more accurately predict prognosis.[10–12] The most clinically meaningful molecular marker is FOXO1 fusion status: fusion-positive tumors (PAX3-FOXO1 or PAX7-FOXO1 rearrangements) often (but not always) show alveolar histology and carry a significantly inferior prognosis: 36% 5-year event-free survival (EFS) compared with 70% for patients with fusion-negative tumors.[9,10,12,13]

Fusion-negative RMS includes most tumors with embryonal histology and represents a heterogenous group that frequently involve RAS-pathway or 11p15 abnormalities.[10,12,13] Within this category, TP53 mutations and the MYOD1L122R mutation define biologically aggressive subsets.[10,13,14] Because of their prognostic significance, MYOD1 and TP53 alterations have been incorporated into recent Children's Oncology Group (COG) clinical trials as exclusion criteria for therapy de-escalation.[6,15]

In addition, histologic spindle cell/sclerosing RMS is now recognized as a heterogeneous molecular group. Most are fusion-negative but a high-risk subset have MYOD1 mutations.[10,13,14] Other spindle cell variants defined by VGLL2, NCOA2, SRF, or other transcription-factor fusions typically occur in infants and portend a more favorable prognosis.[10] By contrast, pleomorphic RMS primarily occurs in adult patients and is biologically distinct from the pediatric forms.[10,16,17]

PATIENT EVALUATION OVERVIEW

RMS occurs in multiple anatomic sites, with the approximate distribution shown in **Table 1**. Because of the variable anatomic presentation, clinicians should maintain an index of suspicion for RMS in children with a mass or symptoms shown in **Table 2**. Rarely (~5%), patients present with an underlying cancer-predisposition syndrome, such as neurofibromatosis, Li-Fraumeni, DICER1, Rubinstein-Taybi, Gorlin basal cell nevus, Beckwith-Wiedemann, or Costello syndrome.[18,19] It is important to recognize any potential cancer predisposition syndrome so that genetic counseling, screening, surveillance, and timely treatment can be offered.[20]

When RMS is suspected, early involvement of a multidisciplinary team is critical. This team should help to guide biopsy and initial imaging to ensure these are performed in accordance with current oncologic standards, as early diagnostic decisions directly affect staging, downstream risk stratification, and ultimately, treatment planning.

Imaging Studies

If there is suspicion for RMS based on clinical presentation or ultrasound imaging, cross-sectional imaging is indicated.

Depending on location and availability, MRI is the optimal modality to assess most primary lesions, with RMS most commonly isointense to muscle on T1-weighted images, and intermediate to high intensity on T2-weighted images.[21] For pelvic tumors, computed tomography (CT) is a reasonable alternative when MRI is not feasible. In addition, CT is excellent for assessing bone involvement and can be performed when osseous invasion is suspected. Cross-sectional imaging of the primary tumor should include the regional draining lymph nodes to guide pathologic nodal evaluation. In the case of extremity tumors, imaging should include the entire limb (**Fig. 1**). Chest CT should be performed as part of staging for the detection of pulmonary metastases, the most common site of distant spread.

When available, either whole-body fluorodeoxyglucose (FDG) -PET/CT or FDG-PET/MRI can be used for the assessment of disease burden.[22,23] PET imaging cannot be relied on to give accurate representation of lymphatic metastasis, and therefore, surgical nodal evaluation, as described in later discussion, is essential.[22,24,25] In addition, although PET/CT is able to evaluate for pulmonary metastasis, its sensitivity remains lower than conventional Chest CT and does not replace diagnostic Chest CT.[23,26] For patients with suspected metastatic disease, bone scan should be performed if FDG-PET is not available.

Table 1
Distribution of rhabdomyosarcoma primary sites

Primary Tumor Site	Percentage
Head and neck	40
Genitourinary	20
Extremities	20
Trunk	10
Other	10

Table 2
Common presenting signs and symptoms by primary site

Primary Site	Symptoms and Signs
Head and neck	Painless or painful swelling Proptosis Ptosis Ophthalmoplegia Headache Vomiting Cranial nerve palsy Other cranial nerve palsies Nasal discharge Nasal/sinus congestion Trismus Systemic hypertension
Limbs/trunk	Asymptomatic swelling
Genitourinary tract/pelvis	Painless scrotal lesions Hematuria Urinary retention/dribbling Vulval nodule Polypoid vaginal lesions Vaginal bleeding/discharge Constipation
Abdomen/liver/biliary	Asymptomatic swelling Abdominal pain Intestinal obstruction Jaundice Cholangitis
Metastatic disease (20% at diagnosis) • Bone • Bone marrow • Lung • Lymph nodes	Otherwise unexplained: Poor feeding Seizures Pain Irritability Pancytopenia

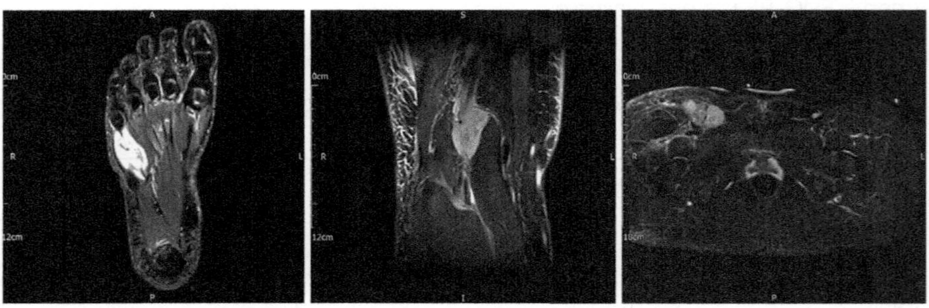

Fig. 1. MRI scans of a 15-year-old girl with a fusion-positive RMS of the right foot and lymph node metastases in the popliteal fossa and groin.

Percutaneous, endoscopic, or incisional biopsy should be the initial surgical procedure in all patients except when primary wide excision of the mass with adequate margins is possible without significant loss of function or excessive morbidity.[8,27] A multidisciplinary discussion should occur before biopsy or upfront resection to obtain consensus on optimal approach. Once tissue is obtained, FOXO1 fusion testing is mandatory in all suspected RMS; this can be performed by fluorescence in situ hybridization or reverse transcription polymerase chain reaction, but modern practice increasingly favors RNA sequencing–based assays, which detect both canonical and rare fusions and avoid false positives in fusion-negative alveolar-appearing tumors.[10,11] Bone marrow biopsy should be performed in all intermediate- and high-risk patients to determine metastatic spread to the marrow.[28] For parameningeal tumors, cerebrospinal fluid cytology should be obtained to detect central nervous system involvement.

Regional lymph nodes should be surgically evaluated with tumors of the extremity, trunk, head and neck, perineal, and perianal regions. These sites carry a higher risk of nodal involvement, and imaging is not able to reliably exclude lymph node metastases, with several large studies demonstrating changes in nodal staging after pathologic confirmation in up to 17% of patients.[29,30] Sentinel lymph node biopsy (SLNB) is more accurate than random lymph node sampling and is the preferred method of nodal evaluation.[29] Indocyanine green (ICG) fluorescence has been increasingly used as an adjunct in SLNB alongside traditional agents, such as Technitium-99 and blue dye.[31–34] In contrast, paratesticular rhabdomyosarcoma (PT-RMS) requires formal retroperitoneal lymph node sampling rather than SLNB for patients over 10 years old or with fusion-positive disease.[25] Specifics on retroperitoneal lymph node sampling are discussed further in the Site-Specific Treatment section (**Fig. 2**).

For patients with abnormal lymph nodes (>1 cm in diameter or PET-avid) visualized on imaging, pathologic confirmation is recommended. If surgical sampling is unobtainable, they should be presumed positive and require radiation therapy to the nodal bed.[25,30]

Staging and Risk Stratification

Staging and risk stratification in RMS is complex, but important, because treatment intensity follows a risk-adapted approach.[35] Patients are assigned a pretreatment

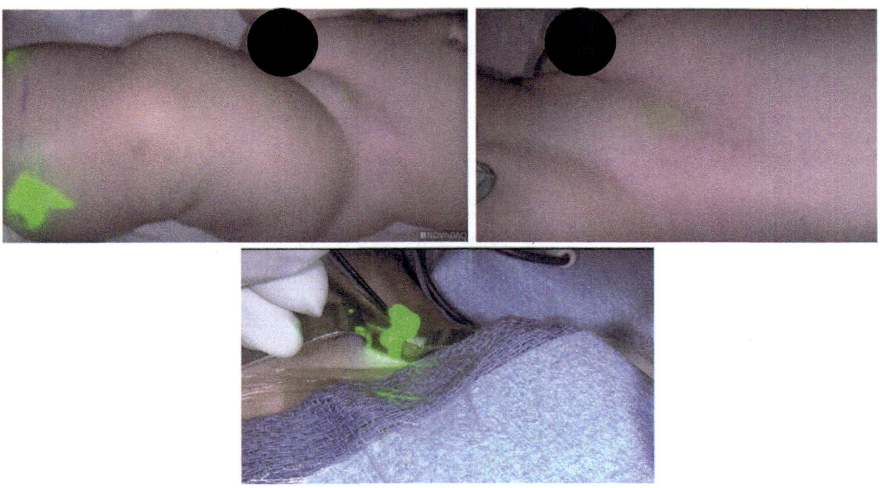

Fig. 2. SLNB using ICG.

stage using the TNM classification (**Table 3**) combined with categorization of the primary tumor site as favorable or unfavorable (**Table 4**). These elements, together, determine the pretreatment stage (**Table 5**), which reflects the anatomic extent of disease before any therapy.[36]

After tissue diagnosis is obtained through either biopsy or upfront resection, a surgicopathologic risk stratification using the Intergroup Rhabdomyosarcoma (IRS) group classification is assigned (**Table 6**). The IRS grouping is a prechemotherapy staging system determined by the extent of the initial surgical resection and the presence of pathologic lymph nodes and distant metastases.

Final risk-group assignment incorporates pretreatment stage, IRS clinical group, tumor biology, and patient age. Both the COG and the European Paediatric Soft Tissue Sarcoma Study Group (EpSSG) now use fusion-based frameworks for risk stratification, derived from contemporary prognostic modeling, and are embedded in their current frontline trials.[37,38] The working COG risk stratification used in modern protocols is summarized in **Table 7**.[6] Ongoing international harmonization efforts through the International Soft Tissue Sarcoma Consortium (INSTRuCT), a collaboration between COG, EpSSG, and other cooperative groups, aim to unify staging, risk stratification, and clinical trial design across regions.[39]

TREATMENT OPTIONS

Treatment of patients with RMS is multimodal, always includes chemotherapy, and usually includes some combination of radiotherapy (RT) and surgery.

Chemotherapy

Chemotherapy is a required component of all RMS treatments, with specific chemotherapy regimen and intensity determined by risk-group assignment (see **Table 7**). COG and EpSSG use similar chemotherapy backbone regimens that differ in the alkylating agent used, with cyclophosphamide used by COG and ifosfamide used by EpSSG. Comparisons between these alkylating agents have shown no significant differences in outcome; however, each gives rise to different potential late effects: ifosfamide is more nephrotoxic, and cyclophosphamide is more gonadotoxic.[40] Targeted agents, including the mTOR (mammalian target of rapamycin) inhibitor temsirolimus, have been evaluated as additions to conventional chemotherapy but have not demonstrated a clear survival benefit to date.[41]

Table 3
TNM staging classification

T1	Tumor confined to tissue of origin
T2	Tumor extends beyond tissue of origin
A	<5 cm in maximum diameter
B	>5 cm in maximum diameter
N0	No nodal involvement
N1	Nodal involvement
NX	Regional lymph nodes not examined; no information
M0	No distant metastases
M1	Distant metastases

Table 4
Favorable/unfavorable prognostic tumor sites

Favorable Primary Tumor Sites	Unfavorable Primary Tumor Sites
Head and neck	Parameningeal
Orbital	Extremities
Genitourinary (now also includes bladder/ prostate in EpSSG but remains unfavorable in COG)	Trunk Chest wall
Biliary (now favorable in EpSSG but remains unfavorable in COG)	Other sites

Although RMS in adults has historically been treated according to adult soft tissue sarcoma paradigms, increasing evidence suggests that adolescents and young adults derive improved outcomes when treated on pediatric-based protocols, underscoring the importance of referral to centers participating in cooperative group trials whenever feasible.[42]

Radiotherapy

In most patients (85%), RT is required to obtain local control at the primary site and is always required for pathologically involved lymph nodes.[43] There are only a few selected groups of patients with low-risk disease where RT can be safely avoided without potentially compromising cure, such as an upfront completely resected PT-RMS or vaginal RMS with a complete chemotherapy response. When RT is omitted in infants to avoid morbidity, local failure rates are increased.[44] Intensity-modulated radiotherapy (IMRT), brachytherapy, and proton-beam RT may achieve adequate tumor control with reduced radiation to normal surrounding tissues.[45] Proton therapy, in particular, is increasingly used in pediatric RMS, when available, owing to its ability to reduce radiation exposure to developing tissues; however, the current data on oncologic outcomes are derived from observational cohorts.[46] Surgeons caring for children with RMS should work closely with radiation oncologists to ensure adequate local control.

Surgical Treatment

Primary resection

Primary upfront resection without biopsy is indicated only when the tumor can be excised with R0 margins without resulting in significant functional deficits, and when

Table 5
Pretreatment staging system

Stage	Site[b]	T Stage[a]	Size[a]	Node Stage[a]	Metastases[a]
1	Favorable	T1 or T2	Any size	N0 or N1 or Nx	M0
2	Unfavorable	T1 or T2	a, ≤5 cm	N0 or Nx	M0
3	Unfavorable	T1 or T2	a, ≤5 cm	N1	M0
			b, >5 cm	N0 or N1 or Nx	
4	Any site	T1 or T2	Any size	N0 or N1 or Nx	M1

[a] Refer to TNM classification.
[b] Refer to **Table 4**.

Table 6
Intergroup Rhabdomyosarcoma Group surgical-pathologic (clinical) grouping classification

IRS-I	Tumor completely removed
IRS-II	a. Microscopic residual tumor b. Involved regional nodes c. Both
IRS-III	Gross residual tumor after incomplete resection or biopsy only
IRS-IV	Distant metastatic disease

multidisciplinary discussion has occurred.[47] Attempting upfront resection with resultant gross residual disease offers no advantage over biopsy alone and should be avoided.[47,48] When feasible, complete resection should include a rim of surrounding tissue with a margin of at least 0.5 cm, provided this can be obtained without unacceptable morbidity.[49,50]

Pretreatment reexcision

Pretreatment reexcision (PRE) is a wide reexcision used to achieve a complete resection (R0 margin) in patients with residual disease after a primary procedure, such as a biopsy or incomplete tumor excision before the initiation of chemotherapy.[51] PRE should only be attempted if there is a very high probability of R0 resection; if this is in doubt, PRE should not be attempted. If an R0 resection is obtained at the PRE operation, the patient is classified as IRS group I, which is associated with improved survival and potential for a decreased intensity of therapy.[52] PRE should only be offered if the entire tumor bed can be resected without loss of function or form and a multidisciplinary discussion has occurred.

Delayed primary excision

Delayed primary excision (DPE) is excision after induction chemotherapy, considered in patients who were not candidates for primary resection or PRE. Although all patients who undergo DPE are recommended to have postoperative RT, a complete R0 resection should be targeted for the greatest reduction in RT dose. A microscopic residual R1 resection will also decrease the dose of adjuvant RT.[53,54] Patients who undergo DPE may experience reduced local failure, supporting multidisciplinary consideration

Table 7
Children's Oncology Group risk-group assignment

Risk Group	Fusion	Status	Stage	Group
Very low risk	Fusion	Negative	1	I
Low risk	Fusion	Negative	1	II, III (orbit only)
	Fusion	Negative	2	I, II
Intermediate risk	Fusion	Negative	1	III (nonorbit)
			2, 3	III
			3	I, II
			4	IV (age <10 y)
	Fusion	Positive	1, 2, 3	I, II, III
High risk	Fusion	Positive	4	IV
	Fusion	Negative	4	IV (age ≥10 y)

of this approach.[55] In comparative analyses, DPE has also been associated with improved local control compared with definitive radiation therapy alone, with lower rates of local recurrence.[56] Debulking operations are not recommended, as there is no evidence that this improves oncologic outcome compared with biopsy alone.[57] Again, DPE should only be undertaken if R0 or R1 margins can be obtained without debilitating functional outcomes.[47]

End of therapy mass

In contrast to DPE, end-of-therapy (EOT) masses are residual radiographic abnormalities identified after completion of all planned chemotherapy and RT, rather than after induction chemotherapy. EOT masses are common, particularly in patients with IRS group III disease.[58] Available evidence demonstrates that routine surgical resection of EOT masses does not improve EFS or OS, and therefore, excision of EOT masses is not indicated.[47,58] Pathologic evaluation of EOT masses most frequently reveals fibrosis and treatment-related necrosis, with viable tumor only identified in half of cases in one series.[59]

Fertility preservation

Fertility-preserving procedures should be considered and offered early during the course of staging and treatment for patients with RMS who are expected to receive gonadotoxic systemic or local therapy. In pubertal patients, sperm or egg storage may be pursued provided that it does not cause undue treatment delay. Otherwise, in both prepubertal and pubertal patients, gonadal cryopreservation is an option. Finally, gonadal transposition is sometimes appropriate for limited indications.[60] All of these options should be discussed as appropriate for the patient and their family in a multidisciplinary setting before treatment.[61,62]

Site-specific treatment

Bladder/prostate. The aim of local treatment of bladder/prostate RMS is oncologic control in conjunction with preservation of bladder and sexual function.[63] Upfront resection is rare, typically bladder dome tumors only. An experienced multidisciplinary team, including pediatric urology, pediatric surgery, oncology, and radiation oncology, must consider the options of DPE with RT, weighing the expected morbidity and benefit of each local control option.[63–66]

Female genital tract. Tumors of the vagina, cervix, and uterus are generally highly chemosensitive, and therefore, upfront surgery is generally not indicated.[67] Patients with favorable histology and biopsy-proven complete response to chemotherapy can often forgo any local therapy, including RT.[67,68] For those with residual disease after chemotherapy, local control via DPE or RT is necessary. Intracavitary brachytherapy is the preferred method of local control.[60,67] DPE should only be considered following extensive multidisciplinary discussion and if an R0 resection is possible.[67]

Paratesticular. PT-RMS should be removed by radical orchiectomy through an inguinal approach.[25,69] The cord should be clamped at the internal ring before mobilization of the tumor. Care is taken not to breach the tunica vaginalis when the tumor, testis, and entire cord up to the internal ring are removed as a single specimen. When scrotal skin is fixed or invaded by tumor, it should be resected en bloc with the specimen; otherwise, there is no indication for hemiscrotectomy. Unlike tumors at other sites, PT-RMS is often resected upfront. PRE without formal hemiscrotectomy or RT is required after incomplete resection to remove tumor-contaminated scrotal and/or cord tissue.[70]

Retroperitoneal lymph node assessment. Accurate staging of nodal metastases in PT-RMS is important because lymph node involvement is frequent (26% in IRS-I and IRS-II trials), and patients with positive nodes require intensified chemotherapy and RT.[71] All patients should have cross-sectional imaging of the retroperitoneal nodes, and patients 10 years of age or older or with fusion-positive disease should also undergo surgical staging of the lymph nodes.[25] A pooled analysis from North America and Europe of 319 patients 10 years of age or older with PT-RMS found that nodal involvement was present in approximately 30% and disease failures were most likely to occur in the nodes. Surgical evaluation of retroperitoneal lymph nodes was the only variable that was associated with EFS and can be performed open or with minimally invasive techniques.[72] There was a 30% lymph node relapse in patients 10 years of age or older who had nodal staging with imaging alone.[25,73–75]

Retroperitoneal lymph node sampling may be performed via an open or minimally invasive approach, including laparoscopic or robotic techniques, provided that oncologic principles are maintained, and an adequate nodal yield is achieved.[25] Although robotic retroperitoneal lymph node sampling has been described in selected series, long-term oncologic equivalence to open or laparoscopic staging has not been definitively established in RMS.[76] ICG has not been established as a standard adjunct for retroperitoneal staging and does not replace systematic nodal sampling in PT-RMS.

COG guidelines suggest retroperitoneal lymph node sampling (between 7 and 12 lymph nodes) taken from multiple areas in the ipsilateral retroperitoneum up to the renal vessels.[75]

Extremity. Aggressive surgical procedures resulting in loss of function are generally not indicated because the efficacy of chemotherapy and RT usually allows sparing of vital structures.[77] SNLB is recommended for accurate nodal staging in all extremity RMS.[29,78] The primary goal of local tumor resection, which is commonly a DPE following induction chemotherapy, is limb-sparing complete (R0) resection. An incision is made along the major axis of the anatomic compartment containing the tumor and must include en bloc resection of previous biopsy and drain sites. When R0 resection cannot be achieved, an R1 (microscopically involved margins) resection with RT usually achieves oncologic control while maintaining optimal functional outcome. Ablative procedures should only be performed after a second opinion from a specialized center. These principles are reinforced in the INSTRuCT surgical guidelines, which emphasize delayed, function-preserving resection, routine SNLB for extremity tumors, and centralized multidisciplinary review for any consideration of ablative surgery.[78]

Bile duct and liver. Patients with bile ducts and liver RMS usually present with jaundice, pruritus, and dilation of the biliary tract. Ultrasonography and MRI with magnetic resonance cholangiopancreatography show the extent of the primary lesion and lymph node involvement, as well as rule out other causes of biliary obstruction. Biopsy rather than primary excisional surgery is recommended because these tumors are expected to have a favorable subtype (fusion-negative/botryoid histopathology) that respond well to chemotherapy.[79] Definitive local control is planned after induction chemotherapy.[79] DPE can be considered, which may require partial hepatectomy and biliary tract reconstruction. The potential benefit of reduced postoperative RT dose following successful DPE must be weighed with the expected surgical morbidity. The long-term effects of RT to the hepatic pedicle are unknown in young patients.[80]

Perianal and perineal. Perineal and perianal RMS are rare but clinically aggressive tumors with reported survival around 50%, reflecting high rates of both nodal involvement and distant relapse.[44,47,81] Because of the proximity to the anal sphincter, urethra, and pelvic floor musculature, complete upfront resection or PRE is seldom feasible without causing major functional morbidity, and these patients typically undergo biopsy followed by chemoradiation for local control.[81] The perineal RMS cohort demonstrates a high incidence of regional lymph node metastases, reinforcing the need for routine nodal evaluation.[81,82] Functional outcomes, including continence and sexual/urinary dysfunction, are significant considerations in long-term survivors.

Metastatic disease

Systematic RT of all metastatic sites is recommended when feasible without disruption of bone marrow function. Recent evidence shows improved OS compared with partial or no irradiation, with 3-year OS rates of 84% versus 54% and 23%, respectively.[83] Nearly half of patients with metastases have single-site disease, and surgical excision may be required to confirm the diagnosis before RT. Those with metastases isolated to lung, lymph nodes, or other sites have improved prognosis compared with those with osseous or bone marrow metastases.[84] Outcomes for patients with bone marrow metastasis are particularly poor and are associated with decreased EFS and OS compared with bone-only metastatic disease.[85] Isolated metastases particularly in the lung may be especially amenable to surgical resection.[86]

FOLLOW-UP

After completion of treatment, the frequency of follow-up assessments is conventionally every 3 to 4 months for the first 2 years followed by every 6 months through year 5.[87] However, there is ongoing debate regarding both the optimal frequency of follow-up visits and the type and intensity of surveillance imaging, reflecting the need to balance early detection of relapse against the cumulative risks of repeated imaging.[88,89] This has led to increasing interest in risk-adapted follow-up strategies to improve the efficiency and value of posttreatment surveillance.[88] Late relapse is uncommon—one COG large study of 2444 patients reported a recurrence rate of 2.9% after 5 years of EFS.[90] Therefore, patients can be referred to the long-term follow-up clinic after 5 years.

Relapse

The most common pattern of relapse in localized RMS is relapse at the primary site (75%) with or without nodal and distant metastases. Relapsed RMS carries a poor prognosis, although 35% of those who relapse following treatment of localized disease remain curable. Relapse of primary metastatic disease is uniformly fatal.

Patients with local relapse should only be treated in centers with experienced multidisciplinary teams for RMS. When treatment with curative intent is deemed feasible after interdisciplinary consultation, the general principle of complete resection should be pursued, and in rare situations, may include radical ablative procedures.[52,91] Cytoreductive surgery combined with hyperthermic intraperitoneal chemotherapy has been reported for abdominal relapse in children with RMS.

When surgical resection is not feasible, biopsies should be considered for genomic profiling so that affected patients can be considered for targeted therapies or early-phase trials.[17,92]

NEW DEVELOPMENTS

As survival outcomes continue to improve, there is increasing recognition of the need to systematically assess functional and patient-reported outcomes following RMS treatment. Recent cooperative-group priorities emphasize that traditional oncologic endpoints alone are insufficient to guide surgical decision making, particularly when multiple local control strategies yield comparable survival.[93,94] Standardized, longitudinal assessment of function, quality of life, and late morbidity will be essential to refine risk-adapted surgical and radiotherapeutic approaches and to identify local control strategies that optimize both cure and long-term patient-centered outcomes.

International, multidisciplinary research teams are increasingly being established to facilitate discovery, share learning, and pool data. The INSTRuCT represents a major collaborative effort among COG, EpSSG, Cooperative Weichteilsarkom Studiengruppe (CWS), and other global groups to harmonize clinical trial design, staging, and risk stratification in RMS.[39] INSTRuCT integrates shared biobanking, centralized data repositories, and coordinated translational research initiatives to accelerate the development of new therapeutic strategies. By unifying historically separate cooperative groups, INSTRuCT has created the framework for international trials and more efficient evaluation of promising biologic agents in this rare disease.

CLINICS CARE POINTS

- Presentation varies widely by age and tumor site– maintain a high index of suspicion for atypical or site-specific symptoms.
- Biopsy and staging should be completed before definitive local therapy, with paratesticular tumors being the only usual exception.
- Regional lymph node evaluation is critical and should be performed for high-risk primary sites, regardless of imaging findings.
- Optimal local control requires a multimodal approach. Surgery should be integrated with chemotherapy and/or radiation to maximize disease control while minimizing morbidity.

DECLARATION OF AI AND AI-ASSISTED TECHNOLOGIES IN THE WRITING PROCESS

During the preparation of this work, the authors used Gen AI. After using this tool/service, the authors reviewed and edited the content as needed and take full responsibility for the content of the publication.

DISCLOSURES

None.

REFERENCES

1. Arndt CAS, Crist WM. Common musculoskeletal tumors of childhood and adolescence. N Engl J Med 1999;341:342–52.
2. McEvoy MT, Siegel DA, Dai S, et al. Pediatric rhabdomyosarcoma incidence and survival in the United States: an assessment of 5656 cases, 2001-2017. Cancer Med 2023;12:3644–56.
3. Bompas E, Campion L, Italiano A, et al. Outcome of 449 adult patients with rhabdomyosarcoma: an observational ambispective nationwide study. Cancer Med 2018;7:4023–35.
4. Rossi S, Nascimento AG, Canal F, et al. Small round-cell neoplasms of soft tissues: an integrated diagnostic approach. Curr Diagn Pathol 2007;13:150–63.
5. Ognjanovic S, Linabery AM, Charbonneau B, et al. Trends in childhood rhabdomyosarcoma incidence and survival in the United States, 1975-2005. Cancer 2009;115:4218–26.

6. Oberoi S, Crane JN, Haduong JH, et al, the Children's Oncology Group Soft Tissue Sarcoma Committee. Children's oncology group's 2023 blueprint for research: soft tissue sarcomas. Pediatr Blood Cancer 2023;70:e30556.
7. Oberlin O, Rey A, Sanchez De Toledo J, et al. Randomized comparison of intensified six-drug versus standard three-drug chemotherapy for high-risk nonmetastatic rhabdomyosarcoma and other chemotherapy-sensitive childhood soft tissue sarcomas: long-Term results from the International Society of Pediatric Oncology MMT95 study. J Clin Oncol 2012;30:2457–65.
8. Oberlin O, Rey A, Brown KLB, et al. Prognostic factors for outcome in localized extremity rhabdomyosarcoma. Pooled analysis from four international cooperative groups. Pediatr Blood Cancer 2015;62:2125–31.
9. Rudzinski ER, Anderson JR, Chi YY, et al. Histology, fusion status, and outcome in metastatic rhabdomyosarcoma: a report from the Children's Oncology Group. Pediatr Blood Cancer 2017. https://doi.org/10.1002/pbc.26645.
10. Hettmer S, Linardic CM, Kelsey A, et al. Molecular testing of rhabdomyosarcoma in clinical trials to improve risk stratification and outcome: a consensus view from European paediatric Soft tissue sarcoma Study Group, Children's Oncology Group and Cooperative Weichteilsarkom-Studiengruppe. Eur J Cancer 2022; 172:367–86.
11. Fan R, Parham DM, Wang LL. An integrative morphologic and molecular approach for diagnosis and subclassification of rhabdomyosarcoma. Arch Pathol Lab Med 2022;146(8):953–9.
12. Dehner CA, Rudzinski ER, Davis JL. Rhabdomyosarcoma: updates on classification and the necessity of molecular testing beyond immunohistochemistry. Hum Pathol 2024;147:72–81.
13. Clay MR, Patel A, Tran Q, et al. Methylation profiling reveals novel molecular classes of rhabdomyosarcoma. Sci Rep 2021. https://doi.org/10.1038/s41598-021-01649-w.
14. Shern JF, Selfe J, Izquierdo E, et al. Genomic classification and clinical outcome in rhabdomyosarcoma: a report from an international consortium. J Clin Oncol 2021;39(26):2859–71.
15. Haduong JH, Heske CM, Allen-Rhoades W, et al. An update on rhabdomyosarcoma risk stratification and the rationale for current and future Children's Oncology Group clinical trials. Pediatr Blood Cancer 2022. https://doi.org/10.1002/PBC.29511.
16. Skapek SX, Anderson J, Barr FG, et al. PAX-FOXO1 fusion status drives unfavorable outcome for children with Rhabdomyosarcoma: a Children's Oncology Group report. Pediatr Blood Cancer 2013;60:1411.
17. Yohe ME, Heske CM, Stewart E, et al. Insights into pediatric rhabdomyosarcoma research: challenges and goals. Pediatr Blood Cancer 2019. https://doi.org/10.1002/PBC.27869.
18. Doros L, Yang J, Dehner L, et al. DICER1 mutations in embryonal rhabdomyosarcomas from children with and without familial PPB-tumor predisposition syndrome. Pediatr Blood Cancer 2012;59:558–60.
19. Ferrari A, Bisogno G, Macaluso A, et al. Soft-tissue sarcomas in children and adolescents with neurofibromatosis type 1. Cancer 2007;109:1406–12.
20. Saletta F, Dalla Pozza L, Byrne JA. Genetic causes of cancer predisposition in children and adolescents. Transl Pediatr 2015;4:67–75.
21. Pl M, H C, BB F, et al. Radiology of soft tissue tumors. Surg Oncol Clin N Am 2014;23:911–36.

22. Wagner LM, Kremer N, Gelfand MJ, et al. Detection of lymph node metastases in pediatric and adolescent/young adult sarcoma: sentinel lymph node biopsy versus fludeoxyglucose positron emission tomography imaging—A prospective trial. Cancer 2017;123:155–60.
23. Federico SM, Spunt SL, Krasin MJ, et al. Comparison of PET-CT and conventional imaging in staging pediatric rhabdomyosarcoma. Pediatr Blood Cancer 2013;60: 1128–34.
24. Vaarwerk B, Breunis WB, Haveman LM, et al. Fluorine-18-fluorodeoxyglucose (FDG) positron emission tomography (PET) computed tomography (CT) for the detection of bone, lung, and lymph node metastases in rhabdomyosarcoma. Cochrane Database Syst Rev 2021. https://doi.org/10.1002/14651858.CD012325.PUB2.
25. Rogers TN, Seitz G, Fuchs J, et al. Surgical management of paratesticular rhabdomyosarcoma: a consensus opinion from the Children's Oncology Group, European paediatric Soft tissue sarcoma Study Group, and the Cooperative Weichteilsarkom Studiengruppe. Pediatr Blood Cancer 2021. https://doi.org/10.1002/pbc.28938.
26. Stanborough R, Demertzis JL, Wessell DE, et al. ACR appropriateness criteria® malignant or aggressive primary musculoskeletal tumor-staging and surveillance: 2022 update. J Am Coll Radiol 2022;19:S374–89.
27. Mitton B, Seeger LL, Eckardt MA, et al. Image-guided percutaneous core needle biopsy of musculoskeletal tumors in children. J Pediatr Hematol Oncol 2014;36: 337–41.
28. Weiss AR, Lyden ER, Anderson JR, et al. Histologic and clinical characteristics can guide staging evaluations for children and adolescents with rhabdomyosarcoma: a report from the children's oncology group soft tissue sarcoma committee. J Clin Oncol 2013;31(26):3226–32. American Society of Clinical Oncology.
29. Jeremiasse B, van der Steeg AFW, Fiocco M, et al, Terwisscha van Scheltinga CEJ. Value of the sentinel node procedure in pediatric extremity rhabdomyosarcoma: a systematic review and retrospective cohort study. Ann Surg Oncol 2021; 28:9048–59.
30. Terwisscha van Scheltinga S, Merks JHM, Guerin F, et al. Surgical lymph node staging in extremity rhabdomyosarcoma: the EpSSG RMS 2005 trial experience. Ann Surg Oncol 2025;32:7751–61.
31. Jeremiasse B, van Scheltinga CEJT, Smeele LE, et al. Sentinel lymph node procedure in pediatric patients with melanoma, squamous cell carcinoma, or sarcoma using near-infrared fluorescence imaging with indocyanine green: a feasibility trial. Ann Surg Oncol 2023;30:2391–8.
32. Jeremiasse B, van den Bosch CH, Wijnen MWHA, et al. Systematic review and meta-analysis concerning near-infrared imaging with fluorescent agents to identify the sentinel lymph node in oncology patients. Eur J Surg Oncol 2020;46: 2011–22.
33. Campwala I, Vignali PDA, Seynnaeve BK, et al. Utility of indocyanine green for sentinel lymph node biopsy in pediatric sarcoma and melanoma. J Pediatr Surg 2024;59:1326–33.
34. Schermerhorn SMV, Vore E, Bondoc AJ, et al. Indocyanine green assists with sentinel lymph node mapping in pediatric and adolescent patients: a pediatric surgical oncology research collaborative prospective observational study. Cancer 2026. https://doi.org/10.1002/cncr.70274.
35. Meza JL, Anderson J, Pappo AS, et al, Children's Oncology Group. Analysis of prognostic factors in patients with nonmetastatic rhabdomyosarcoma treated

on intergroup rhabdomyosarcoma studies III and IV: the Children's Oncology Group. J Clin Oncol 2006;24:3844–51.
36. Crane JN, Xue W, Qumseya A, et al. Clinical group and modified TNM stage for rhabdomyosarcoma: a review from the Children's Oncology Group. Pediatr Blood Cancer 2022. https://doi.org/10.1002/PBC.29644.
37. De Salvo GL, Del Bianco P, Minard-Colin V, et al. Reappraisal of prognostic factors used in the European Pediatric Soft Tissue Sarcoma Study Group RMS 2005 study for localized rhabdomyosarcoma to optimize risk stratification and generate a prognostic nomogram. Cancer 2024;130:2351–60.
38. Hibbitts E, Chi YY, Hawkins DS, et al. Refinement of risk stratification for childhood rhabdomyosarcoma using FOXO1 fusion status in addition to established clinical outcome predictors: a report from the Children's Oncology Group. Cancer Med 2019;8:6437–48.
39. Bisogno G, Sparber-Sauer M, Rodeberg D, et al. The International Soft Tissue Sarcoma Consortium: the baseline analysis of rhabdomyosarcoma data. Cancer 2025. https://doi.org/10.1002/CNCR.35974.
40. Dixon SB, Bjornard KL, Alberts NM, et al. Factors influencing risk-based care of the childhood cancer survivor in the 21st century. CA Cancer J Clin 2018;68: 133–52.
41. Gupta AA, Xue W, Harrison DJ, et al. Addition of temsirolimus to chemotherapy in children,adolescents, and young adults with intermediate-risk rhabdomyosarcoma (ARST1431): a randomised, open-label,phase 3 trial from the Children's Oncology Group. Lancet Oncol 2024;25:912.
42. van der Graaf WTA, Orbach D, Judson IR, et al. Soft tissue sarcomas in adolescents and young adults: a comparison with their paediatric and adult counterparts. Lancet Oncol 2017;18:e166–75.
43. Mandeville HC. Radiotherapy in the management of childhood rhabdomyosarcoma. Clin Oncol 2019;31:462–70.
44. Bradley JA, Kayton ML, Chi YY, et al. Treatment approach and outcomes in infants with localized rhabdomyosarcoma: a report from the Soft Tissue Sarcoma Committee of the children's oncology Group. Int J Radiat Oncol Biol Phys 2018;103:19.
45. Wolden SL, Wexler LH, Kraus DH, et al. Intensity-modulated radiotherapy for head-and-neck rhabdomyosarcoma. Int J Radiat Oncol Biol Phys 2005;61:1432–8.
46. Fukushima H, Mizumoto M, Hosaka S, et al. Systematic review and meta-analysis of photon radiotherapy versus proton beam therapy for pediatric rhabdomyosarcoma: TRP-rhabdomyosarcoma 2024. Int J Clin Oncol 2025;30:1670–7.
47. Polites SF, Rhee DS, Routh JC, et al. Critical elements of pediatric rhabdomyosarcoma surgery. Semin Pediatr Surg 2023. https://doi.org/10.1016/j.sempedsurg.2023.151341.
48. Rogers T, Schmidt A, Buchanan AF, et al. Rhabdomyosarcoma surgical update. Pediatr Blood Cancer 2025. https://doi.org/10.1002/PBC.31496.
49. Lawrence W, Hays DM, Heyn R, et al. Surgical lessons from the Intergroup Rhabdomyosarcoma Study (IRS) pertaining to extremity tumors. World J Surg 1988;12: 676–84.
50. Dasgupta R, Rodeberg DA. Update on rhabdomyosarcoma. Semin Pediatr Surg 2012;21:68–78.
51. Cecchetto G, Guglielmi M, Inserra A, et al, Italian Cooperative Group on Soft-Tissue Sarcomas. Primary re-excision: the Italian experience in patients with localized soft-tissue sarcomas. Pediatr Surg Int 2001;17:532–4.
52. Hayes-Jordan A, Doherty DK, West SD, et al. Outcome after surgical resection of recurrent rhabdomyosarcoma. J Pediatr Surg 2006;41:633–8.

53. Polites SF, Rhee DS, Seitz G, et al. Contemporary surgical management of pediatric non-rhabdomyosarcoma soft tissue sarcoma. Pediatr Blood Cancer 2024. https://doi.org/10.1002/PBC.31257.
54. Rodeberg DA, Wharam MD, Lyden ER, et al. Delayed primary excision with subsequent modification of radiotherapy dose for intermediate-risk rhabdomyosarcoma: a report from the Children's Oncology Group Soft Tissue Sarcoma Committee. Int J Cancer 2015;137:204–11.
55. Jackson CB, Xue W, Gupta AA, et al. Radiation therapy dose escalation failed to improve local control for intermediate-risk rhabdomyosarcoma on ARST1431: a report from the Children's Oncology Group. Int J Radiat Oncol Biol Phys 2025; 123:54–62.
56. Lautz TB, Chi YY, Li M, et al. Benefit of delayed primary excision in rhabdomyosarcoma: a report from the Children's Oncology Group. Cancer 2021;127:275–83.
57. Cecchetto G, Bisogno G, De Corti F, et al, Italian Cooperative Group. Biopsy or debulking surgery as initial surgery for locally advanced rhabdomyosarcomas in children?: the experience of the Italian Cooperative Group studies. Cancer 2007;110:2561–7.
58. Lautz TB, Chi YY, Tian J, et al. Relationship between tumor response at therapy completion and prognosis in patients with Group III rhabdomyosarcoma: a report from the Children's Oncology Group. Int J Cancer 2020;147:1419–26.
59. Rodeberg DA, Stoner JA, Hayes-Jordan A, et al. Prognostic significance of tumor response at the End of Therapy in Group III rhabdomyosarcoma: a report from the children's oncology Group. J Clin Oncol 2009;27:3705–11.
60. De Lambert G, Haie-Meder C, Guérin F, et al. A new surgical approach of temporary ovarian transposition for children undergoing brachytherapy: technical assessment and dose evaluation. J Pediatr Surg 2014;49:1177–80.
61. Lautz TB, Harris CJ, Laronda MM, et al. A fertility preservation toolkit for pediatric surgeons caring for children with cancer. Semin Pediatr Surg 2019. https://doi.org/10.1016/J.SEMPEDSURG.2019.150861.
62. Burns KC, Hoefgen H, Strine A, et al. Fertility preservation options in pediatric and adolescent patients with cancer. Cancer 2018;124:1867–76.
63. Rodeberg DA, Anderson JR, Arndt CA, et al. Comparison of outcomes based on treatment algorithms for rhabdomyosarcoma of the bladder/prostate: combined results from the Children's Oncology Group, German Cooperative Soft Tissue Sarcoma Study, Italian Cooperative Group, and International Society of. Int J Cancer 2011;128:1232–9.
64. Martelli H, Borrego P, Guérin F, et al. Quality of life and functional outcome of male patients with bladder-prostate rhabdomyosarcoma treated with conservative surgery and brachytherapy during childhood. Brachytherapy 2016;15:306–11.
65. Martelli H, Haie-Meder C, Branchereau S, et al. Conservative surgery plus brachytherapy treatment for boys with prostate and/or bladder neck rhabdomyosarcoma: a single team experience. J Pediatr Surg 2009;44:190–6.
66. Arndt C, Rodeberg D, Breitfeld PP, et al. Does bladder preservation (as a surgical principle) lead to retaining bladder function in bladder/prostate rhabdomyosarcoma? Results from Intergroup Rhabdomyosarcoma Study IV. J Urol 2004;171: 2396–403.
67. Lautz TB, Martelli H, Fuchs J, et al. Local treatment of rhabdomyosarcoma of the female genital tract: expert consensus from the Children's Oncology Group, the European Soft-Tissue Sarcoma Group, and the Cooperative Weichteilsarkom Studiengruppe. Pediatr Blood Cancer 2023. https://doi.org/10.1002/PBC.28601.

68. Martelli H, Oberlin O, Rey A, et al. Conservative treatment for girls with nonmetastatic rhabdomyosarcoma of the genital tract: a report from the Study Committee of the International Society of Pediatric Oncology. J Clin Oncol 1999;17:2117–22.
69. Stewart RJ, Martelli H, Oberlin O, et al. Treatment of children with nonmetastatic paratesticular rhabdomyosarcoma: results of the Malignant Mesenchymal Tumors studies (MMT 84 and MMT 89) of the International Society of Pediatric Oncology. J Clin Oncol 2003;21:793–8.
70. Seitz G, Dantonello TM, Kosztyla D, et al, Cooperative Soft Tissue Sarcoma Study Group. Impact of hemiscrotectomy on outcome of patients with embryonal paratesticular rhabdomyosarcoma: results from the Cooperative Soft Tissue Sarcoma Group Studies CWS-86, 91, 96 and 2002P. J Urol 2014;192:902–7.
71. Lawrence W, Hays DM, Heyn R, et al. Lymphatic metastases with Childhood rhabdomyosarcoma A report from the Intergroup rhabdomyosarcoma Study. Cancer 1987;60(4):910–5.
72. Walterhouse DO, Barkauskas DA, Hall D, et al. Demographic and treatment variables influencing outcome for localized paratesticular rhabdomyosarcoma: results from a pooled analysis of North American and European cooperative groups. J Clin Oncol 2018;36:3466–76.
73. Weiner GJ. Building better monoclonal antibody-based therapeutics. Nat Rev Cancer 2015;15:361–70.
74. Tomaszewski JJ, Sweeney DD, Kavoussi LR, et al. Laparoscopic retroperitoneal lymph node dissection for high-risk pediatric patients with paratesticular rhabdomyosarcoma. J Endourol 2010;24:31–4.
75. Routh JC, Dasgupta R, Chi YY, et al. Impact of local control and surgical lymph node evaluation in localized paratesticular rhabdomyosarcoma: a report from the Children's Oncology Group Soft Tissue Sarcoma Committee. Int J Cancer 2020; 147:3168–76.
76. Mansfield SA, Murphy AJ, Talbot L, et al. Alternative approaches to retroperitoneal lymph node dissection for paratesticular rhabdomyosarcoma. J Pediatr Surg 2020;55:2677–81.
77. Donaldson SS, Meza J, Breneman JC, et al, Children's Oncology Group Soft Tissue Sarcoma Committee formely Intergroup Rhabdomyosarcoma Group Representing the Children's Oncology Group and the Quality Assurance Review Center. Results from the IRS-IV randomized trial of hyperfractionated radiotherapy in children with rhabdomyosarcoma - a report from the IRSG. Int J Radiat Oncol Biol Phys 2001;51:718–28.
78. Morris CD, Tunn PU, Rodeberg DA, et al. Surgical management of extremity rhabdomyosarcoma: a consensus opinion from the Children's Oncology Group, the European Pediatric Soft-Tissue Sarcoma Study Group, and the Cooperative Weichteilsarkom Studiengruppe. Pediatr Blood Cancer 2023. https://doi.org/10.1002/PBC.28608.
79. Guérin F, Rogers T, Minard-Colin V, et al. Outcome of localized liver-bile duct rhabdomyosarcoma according to local therapy: a report from the European Paediatric Soft-Tissue Sarcoma Study Group (EpSSG)-RMS 2005 study. Pediatr Blood Cancer 2019. https://doi.org/10.1002/PBC.27725.
80. Spunt SL, Lobe TE, Pappo AS, et al. Aggressive surgery is unwarranted for biliary tract rhabdomyosarcoma. J Pediatr Surg 2000;35:309–16.
81. Dasgupta R, Xue W, Dixon AH, et al. Outcomes for patients with perineal and perianal rhabdomyosarcoma: a report from the Children's Oncology Group Soft Tissue Sarcoma Committee. Pediatr Blood Cancer 2024. https://doi.org/10.1002/PBC.31303.

82. Martynov I, Tobi L, Strömer A, et al. Prevalence of locoregional and distant lymph node metastases in children and adolescents/young adults with soft tissue sarcomas: a Bayesian meta-analysis of proportions. eClinicalMedicine 2025. https://doi.org/10.1016/j.eclinm.2025.103390.
83. Cameron AL, Elze MC, Casanova M, et al. The impact of radiation therapy in children and adolescents with metastatic Rhabdomyosarcoma. Int J Radiat Oncol Biol Phys 2021;111:968–78.
84. Mercolini F, Sparber-Sauer M, Mascarenhas L, et al. Single site metastatic rhabdomyosarcoma: an INternational Soft Tissue saRcoma ConsorTium (INSTRuCT) pooled analysis. Eur J Cancer 2025. https://doi.org/10.1016/j.ejca.2025.115793.
85. Schloemer NJ, Xue W, Qumseya A, et al. Prognosis of children and young adults with newly diagnosed rhabdomyosarcoma metastatic to bone marrow treated on Children's Oncology Group studies. Pediatr Blood Cancer 2023. https://doi.org/10.1002/pbc.30701.
86. Vasquez JC, Luo LY, Hiniker SM, et al. Rhabdomyosarcoma with isolated lung metastases: a report from the Soft Tissue Sarcoma Committee of the Children's Oncology Group. Pediatr Blood Cancer 2023. https://doi.org/10.1002/pbc.30293.
87. Gupta AA, Xue W, Harrison DJ, et al. Addition of temsirolimus to chemotherapy in children, adolescents, and young adults with intermediate-risk rhabdomyosarcoma (ARST1431): a randomised, open-label, phase 3 trial from the Children's Oncology Group. Lancet Oncol 2024;25:912–21.
88. Vaarwerk B, Mallebranche C, Affinita MC, et al. Is surveillance imaging in pediatric patients treated for localized rhabdomyosarcoma useful? The European experience. Cancer 2020;126:823–31.
89. Casanova M, Bergamaschi L, Chiaravalli S, et al. Relapse after non-metastatic rhabdomyosarcoma: the impact of routine surveillance imaging on early detection and post-relapse survival. Pediatr Blood Cancer 2023. https://doi.org/10.1002/PBC.30095.
90. Kreimer S, Xue W, Qumseya A, et al. Late events occurring after 5 years in pediatric rhabdomyosarcoma: a report from the Children's Oncology Group. Pediatr Blood Cancer 2025;72:e31421.
91. Dantonello TM, Int-Veen C, Schuck A, et al. Survival following disease recurrence of primary localized alveolar rhabdomyosarcoma. Pediatr Blood Cancer 2013;60:1267–73.
92. Chen C, Dorado Garcia H, Scheer M, et al. Current and future treatment strategies for rhabdomyosarcoma. Front Oncol 2019. https://doi.org/10.3389/FONC.2019.01458.
93. Pio L, Lobos P, Abib S, et al. International patterns and disparities in functional sequelae (FUSE) follow-up after pediatric solid tumor resection: a report from the international Society of Pediatric Surgical Oncology. Surgery (United States) 2026;190:109832.
94. van Gorp M, Grootenhuis MA, Darlington AS, et al. Patient reported outcomes and measures in children with Rhabdomyosarcoma. Cancers (Basel) 2023. https://doi.org/10.3390/CANCERS15020420.

Non-rhabdomyosarcoma Soft Tissue Sarcoma

Daniel S. Rhee, MD, MPH[a,*], David A. Rodeberg, MD[b]

KEYWORDS

- Pediatric non-rhabdomyosarcoma • Pediatric soft tissue sarcoma
- Synovial sarcoma • Infantile fibrosarcoma • Desmoplastic small round cell tumor
- Malignant peripheral nerve sheath tumor

KEY POINTS

- Non-rhabdomyosarcoma soft tissue sarcomas (NRSTSs) comprise a heterogeneous group of many rare distinct tumor subtypes.
- Studying NRSTS together in large clinical trials has allowed identification of important prognostic factors, risk stratification, and optimal treatment regimens.
- Surgery is essential in the treatment of NRSTS and low-grade tumors can be treated with surgery alone, whereas intermediate or high grade require multi-modal therapy.
- Improving outcomes for patients with advanced or metastatic disease remain a challenge given their variable or uncertain chemosensitivity. New therapeutic concepts are needed.

INTRODUCTION

Non-rhabdomyosarcoma soft tissue sarcomas (NRSTSs) comprise a heterogeneous group of tumors with over 50 distinct histology subtypes. These tumors are presumed to be mesenchymal in origin from a diverse array of tissues including synovium, fat, muscle, endothelium, lymphatics, and fascia. Classification is often according to the normal tissue types from which they are derived. These tumors can arise in any anatomic location, and their biologic behavior can vary widely from indolent to highly malignant. This creates diagnostic and treatment challenges best managed by experienced multi-disciplinary teams in centers that can also offer the opportunity to enroll patients in clinical trials. To facilitate performing clinical trials, NRSTS subtypes have been combined into broad categories. These trials have been successful in identifying prognostic factors and optimizing treatment strategies for this diverse group of

[a] Division of Pediatric Surgery, Department of Surgery, Memorial Sloan Kettering Cancer Center, 1275 York Avenue, New York, NY 10065, USA; [b] Division of Pediatric Surgery, Department of Surgery, Kentucky Children's Hospital, 740 S. Limestone, Second floor, Wing D, Room J201, Lexington, KY 40536, USA
* Corresponding author.
E-mail address: Drhee1@jhmi.edu

Surg Oncol Clin N Am 35 (2026) 749–764
https://doi.org/10.1016/j.soc.2026.03.003 **surgonc.theclinics.com**

Abbreviations	
ALK	Anaplastic lymphoma kinase
ANNUBP	Atypical Neurofibromatous Neoplasm with Uncertain Biologic Potential
CT	Computed tomography
DSRCT	Desmoplastic small round cell tumor
EFS	Event-free survival
IFS	Infantile fibrosarcoma
IMT	Inflammatory myofibroblastic tumors
MPNST	Malignant peripheral nerve sheath tumor
NRSTS	Non-rhabdomyosarcoma soft tissue sarcoma
OS	Overall survival
PRE	Primary re-excision
STS	Soft tissue sarcoma

tumors. As the genetics and tumor biology of the various subtypes are further refined, the optimal treatment strategies will continue to evolve.

Soft tissue sarcomas (STS) account for 7% of pediatric cancers in patients less than 20 years of age, with the main 2 categories being rhabdomyosarcoma and NRSTS. NRSTS comprises 50% to 60% of STSs, and there are 500 to 600 new cases per year in this age cohort.[1,2] Age distribution is bimodal, with one peak before the age of 4 years and a second larger peak in adolescents and young adults. Infantile fibrosarcoma (IFS) and malignant rhabdoid tumors are more common in infancy, whereas in older patients, synovial sarcoma (SS), undifferentiated sarcoma, and malignant peripheral nerve sheath tumor (MPNST) are more common.[3–5] Generally, males and females are equally affected except for desmoplastic small round blue cell tumors that predominantly occur in males (90%).

Specific genetic and translocation aberrations play a critical role in the development of multiple NRSTS subtypes. The identification of these translocations has not only improved diagnostic precision but also opened the door to targeted therapeutic strategies[6] (**Table 1**). Although most NRSTSs arise sporadically, several inherited cancer predisposition syndromes significantly increase risk. For example, neurofibromatosis type 1, caused by mutations in the NF1 gene, is strongly associated with MPNSTs.[7,8]

Table 1
Genetic alteration of selected non-rhabdomyosarcoma soft tissue sarcomas

Histology	Genetic Aberrations
Synovial sarcoma	t(X;18) (p11;q11) SSX-SYT
Infantile fibrosarcoma	t(12;15) (p13,q25)ETV-NTRK3
Desmoplastic small round cell tumor	t(11;22) (p13;q12) EWSR1-WT1
Hemangiopericytoma	t(12;19) (q13;q13.3) and t(13;22) (q22;q13.3)
Extraosseous Ewing sarcoma	t(11;22) (2q4;q12) EWSR1-FLI1
Malignant rhabdoid tumor	Inactivation SMARCB1
Dermatofibrosarcoma protuberans	t(17;22) (q22;q13) COLIAI-PDGFb
Alveolar soft part sarcoma	t(X;17) (p11.2;q25) ASPL-TFE3
Malignant peripheral nerve sheath tumor	17q11.2, loss or rearrangement of 10p, 11q, 17q, 22q NF1
Inflammatory myofibroblastic tumor	2p23 rearrangement ALK

Similarly, Li Fraumeni syndrome, an autosomal dominant disorder resulting from mutations in the p53 tumor suppressor gene, predisposes individuals to a wide spectrum of malignancies, including multiple soft tissue sarcoma subtypes, bone sarcoma, breast carcinoma, brain tumors, and leukemia.[9] Familial adenomatous polyposis is linked to elevated risk of colon cancer and desmoid tumors.[10] Other syndromes increasing risk of NRSTS include Werner syndrome, Gorlin syndrome, germline mutations in RB1 (leiomyosarcoma), and SMARCB1 (malignant rhabdoid tumor).[11,12] Beyond genetic factors, environmental and external exposures further amplify risk. Prior history of therapeutic radiation is a well-established contributor, particularly when sarcomas arise within previously irradiated fields. Viral infections also play a role; for instance, Epstein-Barr virus infection in patients with human immunodeficiency virus has been linked to leiomyosarcoma. Chronic conditions such as longstanding lymphedema can lead to lymphangiosarcoma.[13,14] Importantly, children with history of cancer face a greater than 9 fold risk of developing a sarcoma than the general population, especially within prior radiation fields.[15,16]

Clinical Presentation and Diagnostic Evaluation

NRSTSs typically present as a painless mass, most commonly arising from the extremities or trunk. Symptoms can occur based on size and location and include pain, numbness, or weakness when adjacent to neurovascular structures. Intraabdominal lesions can lead to abdominal pain or obstructive findings, and thoracic lesions can lead to respiratory symptoms. Systemic findings such as fever, weight loss, anorexia, or anemia are rare but may occur with widely metastatic disease. Symptoms are often subtle and delays from symptom onset to diagnosis are common.[17]

Evaluation begins with a comprehensive history including family history, predisposing conditions, and physical examination. Plain radiographs can show bony destruction or calcifications present within the tumor seen with SS. Ultrasound can be useful to differentiate cystic and solid masses and to give further information regarding the depth of the mass, involvement of adjacent structures, and proximity to vascular structures as well as vascularity of the tumor itself. Cross-sectional imaging is required to better characterize the mass in relation to its surrounding structures. MRI is the preferred modality for extremity and trunk lesions as it provides a superior view of muscle and soft tissue structures. Computed tomography (CT) is the preferred imaging for abdominal or pelvic tumors and for evaluation for lung metastasis. Fluorodeoxyglucose PET is increasingly used for further assessment of regional and metastatic spread.[18,19] Metastatic disease occurs in 15% of patients with the lungs being the most common distant metastatic site, although metastases may also occur in the bone, liver, subcutaneous tissue, and brain. Bone marrow involvement is rare.[4,20]

An adequate tissue biopsy is essential for histologic, immunocytochemical, as well as molecular studies. Core needle biopsies or incisional biopsies are recommended; however, upfront resection with negative margins may be appropriate for small or superficial lesions. Fine need aspiration does not provide adequate material and is not recommended. Careful planning is required for biopsy to ensure adequate viable tissue is obtained and biopsy tracts are placed where they can be excised with the definitive operation. Intrathoracic or intraabdominal masses may be best approached with percutaneous image-guided core needle biopsies, or minimally invasive or open biopsy as appropriate.

Regional lymph node metastases occur in about 4% to 8% of NRSTS; however, higher rates of lymph node involvement are seen in epithelioid (18%), clear cell sarcomas (14%), undifferentiated sarcoma (14%), angiosarcomas (17%), and extracranial malignant rhabdoid tumor (17%).[4,21–24] Positive regional lymph node involvement is more likely with high pathologic grade primary tumors and patients with distant metastasis.[25] Clinically or radiographically positive or indeterminate regional lymph nodes should be biopsied to definitively confirm the presence or absence of pathologic nodal disease. This can be done through targeted nodal sampling or ultrasound guided core needle biopsy. For clinically negative nodes, regional node sampling should be considered in clear cell sarcoma, epithelioid sarcoma, angiosarcoma, and extracranial malignant rhabdoid tumor given their higher rates of nodal disease. Sentinel lymph node biopsy is an effective and preferred method over random lymph node sampling. Standard tracers include radiocolloids (technetium-99m), blue dye, and indocyanine green. Tracers should be injected in the same drainage route as the primary tumor, typically peritumoral in the subcutaneous or intradermal space. Regional nodal staging should occur before the start of chemotherapy.[22]

Staging and Risk Stratification

Key prognostic factors for NRSTS include the site of primary tumor, tumor size, tumor grade and histology, depth of tumor invasion, presence of metastases, completeness of tumor resection or resectability, and use of radiation therapy (RT).[26,27] In adults, the staging system for STS utilized in the United States is the American Joint Committee on Cancer (AJCC) staging which is based on site of origin and utilizes the standard tumor, node, metastasis (TNM) classification, with the addition of tumor grade.28 However, this system has not been validated in pediatric studies. Tumor grade is based upon tumor histology, degree of cellularity, cellular pleomorphism, invasive growth, degree of necrosis, and mitotic activity.[29] Low-grade tumors are mostly localized and rarely metastasize, whereas high-grade lesions show a more aggressive behavior with increased risk of metastatic spread. The Pediatric Oncology Group grading system and the Fédération National des Centres de Lutte Contre le Cancer are the 2 primary grading systems utilized for NRSTS.

General Treatment Strategies

Ongoing challenges in understanding optimal NRSTS management strategies include inconsistency in initial evaluation and care, wide variations in treatment delivery, difficulty in accurate histologic diagnosis, and poor application of appropriate tumor molecular characterization.[30] Because of this, treatment should be coordinated by experienced multidisciplinary teams at institutions with the ability to enroll patients in clinical trials.

A clinical trial evaluating a risk-based treatment strategy for NRSTS was prospectively studied through the Children's Oncology Group where patients less than 30 years of age were assigned risk groups by presence of metastasis, tumor resectability and margin status, and tumor size and grade (**Fig. 1**). Patients were assigned into 1 of 3 risk groups and underwent risk adapted therapy with survival results as seen in **Table 2**. The principal components of the risk-based therapy are described in the subsequent sections.

Surgical treatment

NRSTSs are frequently resistant to chemotherapy, and therefore surgery is the predominant therapy for most subtypes. Tumor resectability and completeness of resection have major prognostic implications on outcomes for nearly all tumor histologies. The goal of surgery is complete resection of the tumor with negative margins. In the Children's Oncology Group ARST0332 study, completeness of resection resulted in the best outcomes with R0 resections achieving 5 year event free survival (EFS) 83.6% and 5 year overall survival (OS) 92.8% compared to R1 (66.2% and 79.7%)

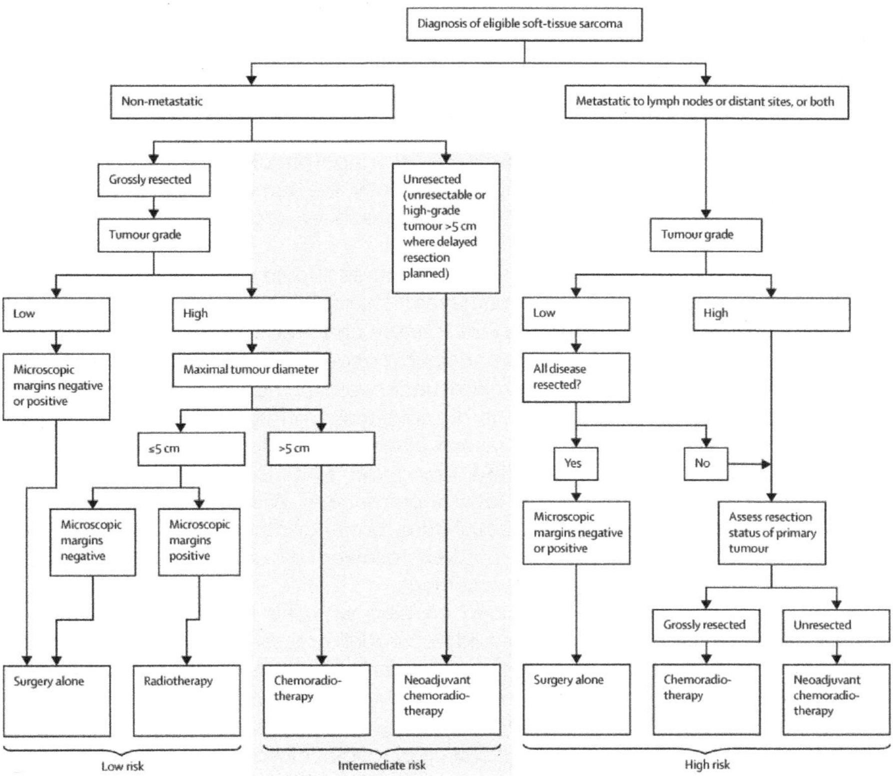

Fig. 1. Risk stratification and treatment paradigm for NRSTS. (*From* Rajkumar Venkatramani et al. Synovial Sarcoma in Children, Adolescents, and Young Adults: A Report From the Children's Oncology Group ARST0332 Study. J Clin Oncol 2021;39, 3927–3937. https://doi.org/10.1200/JCO.21.01628.)

and R2 (49.2% and 62.7%), respectively.[4,31] Upfront primary resection should be considered for small, superficial tumors amenable to complete resection without excess morbidity. This is often a suitable approach for low-grade tumors or high-grade tumors of 5 cm or less. Preoperative imaging to determine the tumor's relationship to critical structures including neurovascular structures, bones, joints, and spine,

Table 2
Risk stratification of non-rhabdomyosarcoma soft tissue sarcomas and outcomes from the Children's Oncology Group ARST0332 Trial

Risk Group	Criteria	% Cohort	5 y EFS	5 y OS
Low risk	Nonmetastatic tumors, R0 resection, R1 for low-grade tumor, or R1 for high grade $\leq$ 5 cm	42.0%	88.9%	96.2%
Intermediate risk	Nonmetastatic tumors, R0 or R1>5 cm for high-grade tumor, or unresected tumor of any grade or size	42.9%	65.0%	79.2%
High risk	Metastatic disease	15.1%	21.2%	35.5%

as well as general location in the body, will aid in surgical decision making. Patients with positive or unknown margin status should be considered for primary re-excision (PRE) if negative margins can be achieved without excess morbidity.[31,32] PRE is intended to achieve a wide resection while still preserving function and should include the scar and the superficial and deep tissues left behind during the previous surgery.[32] PRE should also be performed after a non-oncologic NRSTS procedure such as a "shelling out" of the tumor. Frequently the tumor will infiltrate beyond the pseudocapsule and microscopic disease has been reported in up to 48% of patients.[31]

Larger tumors and those abutting critical structures should undergo biopsy and histologic confirmation followed by neoadjuvant chemotherapy and/or radiation and delayed excision if possible. Neoadjuvant therapy can improve the ability to achieve negative margins with 82% of patients achieving negative margins after neoadjuvant therapy compared to 57% of those who underwent immediate primary resection without neoadjuvant therapy.[4] There is no consensus on optimal margin distance, although 0.5 cm margin or a closer fascial plane is considered sufficient. For low-risk patients with completely resected low-grade NRSTS, margins greater than 1 mm may be sufficient to prevent local recurrence.[33] Wide margins may not be possible in locations close to neurovasculature, bone, or other important structures. Specimens should be oriented and marked followed by communication with the pathologist to allow proper margin assessment.

Prior biopsy tracts should be excised en bloc with the tumor. When aiming to achieve an R0 resection, dissection should be through grossly normal tissue achieving an envelope of normal tissue entirely surrounding the tumor. Radical excision or resecting entire anatomic compartments is not usually required. Frozen section can be used to evaluate the tumor bed after resection when there is concern for microscopic residual disease. Titanium clips can be placed at close tumor margins or in uncertain areas to help guide external beam radiation. For tumors abutting bone or fascia, the adjacent periosteum or fascia should be excised. In patients for whom brachytherapy will be delivered, it is often beneficial to leave a drain to avoid fluid collections that will negatively interfere with subsequent therapies.

Wound complications are noted in 2% to 10% of patients after surgical excision. However, the use of neoadjuvant RT is associated with increased rates of wound complications ranging from 22% to 35%.[34] The addition of pazopanib, a tyrosine kinase inhibitor, was shown in ARST1321 to further increase wound issues. Patients with addition of pazopanib to RT and chemotherapy had a 2 fold increased (to 50%) wound complication rate compared to 22% without pazopanib. However, grade III complications (requiring intervention) occurred in 26% which is considered comparable to contemporary literature for patients undergoing preoperative RT.[35] Surgeons may elect to utilize muscle flaps, pedicled myocutaneous flaps, and free flaps to provide well-vascularized tissue for coverage. Seromas are common and drains should be left if concerned intraoperatively. In abdominal tumors, adhesive bowel obstructions or intestinal damage may occur.

Medical treatment

Many NRSTSs are not sensitive to chemotherapy and patients with high-risk or metastatic disease continue to have dismal outcomes, with 5 year EFS of 21%. Novel treatment approaches are needed.[4] SS, unclassified sarcoma, and embryonal sarcoma of the liver show good pathologic response to chemotherapy. Other histologies such as alveolar soft-part sarcoma or clear cell sarcoma are highly resistant to chemotherapy.[36–38] The most common chemotherapy backbone for NRSTS is ifosfamide-doxorubicin. Neoadjuvant chemotherapy is indicated for metastatic disease or unresectable localized tumors to improve resectability, and neoadjuvant combined chemoradiotherapy may yield higher response rates in selected cases. Adjuvant chemotherapy may be indicated for high-grade or larger tumors, but can be omitted in low-risk completed resected tumors less than 5 cm in size.[4,39,40]

Biologic therapies are therapeutic options for pediatric NRSTS. These include tyrosine kinase inhibitors (pazopanib), neurotrophic tyrosine receptor kinase (NTRK) inhibitors (larotractinib, entrectinib) for IFS, EZH2 inhibitors (tazemetostat) for epithelioid sarcoma, anaplastic lymphoma kinase (ALK) inhibitors (crizotinib) for inflammatory myofibroblastic tumors (IMT), and mitogen-activated extracellular signal-regulated kinase (MEK) inhibitors (selumetinib) for MPNST.[41] ARST1321 found pazopanib added to neoadjuvant chemoradiotherapy in children and adults with intermediate or high-grade NRSTS produced a significantly greater near pathologic response ($\geq$90% necrosis), leading to early termination of the study. Three year EFS and OS for all patients in the intent to treat analysis were 52.5% and 75.7% for the pazopanib group and 50.6% and 65.4% in the non-pazopanib group, respectively. These outcomes were not statistically significant although the study was not powered to evaluate these end points.[35,42,43]

Radiation therapy

RT can be used for definitive local control for unresectable tumors as well as for resected tumors with positive margins. RT should be considered for patients with high risk of local failure including marginally resected high-grade tumors of any size, high-grade tumors greater than 5 cm, and initially unresected disease. Neoadjuvant RT can also be used to aid in achieving negative margins with delayed resection. For patients enrolled on the clinical trial ARST0332 who received neoadjuvant chemoradiotherapy, greater than 90% underwent an R0 or R1 resection. Neoadjuvant chemoradiotherapy also allowed smaller RT tissue volumes and lower radiation doses than postoperative RT. Resection following radiation should be performed after 4 to 6 weeks to allow sufficient time for radiation-associated inflammation to resolve without allowing fibrosis to occur.[4,44] Radiation field size and dose is dependent on patient and tumor factors and the surgical procedure. Radiation doses range between 45 and 50 Gy in the preoperative period with an option to boost postoperatively to 10 to 20 Gy. In the postoperative setting, RT dosing is generally between 55 and 60 Gy.[45] Radiation margins are typically 2 to 4 cm longitudinally and encompass fascial planes axially. Given their incomplete growth and development, long-term side-effects of RT in children include limb length discrepancy, joint dysfunction, and cosmetic deformity.[46] Radiation techniques including proton-beam, 3 dimensional conformal RT, or intensity-modulated RT can facilitate normal tissue sparing and decreasing fibrosis or growth impairment.

Management of pulmonary metastatic disease

The most common site of distant metastases in NRSTS is the lungs which comprise 71% of all metastatic disease.[4] Surgical biopsy may be indicated at time of diagnosis when pulmonary lesions are indeterminate to allow appropriate staging and treatment. As many NRSTSs are not responsive to chemotherapy, pulmonary metastatectomy plays an important therapeutic role and should be considered when complete resection is anticipated.[47,48] The number and location of lesions can determine whether a minimally invasive or open approach is most appropriate. Non-anatomic wedge resections should be utilized to minimize excision of adjacent normal parenchyma. Larger anatomic resections may be required in select cases but should consider the ability to achieve complete resection, control of the primary tumor, and the patient's ability to tolerate the resection.

Management of Selected Non-rhabdomyosarcoma Soft Tissue Sarcoma Histologic Subtypes

Infantile fibrosarcoma

IFS is the most common STS in children under 2 years of age but has been known to occur up to 4 years of age. These tumors most commonly occur in the extremities, but may also occur on the neck, mediastinum, and retroperitoneum.[49,50] IFSs are often identified prenatally or at birth and can be mistaken as congenital or infantile hemangiomas.[51] They can grow rapidly, are rarely metastatic, and are classified as tumors of intermediate malignancy. It is characterized by t(12;15) (p13;q25) translocation coding for ETV6-NTRK3 gene fusion, which differentiates them from the adult fibrosarcoma variant.[52]

Complete surgical resection is curative in most patients. Neoadjuvant chemotherapy with a delayed primary resection can facilitate complete excision, limb sparing, and improve functional outcomes by avoiding mutilating surgery. Effective chemotherapy agents include vincristine, ifosfamide, dactinomycin, and cyclophosphamide. Targeted therapy with larotrectinib, an NTRK inhibitor, has been shown to be effective with TRK fusion-positive IFS and should be considered as an option for frontline therapy in these tumors.[53,54] Radiotherapy is not typically used for IFS due to concerns for long-term effects in this very young population. The prognosis of patients with IFS is generally quite good, with OS as high as 80% to 95%. There have also been several cases of spontaneous regression, or regression following partial resection, suggesting potential transformation to mature hemangiomatous tissue with time.[55,56]

Synovial sarcoma

SS is the most common NRSTS subtype (~25% of all NRSTSs). It carries the t(X;18) (p11.2;q11.2) chromosomal translocation and the SYT::SSX fusion transcript. SS is more commonly seen in patients older than 10 years of age with a median age of 13 years. Eighty percent are located on the extremities. The cystic appearance on imaging can be misleading suggesting a benign lesion; however, most SS are considered intermediate-to-high-grade tumors. Tumors larger than 5 cm have a higher risk of metastatic disease (15%), most commonly to the lungs (40%).[57,58]

Completely resected SS less than 5 cm can be managed with surgery alone, regardless of grade.[59] However, tumor size greater than 5 cm is associated with worse EFS and warrants neoadjuvant chemotherapy or radiation.[60] SS is more sensitive to chemotherapy than many other NRSTS (40%–65% response rate); however, the use of adjuvant chemotherapy does not always improve OS but may improve surgical resectability. Data from ARST0332 showed 5 year OS vary by risk group, with 98%, 89%, and 13% OS for low, intermediate, and high-risk patients, respectively. Long-term follow-up is of utmost importance, as SS tends to recur locally but can present with metastatic disease beyond 5 years.[61]

Malignant peripheral nerve sheath tumor

MPNSTs comprise 5% of STS in patients younger than 20 years. MPNST can arise spontaneously or occur in children with neurofibromatosis type 1 (NF1). The lifetime risk of patients with NF1 developing MPNST is approximately 8% to 13%; however, 20% to 55% of patients with MPNST have NF1.[62]

MPNSTs are highly aggressive tumors that present as a firm mass, most commonly in the trunk or extremities. Since they often arise in association with major nerve trunks and peripheral nerve branches, they may present with pain or neurologic deficits. In patients with NF1, there can be a multi-step, stepwise malignant transformation from benign neurofibromas to Atypical Neurofibromatous Neoplasm with Uncertain Biologic Potential (ANNUBP), characterized by nuclear atypia, hypercellularity, variable loss of neurofibroma architecture, and/or mitotic activity.[63] Accurately differentiating ANNUBP from MPNST is important since it is thought to have a lower risk of recurrence and therefore requires less aggressive resection. Finally, ANNUBP progress to high-grade MPNST, driven by cumulative genetic mutations, including NF1 loss, CDKN2A deletion, and PRC2 mutations.[64] This transformation is frequently heralded by the onset of pain or rapid growth in a preexisting plexiform neurofibroma thus raising concern for development of MPNST. MRI is the preferred imaging modality, but PET/CT may help differentiate this progression from benign neurofibroma, to ANNUBP and finally MPNST. At presentation, distant metastasis occurs in 10% where the most common location is lung. Complete surgical resection, whenever possible, is the cornerstone of treatment and improved outcomes are seen when an R0 or R1 resection is achieved.[65] RT may be effective in the setting of microscopic residual disease, but evidence to support its efficacy is limited.[66,67] Neoadjuvant chemotherapy may improve surgical resectability although MPNSTs have a poor response (23% overall response rate) to standard sarcoma chemotherapy[65] (**Fig. 2**A, B). Among NRSTSs, MPNST has the worst prognosis with 5 year OS 43% to 69%. Patients with low-risk disease have significantly better outcomes (5 year EFS and OS 88% and 83%, respectively) compared to intermediate (52% and 68%) and high-risk disease (0% for both).[65]

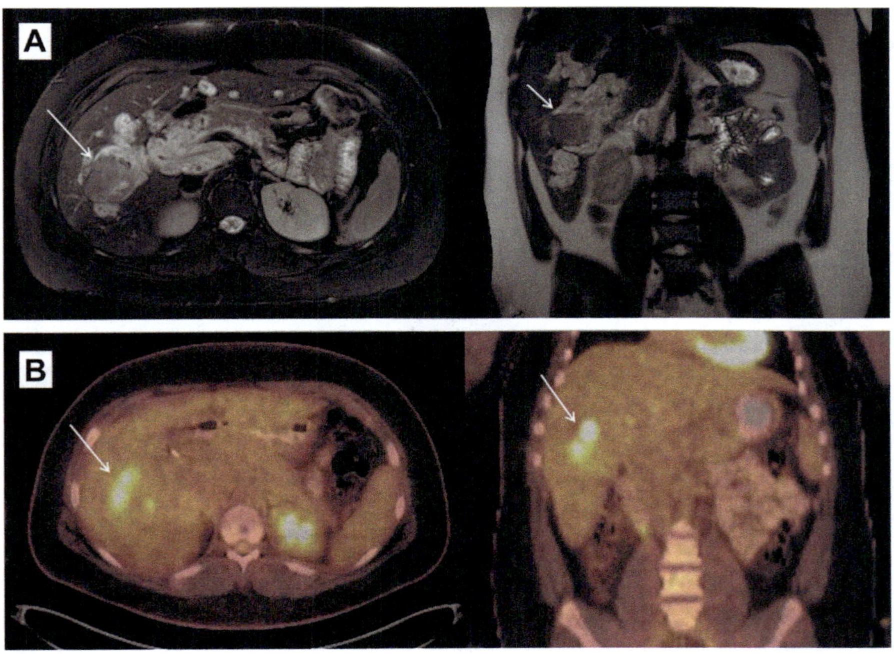

Fig. 2. MPNST in a 16 year old boy. (*A*) MRI findings of MPNST (*arrow*) arising from within a large plexiform neurofibroma in the liver. (*B*) 18F-FDG PET-CT shows a discrete nodular lesion (*arrow*) in the background of periportal plexiform neurofibroma.

Desmoplastic small round cell tumor

Desmoplastic small round cell tumors (DSRCTs) are most commonly seen in adolescents and young adults and display a significant male predominance (90%). These tumors are locally aggressive and usually arise from peritoneal surfaces. They can also arise from the kidney or other solid organs.[68] They often present as multiple peritoneal tumor implants or omental masses, which can be adherent to or invade adjacent structures. These are characterized by the translocation t(11;22) (p13;q12) and the EWSR1-WT1 gene fusion.[69] Lymph node involvement as well as metastasis to the liver, lung, bone, bone marrow, and kidney can occur.

These tumors are highly chemosensitive to Ewing sarcoma type chemotherapy. The most common chemotherapy regimen is vincristine/doxorubicin/cyclophosphamide and ifosfamide/etoposide which alternates between 2 drug combinations. After neoadjuvant chemotherapy, gross tumor resection with cytoreductive surgery is an essential component of treatment and is associated with improved outcomes. This can be followed by whole abdominal RT.[68,70] In addition to cytoreductive surgery, use of hyperthermic intraperitoneal chemotherapy and intraperitoneal instillation of antibody 131I-8H9 are being explored in highly specialized centers.[71,72] Radioembolotherapy with yttrium-90 microspheres can be used to treat hepatic metastasis.[73] Treatment of DSRCT should be centralized, and prospective randomized international trials are necessary for judging effects of new treatment regimens. The overall prognosis remains poor with an estimated survival of 15% at 5 years but with multi-modality approach, survival can be improved to 30% to 40% at 5 years.[74]

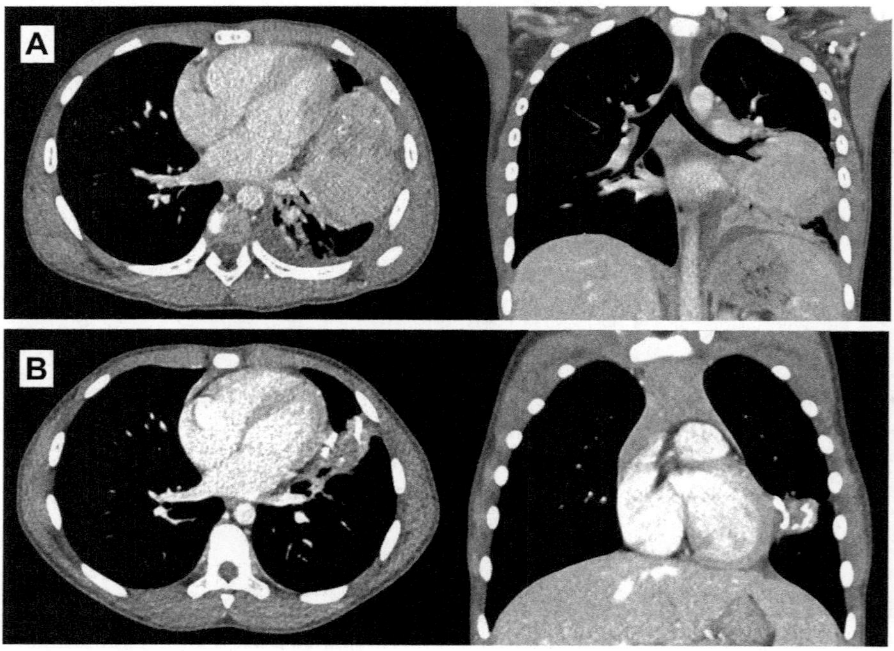

Fig. 3. IMT in a 9 year old girl. (*A*) Initial tumor extension with involvement of upper and lower lobes. (*B*) Response after tumor biopsy and treatment with crizotinib.

Inflammatory myofibroblastic tumors

IMTs are tumors of intermediate malignancy. These are locally invasive and occur most frequently in the lung followed by the abdominal cavity. Metastatic spread is rare (5%–7%).[75,76] IMT mainly affects children with a median age of 9 to 11 years. Presenting symptoms are common and include pain or respiratory symptoms. One-third of patients with IMT experience systemic symptoms (fever, weight loss, malaise, anemia).[76] In 50% to 60% of cases, IMT is characterized by a rearrangement of the ALK gene located on chromosome 2p23 with various gene partners including ROS proto-oncogene 1, receptor tyrosine kinase (ROS1), rearranged during transfection (RET), and NTRK, and platelet derived growth factor receptor (PDGFR)β.[77,78] Overall prognosis is excellent with reported 5 year EFS of 80% to 83% and OS greater than 95%.[75,76]

Complete surgical resection, when feasible, is the mainstay for treatment. For patients who undergo R0/R1 resection, surgery alone may be adequate. However, unresectable tumors should be biopsied followed by systemic therapy with the goal to reduce tumor size and improve the feasibility of resection.[59] Aggressive attempts to obtain a complete resection may not be warranted as prior studies have shown no difference in recurrence with gross or microscopic margins.[75] Chemotherapy may be used as neoadjuvant therapy although responses are variable. Successful use of steroids or nonsteroidal anti-inflammatory drug (NSAIDs) have also been reported.[76] Patients with ALK + tumors can be treated with an ALK inhibitor such as crizotinib and ceritinib (**Fig. 3**A, B). The increasing availability of targeted therapies with tyrosine kinase inhibitors including ROS1 and NTRK inhibitors offers promising options for those with the corresponding molecular abnormality.[59,76,79]

SUMMARY

NRSTS is a diverse group of STSs with a wide range of behavior, presentation, and response to treatment. As most NRSTSs are not responsive to chemotherapy, surgery remains the cornerstone of treatment of NRSTS and excellent outcomes for low-risk tumors can be achieved with surgery alone. However, the prognosis for high risk, metastatic, or advanced tumors remains poor despite aggressive multimodal treatment and new treatment modalities are needed to improve outcomes for these challenging patients. Studying NRSTS as a combined classification in cooperative group trials has been successful in identifying prognostic factors and improving treatment strategies. As the genetics and tumor biology of the various sarcoma subtypes are further refined, the optimal treatment strategies will continue to evolve.

CLINICS CARE POINTS

- Despite the significant heterogeneity in NRSTS, studying NRSTS together in large clinical trials has allowed approrpriate risk stratification to guide risk-adapted therapy.
- Surgical resection of NRSTS to negative margins when possible is essential for achieving cure.
- Patients with high risk disease have poor outcomes despite multi-modal therapy approaches and new treatment modalities are needed.

DISCLOSURES

The authors have nothing to disclose.

REFERENCES

1. Ferrari A, Sultan I, Huang TT, et al. Soft tissue sarcoma across the age spectrum: a population-based study from the surveillance epidemiology and end results database. Pediatr Blood Cancer 2011;57(6):943–9.
2. National Cancer Institute. NCCR*Explorer: an interactive website for NCCR cancer statistics. Bethesda (MD): National Cancer Institute; 2025. Available online.
3. Weiss AR, Harrison DJ. Soft tissue sarcomas in adolescents and young adults. J Clin Oncol 2024;42(6):675–85.
4. Spunt SL, Million L, Chi YY, et al. A risk-based treatment strategy for non-rhabdomyosarcoma soft-tissue sarcomas in patients younger than 30 years (ARST0332): a Children's Oncology Group prospective study. Lancet Oncol 2020;21(1):145–61.
5. Waxweiler TV, Rusthoven CG, Proper MS, et al. Non-Rhabdomyosarcoma soft tissue sarcomas in children: a surveillance, epidemiology, and end results analysis validating COG risk stratifications. Int J Radiat Oncol Biol Phys 2015;92(2): 339–48.
6. Black JO, Al-Ibraheemi A, Arnold MA, et al. The pathologic diagnosis of pediatric soft tissue tumors in the era of molecular medicine: the sarcoma pediatric pathology research interest group perspective. Arch Pathol Lab Med 2024;148(1): 107–16.
7. Bates JE, Peterson CR, Dhakal S, et al. Malignant peripheral nerve sheath tumors (MPNST): a SEER analysis of incidence across the age spectrum and therapeutic interventions in the pediatric population. Pediatr Blood Cancer 2014;61(11): 1955–60.
8. Evans DGR, Huson SM, Birch JM. Malignant peripheral nerve sheath tumours in inherited disease. Clin Sarcoma Res 2012;2(1):17.
9. Scollon S, Anglin AK, Thomas M, et al. A comprehensive review of pediatric tumors and associated cancer predisposition syndromes. J Genet Couns 2017; 26(3):387–434.
10. Groen EJ, Roos A, Muntinghe FL, et al. Extra-intestinal manifestations of familial adenomatous polyposis. Ann Surg Oncol 2008;15(9):2439–50.
11. Grant CN, Rhee D, Tracy ET, et al. Pediatric solid tumors and associated cancer predisposition syndromes: workup, management, and surveillance. A summary from the APSA Cancer Committee. J Pediatr Surg 2022;57(3):430–42.
12. Dermawan JK, Abramson DH, Chiang S, et al. The impact of Li-Fraumeni and germline retinoblastoma mutations on leiomyosarcoma initiation, outcomes, and genetic testing recommendations. Clin Cancer Res 2024;30(20):4780–90.
13. McClain KL, Joshi VV, Murphy SB. Cancers in children with HIV infection. Hematol Oncol Clin North Am 1996;10(5):1189–201.
14. Farzaliyev F, Hamacher R, Steinau Professor HU, et al. Secondary angiosarcoma: a fatal complication of chronic lymphedema. J Surg Oncol 2020;121(1):85–90.
15. Tringale KR, Casey DL, Niyazov G, et al. Second cancer risk in childhood cancer survivors treated with intensity-modulated radiation therapy: an updated analysis of more than 10 years of follow-up. Pediatr Blood Cancer 2022;69(5):e29600.
16. Casey DL, Friedman DN, Moskowitz CS, et al. Second cancer risk in childhood cancer survivors treated with intensity-modulated radiation therapy (IMRT). Pediatr Blood Cancer 2015;62(2):311–6.
17. Haimi M, Peretz Nahum M, Ben Arush MW. Delay in diagnosis of children with cancer: a retrospective study of 315 children. Pediatr Hematol Oncol 2004; 21(1):37–48.

18. Kao SC. Overview of the clinical and imaging features of the most common non-rhabdomyosarcoma soft-tissue sarcomas. Pediatr Radiol 2019;49(11):1524–33.
19. Khalatbari H, Shulkin BL, Parisi MT. PET/CT and PET/MR in soft tissue sarcoma: an update. Semin Nucl Med 2024;54(3):313–31.
20. Pappo AS, Rao BN, Jenkins JJ, et al. Metastatic nonrhabdomyosarcomatous soft-tissue sarcomas in children and adolescents: the St. Jude Children's Research Hospital experience. Med Pediatr Oncol 1999;33(2):76–82.
21. Alvarez E, He J, Spunt SL, et al. Lymph node metastases in paediatric and young adult patients with non-rhabdomyosarcoma soft tissue sarcoma (NRSTS): findings from Children's Oncology Group (COG) study ARST0332. Eur J Cancer 2023;180:89–98.
22. Terwisscha van Scheltinga S, Schoot RA, Routh JC, et al. Lymph node staging and treatment in pediatric patients with soft tissue sarcomas: a consensus opinion from the children's oncology group, European paediatric soft tissue sarcoma study group, and the cooperative Weichteilsarkom Studiengruppe. Pediatr Blood Cancer 2025;72(4):e31538.
23. Brennan B, De Salvo GL, Orbach D, et al. Outcome of extracranial malignant rhabdoid tumours in children registered in the European Paediatric Soft Tissue Sarcoma Study Group Non-Rhabdomyosarcoma Soft Tissue Sarcoma 2005 Study-EpSSG NRSTS 2005. Eur J Cancer 2016;60:69–82.
24. Enault M, Minard-Colin V, Corradini N, et al. Extracranial rhabdoid tumours: results of a SFCE series of patients treated with a dose compression strategy according to European Paediatric Soft tisue sarcoma study group recommendations. Eur J Cancer 2022;161:64–78.
25. Orbach D, Carton M, Heinz AT, et al. Regional lymph node invasion in pediatric non-rhabdomyosarcoma soft tissue sarcoma: an international cohort study from the International Soft Tissue Sarcoma Consortium. eClinicalMedicine 2025;87: 103409.
26. Spunt SL, Poquette CA, Hurt YS, et al. Prognostic factors for children and adolescents with surgically resected nonrhabdomyosarcoma soft tissue sarcoma: an analysis of 121 patients treated at St Jude Children's Research Hospital. J Clin Oncol 1999;17(12):3697–705.
27. Spunt SL, Hill DA, Motosue AM, et al. Clinical features and outcome of initially unresected nonmetastatic pediatric nonrhabdomyosarcoma soft tissue sarcoma. J Clin Oncol 2002;20(15):3225–35.
28. AJCC cancer staging manual. In: Amin MB, Edge SB, Greene FL, et al, editors. 6th edition. New York: Springer; 2017.
29. Parham DM, Webber BL, Jenkins JJ, et al. Nonrhabdomyosarcomatous soft tissue sarcomas of childhood: formulation of a simplified system for grading. Mod Pathol 1995;8(7):705–10.
30. Ferrari A, Orbach D, Sparber-Sauer M, et al. The treatment approach to pediatric non-rhabdomyosarcoma soft tissue sarcomas: a critical review from the INternational soft tissue SaRcoma ConsorTium. Eur J Cancer 2022;169:10–9.
31. Chui CH, Spunt SL, Liu T, et al. Is reexcision in pediatric nonrhabdomyosarcoma soft tissue sarcoma necessary after an initial unplanned resection? J Pediatr Surg 2002;37(10):1424–9.
32. Sparber-Sauer M, Ferrari A, Spunt SL, et al. The significance of margins in pediatric non-rhabdomyosarcoma soft tissue sarcomas: consensus on surgical margin definition harmonization from the INternational soft tissue SaRcoma ConsorTium (INSTRuCT). Cancer Med 2023;12(10):11719–30.

33. Douglass DP, Coffin CM, Randall RL, et al. Clinical features and outcomes of young patients with low-grade non-rhabdomyosarcoma soft tissue sarcomas treated with a risk-based strategy: a report from Children's Oncology Group study ARST0332. Pediatr Blood Cancer 2024;71(8):e31062.
34. O'Sullivan B, Davis AM, Turcotte R, et al. Preoperative versus postoperative radiotherapy in soft-tissue sarcoma of the limbs: a randomised trial. Lancet 2002;359(9325):2235–41.
35. Kayton ML, Weiss AR, Xue W, et al. Neoadjuvant pazopanib in nonrhabdomyosarcoma soft tissue sarcomas (ARST1321): a report of major wound complications from the Children's Oncology Group and NRG oncology. J Surg Oncol 2023;127(5):871–81.
36. Pratt CB, Pappo AS, Gieser P, et al. Role of adjuvant chemotherapy in the treatment of surgically resected pediatric nonrhabdomyosarcomatous soft tissue sarcomas: a Pediatric Oncology Group Study. J Clin Oncol 1999;17(4):1219.
37. Ferrari A. Role of chemotherapy in pediatric nonrhabdomyosarcoma soft-tissue sarcomas. Expert Rev Anticancer Ther 2008;8(6):929–38.
38. Ferrari A, De Salvo GL, Brennan B, et al. Synovial sarcoma in children and adolescents: the European Pediatric Soft Tissue Sarcoma Study Group prospective trial (EpSSG NRSTS 2005). Ann Oncol 2015;26(3):567–72.
39. Ferrari A, van Noesel MM, Brennan B, et al. Paediatric non-rhabdomyosarcoma soft tissue sarcomas: the prospective NRSTS 2005 study by the European Pediatric Soft Tissue Sarcoma Study Group (EpSSG). Lancet Child Adolesc Health 2021;5(8):546–58.
40. Heinz AT, Schönstein A, Koscielniak E, et al. Children and adolescents with localised non-rhabdomyosarcoma soft tissue sarcoma: results of the CWS-96 and CWS-2002P prospective trials with reclassification of the trial data incorporating the recent soft tissue sarcoma registry. Pediatr Blood Cancer 2025;11:e32159.
41. Harris CJ, Waters AM, Tracy ET, et al. Precision oncology: a primer for pediatric surgeons from the APSA cancer committee. J Pediatr Surg 2020;55(9):1706–13.
42. Weiss AR, Chen YL, Scharschmidt TJ, et al. Outcomes after preoperative chemoradiation with or without pazopanib in non-rhabdomyosarcoma soft tissue sarcoma: a report from Children's Oncology Group and NRG oncology. J Clin Oncol 2023;41(31):4842–8.
43. Weiss AR, Chen YL, Scharschmidt TJ, et al. Pathological response in children and adults with large unresected intermediate-grade or high-grade soft tissue sarcoma receiving preoperative chemoradiotherapy with or without pazopanib (ARST1321): a multicentre, randomised, open-label, phase 2 trial. Lancet Oncol 2020;21(8):1110–22.
44. Polites SF, Rhee DS, Seitz G, et al. Contemporary surgical management of pediatric non-rhabdomyosarcoma soft tissue sarcoma. Pediatr Blood Cancer 2024;71(11):e31257.
45. Delaney TF, Chen YLE. Positive surgical margins in soft tissue sarcoma treated with preoperative radiation: is a postoperative boost necessary: in Regard to Al Yami et al. (Int J Radiat Oncol Biol Phys 2010;77:1191-1197). Int J Radiat Oncol Biol Phys 2011;80(3). https://doi.org/10.1016/j.ijrobp.2011.02.030.
46. Tinkle CL, Fernandez-Pineda I, Sykes A, et al. Nonrhabdomyosarcoma soft tissue sarcoma (NRSTS) in pediatric and young adult patients: results from a prospective study using limited-margin radiotherapy. Cancer 2017;123(22):4419–29.
47. Stanelle EJ, Christison-Lagay ER, Wolden SL, et al. Pulmonary metastasectomy in pediatric/adolescent patients with synovial sarcoma: an institutional review. J Pediatr Surg 2013;48(4):757–63.

48. Croteau NJ, Heaton TE. Pulmonary metastasectomy in pediatric solid tumors. Children (Basel) 2019;6(1). https://doi.org/10.3390/children6010006.
49. Sultan I, Casanova M, Al-Jumaily U, et al. Soft tissue sarcomas in the first year of life. Eur J Cancer 2010;46(13):2449–56.
50. Sulkowski JP, Raval MV, Browne M. Margin status and multimodal therapy in infantile fibrosarcoma. Pediatr Surg Int 2013;29(8):771–6.
51. Hayek SN, Janom HH, Ibrahim A, et al. Infantile fibrosarcoma misdiagnosed as vascular tumors. Hand (N Y) 2013;8(4):464–8.
52. Knezevich SR, McFadden DE, Tao W, et al. A novel ETV6-NTRK3 gene fusion in congenital fibrosarcoma. Nat Genet 1998;18(2):184–7.
53. Hong DS, DuBois SG, Kummar S, et al. Larotrectinib in patients with TRK fusion-positive solid tumours: a pooled analysis of three phase 1/2 clinical trials. Lancet Oncol 2020;21(4):531–40.
54. Laetsch TW, Voss S, Ludwig K, et al. Larotrectinib for newly diagnosed infantile fibrosarcoma and other pediatric NTRK fusion-positive solid tumors (Children's Oncology Group ADVL1823). J Clin Oncol 2025;43(10):1188–97.
55. Orbach D, Sparber-Sauer M, Corradini N, et al. Infantile fibrosarcoma: is spontaneous regression possible? Pediatr Blood Cancer 2023;70(11):e30623.
56. Orbach D, Brennan B, De Paoli A, et al. Conservative strategy in infantile fibrosarcoma is possible: the European paediatric soft tissue sarcoma study group experience. Eur J Cancer 2016;57:1–9.
57. Sultan I, Rodriguez-Galindo C, Saab R, et al. Comparing children and adults with synovial sarcoma in the surveillance, epidemiology, and end results program, 1983 to 2005: an analysis of 1268 patients. Cancer 2009;115(15):3537–47.
58. Pappo AS, Fontanesi J, Luo X, et al. Synovial sarcoma in children and adolescents: the St Jude Children's research hospital experience. J Clin Oncol 1994;12-(11):2360–6.
59. Ferrari A, Brennan B, Casanova M, et al. Pediatric non-rhabdomyosarcoma soft tissue sarcomas: standard of care and treatment recommendations from the European paediatric soft tissue sarcoma study group (EpSSG). Cancer Manag Res 2022;14:2885–902.
60. Ferrari A, Chi YY, De Salvo GL, et al. Surgery alone is sufficient therapy for children and adolescents with low-risk synovial sarcoma: a joint analysis from the European paediatric soft tissue sarcoma study group and the Children's Oncology Group. Eur J Cancer 2017;78:1–6.
61. Venkatramani R, Xue W, Randall RL, et al. Synovial sarcoma in children, adolescents, and young adults: a report from the Children's Oncology Group ARST0332 study. J Clin Oncol 2021;39(35):3927–37.
62. Carli M, Ferrari A, Mattke A, et al. Pediatric malignant peripheral nerve sheath tumor: the Italian and German soft tissue sarcoma cooperative group. J Clin Oncol 2005;23(33):8422–30.
63. Miettinen MM, Antonescu CR, Fletcher CDM, et al. Histopathologic evaluation of atypical neurofibromatous tumors and their transformation into malignant peripheral nerve sheath tumor in patients with neurofibromatosis 1-a consensus overview. Hum Pathol 2017;67:1–10.
64. Yu Y, Wei C, Yue M, et al. From benign neurofibromas to malignant peripheral nerve sheath tumors (MPNST): a gaming among multiple factors. Cellular oncology (Dordrecht, Netherlands) 2025;48(4):841–57.
65. Crane JN, Xue W, Qumseya A, et al. Malignant peripheral nerve sheath tumors: a report from children's oncology group study ARST0332. J Natl Cancer Inst 2026;1–10.

66. Kahn J, Gillespie A, Tsokos M, et al. Radiation therapy in management of sporadic and neurofibromatosis type 1-associated malignant peripheral nerve sheath tumors. Front Oncol 2014;4:324.
67. Ferrari A, Bergamaschi L, Chiaravalli S, et al. Malignant peripheral nerve sheath tumor in children and adolescents: local treatment in a retrospective single-center experience. Pediatr Blood Cancer 2025;72(8):e31813.
68. Hayes-Jordan A, LaQuaglia MP, Modak S. Management of desmoplastic small round cell tumor. Semin Pediatr Surg 2016;25(5):299–304.
69. Sawyer JR, Tryka AF, Lewis JM. A novel reciprocal chromosome translocation t(11;22)(p13;q12) in an intraabdominal desmoplastic small round-cell tumor. Am J Surg Pathol 1992;16(4):411–6.
70. Lal DR, Su WT, Wolden SL, et al. Results of multimodal treatment for desmoplastic small round cell tumors. J Pediatr Surg 2005;40(1):251–5.
71. Hayes-Jordan A, Green H, Lin H, et al. Cytoreductive surgery and hyperthermic intraperitoneal chemotherapy (HIPEC) for children, adolescents, and young adults: the first 50 cases. Ann Surg Oncol 2015;22(5):1726–32.
72. Modak S, Zanzonico P, Grkovski M, et al. B7H3-Directed intraperitoneal radioimmunotherapy with radioiodinated omburtamab for desmoplastic small round cell tumor and other peritoneal tumors: results of a phase I study. J Clin Oncol 2020;38(36):4283–91.
73. Subbiah V, Murthy R, Anderson PM. [90Y]yttrium microspheres radioembolotherapy in desmoplastic small round cell tumor hepatic metastases. J Clin Oncol 2011;29(11):e292–4.
74. Subbiah V, Lamhamedi-Cherradi SE, Cuglievan B, et al. Multimodality treatment of desmoplastic small round cell tumor: chemotherapy and complete cytoreductive surgery improve patient survival. Clin Cancer Res 2018;24(19):4865–73.
75. Rich BS, Fishbein J, Lautz T, et al. Inflammatory myofibroblastic tumor: a multi-institutional study from the pediatric surgical oncology research collaborative. Int J Cancer 2022;151(7):1059–67.
76. Casanova M, Brennan B, Alaggio R, et al. Inflammatory myofibroblastic tumor: the experience of the European pediatric soft tissue sarcoma study group (EpSSG). Eur J Cancer 2020;127:123–9.
77. Coffin CM, Hornick JL, Fletcher CDM. Inflammatory myofibroblastic tumor: comparison of clinicopathologic, histologic, and immunohistochemical features including ALK expression in atypical and aggressive cases. Am J Surg Pathol 2007;31(4):509–20.
78. Mossé YP, Voss SD, Lim MS, et al. Targeting ALK with crizotinib in pediatric Anaplastic large cell lymphoma and inflammatory myofibroblastic tumor: a Children's Oncology Group Study. J Clin Oncol 2017;35(28):3215–21.
79. Schoot RA, Orbach D, Minard Colin V, et al. Inflammatory myofibroblastic tumor with ROS1 gene fusions in children and young adolescents. JCO Precis Oncol 2023;7:e2300323.

Primary Bone Tumors

Osteosarcoma and Ewing Sarcoma

Thomas J. Scharschmidt, MD[a,*], Rajul Gupta, MD[b],
Kate Harrison, MD[c], Odion Binitie, MD[c]

KEYWORDS

• Osteosarcoma • Ewing sarcoma • Bone tumor

KEY POINTS

- Limb salvage surgery is increasingly popular for childhood bone sarcomas, given the recent surgical advances.
- ^{18}FluoroDeoxyGlucose (FDG)-PET is increasingly popular for childhood bone sarcoma imaging, and can potentially replace other historic modalities like bone scan for osteosarcoma and Ewing sarcoma.
- Given the survival plateau with the conventional chemotherapy-only approach, multiple new therapeutic options are being explored for frontline therapy, metastatic disease, and relapsed/refractory disease.

INTRODUCTION

Osteosarcoma and Ewing sarcoma are the 2 most common primary malignant bone tumors in children and adolescents, characterized by aggressive biology, complex multimodal treatment, and limited improvement in survival over recent decades. Osteosarcoma demonstrates a bimodal age distribution, a strong association with cancer predisposition syndromes, and diverse histologic subtypes, whereas Ewing sarcoma is defined by EWSR1-ETS fusion–driven molecular pathology and occurs predominantly in the second decade of life. Contemporary diagnosis relies on high-quality imaging—including radiographs, MRI, and FDG-PET/CT—to define local extent, identify metastatic disease, and guide biopsy. Standard management of both tumors includes neoadjuvant multiagent chemotherapy followed by surgery and adjuvant systemic therapy; radiation therapy is reserved for unresectable disease or close/positive margins in Ewing sarcoma. Advances in limb-salvage surgery, 3D-printed reconstructions, carbon-fiber implants, and targeted intraoperative

[a] Division of Musculoskeletal Oncology, Nationwide Children's Hospital, and The Ohio State University, Columbus, OH, USA; [b] Division of Musculoskeletal Oncology, Nationwide Children's Hospital, Columbus, OH, USA; [c] Department of Sarcoma, Moffitt Cancer Center, Tampa, FL, USA
* Corresponding author.
E-mail address: thomas.scharschmidt@nationwidechildrens.org

Surg Oncol Clin N Am 35 (2026) 765–783
https://doi.org/10.1016/j.soc.2026.04.010 surgonc.theclinics.com

Abbreviations	
COG	Children's Oncology Group
MAP	methotrexate, adriamycin, and cisplatin
NOS	not otherwise specified
VDC/IE	vincristine, doxorubicin, and cyclophosphamide alternating with ifosfamide and etoposide
VFET	vascularized fibular epiphyseal transfer
VIDE	vincristine, ifosfamide, doxorubicin, and etoposide

technologies continue to expand surgical options while optimizing local control. Despite improvements in surgical techniques and treatment delivery, outcomes for metastatic, relapsed, and chemotherapy-refractory disease remain poor. Ongoing clinical trials investigating tyrosine kinase inhibitors, immune-based treatments, and novel delivery platforms—including antibody–drug conjugates, mRNA nanoparticles, and chimeric antigen receptor (CAR)-T cell therapies—represent key avenues for future progress. Greater integration of molecular diagnostics, radiomics, and advanced surgical technology will be central to overcoming the current therapeutic plateau for these sarcomas.

- Osteosarcoma
- Ewing sarcoma
- Neoadjuvant chemotherapy
- Limb salvage surgery
- Targeted therapy

OSTEOSARCOMA

Epidemiology

Conventional osteosarcoma (OSA) is the most common primary bone sarcoma, with an incidence of 3 cases per million per year. The incidence is highest in adolescents, with 8 to 11 cases per million. Another peak in OSA incidence is observed in individuals aged 60 years and older. Younger patients develop tumors predominantly in the extremities, but elderly patients have a higher frequency of developing axial tumors.[1,2] Extremity OSA is commonly seen in the distal femur (32%), proximal tibia (15%), proximal humerus (8%), and proximal femur (5%).[3] In elderly individuals, OSAs in the axial skeleton are more frequently seen than in adolescents.

OSA occurs more frequently in males than in females, with a ratio of 1.4:1.[4] Children less than 10 years of age at diagnosis have a higher incidence of cancer predisposition syndromes.

Predisposing Factors for Osteosarcoma

Predisposing factors for OS include the following:

1. Prior radiation therapy

   Approximately 50% to 60% of radiation-induced sarcomas are OSAs and carry a poor prognosis. Radiation-induced osteosarcoma, though rare, is increasing in incidence as cancer survival improves.[5] Tumors generally occur at least 4 years after radiation, and at a mean of about 14 years post-radiation exposure.[6] Radiation-induced OSA is seen in the calvarium, chest wall, and irradiated long bones.[5,7] These secondary tumors are far more aggressive than their primary tumors.[7]
2. Paget's disease of bone

OSA in Paget's disease occurs in less than 1% but increases to 10% in polyostotic disease.[8] Pagetoid OSA frequently affects individuals more than 60 years of age and is responsible for more than 50% of cases in elderly patients. The tumors are osteoblastic and may be metachronous.[5] These tumors typically affect the pelvis, proximal femur, and proximal humerus, but often spare the spine[9] with a poor prognosis.

3. Fibrous dysplasia, Mccune-Albright syndrome, and Mazabraud syndrome
   OSA, followed by chondrosarcoma and fibrosarcoma, are the most common malignancies observed with fibrous dysplasia and associated syndromes.[9] These malignancies usually develop in the third to fourth decade of life and are common in the craniofacial bones, the femur, and the tibia[10] with a poor response to chemotherapy.
4. Genetic syndromes: **Table 1** details hereditary syndromes associated with osteosarcoma.

Classification and Pathology

The World Health Organization classifies OSA into low-grade central, OSA-not otherwise specified (NOS), parosteal, periosteal, high-grade surface, and secondary subtypes. OSA-NOS is further subdivided into conventional, small cell, and telangiectatic subtypes. Conventional OSA has been further subdivided into histologic subtypes, including chondroblastic, fibroblastic, and osteoblastic osteosarcoma, without prognostic differences. Chief histologic features include permeative growth, cellular atypia, neoplastic bone (some deposited on normal trabeculae, and the presence of benign giant cells). High-grade surface OSA shares these pathologic features.[18] Parosteal OSAs mainly occur in the posterior distal femoral metaphysis, with 3 out of every 4 cases reported at this site.[19] Parosteal OSA is a surface lesion that grows mainly into soft tissue but invades bone about 25% of the time. Periosteal OSAs, contrastingly, occur mainly on the anterior tibial shaft[20] and are intimately associated with the bone. Both these lesions have a malignant cartilage cap.

Imaging

Plain radiographs are the first imaging investigation. Osteoid, a pure lytic appearance, chondroid matrix, or mixed matrix can be observed. Borders are ill defined, with endosteal scalloping, and a broad, ill-defined or moth-eaten transition zone. A periosteal reaction is often likened to a sunburst appearance, and a Codman triangle is frequently observed. Pathologic fractures and soft tissue masses may be encountered. Osseous metastasis may occasionally be seen (**Figs. 1** and **2**).

Contrast MRI of the affected part (including the entire involved bone) details the anatomy and provides information about neurovascular, physeal, and joint space involvement. Imaging should contain the primary tumor and screen for skip lesions or osseous metastasis. On T1 images, the tumor appears hypointense and heterogeneous, with matrix signal reflective of the type of matrix formation. Involved bone marrow has a lower signal on T1-weighted images and can be delineated against the bright signal of healthy bone marrow. T2 images are excellent for determining tumor spread into extraosseous anatomic compartments and the tumor's relationship to neurovascular structures but overestimate the extent of intramedullary tumor. Necrotic areas do not enhance on contrast administration.[21]

Staging

Chest computed tomography (CT) scans are performed without contrast to screen for pulmonary nodules. Whole-body 18F-PDG PET/CT is also very important in staging

Table 1
Hereditary syndromes associated with osteosarcoma

Inheritance	Syndrome	Gene/Key Features	OSA Characteristics	Prognosis/Notes
Autosomal dominant	Li-Fraumeni syndrome[11]	TP53 mutation; multiple malignancies	Mean age ~14; axial and periosteal sites; chondroblastic histology more common	Similar PFS to sporadic OSA; lower overall survival due to secondary malignancies
Autosomal dominant	Hereditary retinoblastoma[12]	RB1 mutation on chromosome 13; high survival of primary tumor	300–600× increased OSA risk; craniofacial sites; often in irradiated areas	Good histologic response; difficult margins in craniofacial cases; 20% develop additional malignancies
Autosomal dominant	Diamond-Blackfan anemia[13,14]	Bone marrow failure syndrome	Very rare OSA; poor outcomes	High mortality from therapy complications or pulmonary metastases; other cancers more common
Autosomal recessive	Rothmund-Thomson syndrome[15]	RECQL4 mutation; rash, short stature, sparse hair	~1/3 develop OSA; long bones affected	Prognosis similar to sporadic OSA; doxorubicin mucositis dose limiting
Autosomal recessive	RAPADILINO syndrome[16]	RECQL4-related; no facial rash	Increased malignancy risk, especially with growth hormone therapy	Similar cancer predisposition to RTS
Autosomal recessive	Werner syndrome[17]	Adult progeria; premature aging	OSA at atypical sites; onset age 35–57	Increased frequency compared to general population
Autosomal recessive	Bloom syndrome	BLM mutation; common in Ashkenazi Jewish population	Wilms tumor and OSA in childhood; leukemia/lymphoma in adolescence	Multiple malignancies; rarely survive past 40

Abbreviations: PFS, progression free survival; RTS, Rothmund-Thomson syndrome.

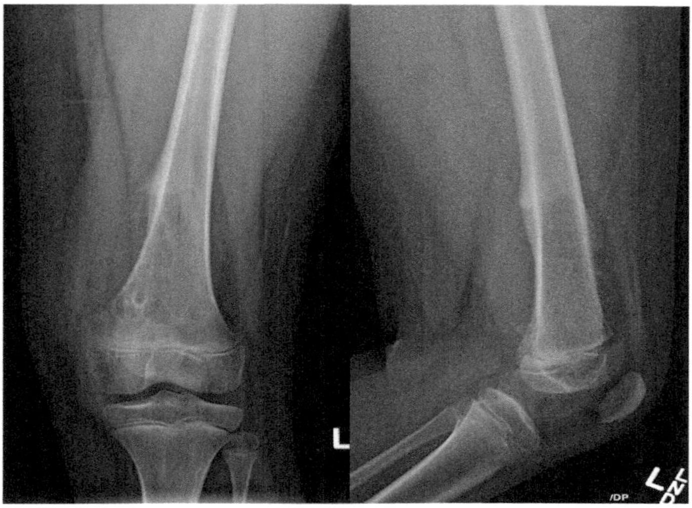

Fig. 1. Plain radiographs of a distal femoral osteosarcoma demonstrating a typical Codman triangle.

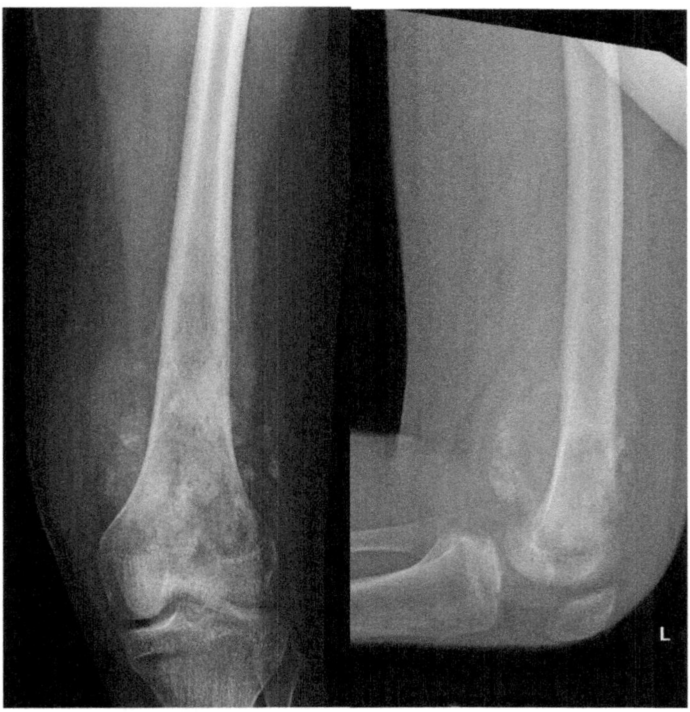

Fig. 2. Plain radiographs of a distal femoral osteosarcoma demonstrating a sunburst appearance, soft tissue mass, and mixed lytic and sclerotic matrix.

and surveillance.[22] It readily demonstrates skip lesions and pulmonary nodules (if >1 cm). Pre and post chemotherapy metabolic activity of the tumor correlates with histologic response and has prognostic value. Finally, whole-body PET/CT is useful for monitoring and surveillance.[23] Bone scans are generally helpful only for a hypometabolic lesion, which can be identified in the CT images in the PET/CT scan. Therefore, many institutions opt for a whole-body PET/CT scan instead of a bone scan[23] (**Fig. 3**A, B).

Biopsy

Biopsy is performed in accordance with biopsy principles elucidated by Jaffe and Malawar.[24,25] Biopsy should be performed in the treating sarcoma center, as an improperly done biopsy can jeopardize limb salvage. Open surgical biopsy remains the gold standard, yielding a diagnostic specimen in more than 95% of cases. Image-guided core needle biopsy achieves a diagnostic yield of 75% to 85%. Low-grade central OSA is a diagnostic challenge, being difficult to distinguish from benign tumors. Open biopsy has better results diagnostic success for low-grade central OSA than core needle biopsy.[26]

Open biopsy tracts are much more frequently seeded with tumor cells than image guided core needle biopsy.[27] Current Children's Oncology Group (COG) recommendations require sampling of 2 to 3 mm^3 of tissue, which is equivalent to 15 to 20 soft tissue cores or 7 to 10 bony cores. Specimens must be sent fresh to the pathology laboratory, where they will be allocated to frozen, touch, fresh-frozen, and formalin-preserved fractions. Preservation of tissue architecture is paramount, and the tissue sample must be handled with care to avoid crushing. Hemostasis is essential, since

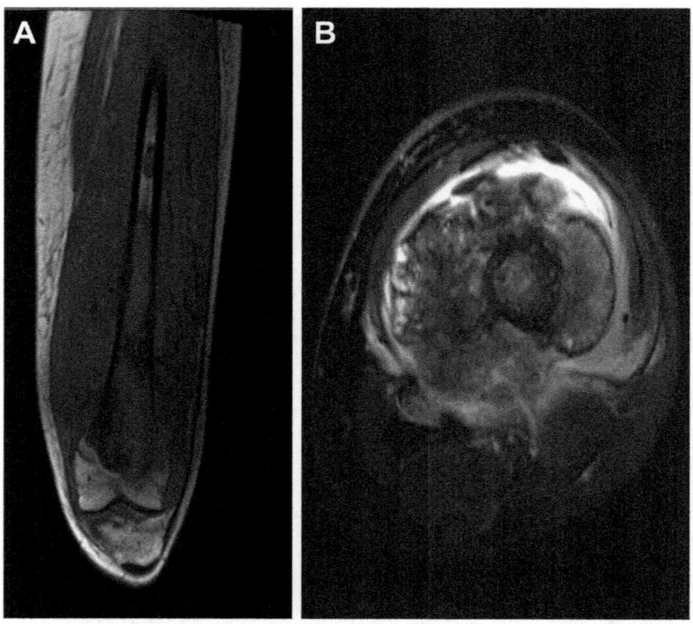

Fig. 3. (*A*) Coronal T1-weighted MRI images demonstrating right distal femoral osteosarcoma of the same patient depicted in **Fig. 2**. Medullary extent can be visualized, and a skip lesion can be seen. (*B*) T2 Fat suppressed images demonstrate the soft tissue extension, as well as the relation to the soft tissue mass.

hematoma spread may cause tumor dissemination.[28] A hemostatic agent (such as bone wax) should be used to occlude the bone after the specimen is taken to minimize bleeding and contamination of surrounding tissues.

Neoadjuvant Chemotherapy

Neoaduvant chemotherapy (NACT) is standardized for high-grade tumors via COG protocols and guidelines. Two cycles of methotrexate, adriamycin, and cisplatin (MAP), administered every 3 weeks, remains the recommended neoadjuvant regimen. Interval compression from 3 to 2 weeks has not improved outcomes, nor has the addition of ifosfamide.[29] Human epidermal growth factor receptor-2 (HER-2)-expressing metastatic OSA does not benefit from the addition of targeted agents such as trastuzumab.[30] Despite preclinical evidence of efficacy, the addition of zolendronic acid did not improve outcomes in a French trial that chiefly enrolled adult patients.[31] Increasing the number of neoadjuvant cycles may improve the histologic response rate, but it has not been demonstrated to increase survival.[32]

Histologic Response

Multiple systems have been used to grade histologic response after neoadjuvant chemotherapy. **Table 2** summarizes these systems.

What is considered a "good response" and how percent necrosis impacts prognosis are matters of debate. Richardson and colleagues in a national cancer database study demonstrated that there is no survivorship advantage in patients with greater than 95% necrosis and 90% to 95% necrosis. Moreover, there was little difference in survival among patients with necrosis of less than 90%.[33] However, Parambil and colleagues urged the exploration of other thresholds, and in their study demonstrated that event free survival (EFS) was best predicted by 85.5% tumor necrosis in localized OSA.[37] On the contrary, Bielack and colleagues demonstrated that necrosis in osteosarcoma is a graded phenomenon, with increased necrosis resulting in better survival.[38] This issue is further confounded by Kang and colleagues, who demonstrated low interobserver but high intraobserver variability in necrosis rate after NACT in OSA.[39] A recent study demonstrated objective and reproducible results using a deep-learning model, which showed high correlation with the reported necrosis rate as determined by an expert pathologist and could successfully predict survival.[40] Most centers agree that greater than 90% necrosis represents a good histologic response to NACT.

Adjuvant Chemotherapy

While it is appropriate to continue the MAP regimen in good responders, efforts to improve survival in poor responders by adding ifosfamide and etoposide to MAP have not yielded any improvement in survival.[41] The addition of mifamurtide in the adjuvant setting has been reported.[42,43] Other adjuvant agents are in clinical trials, with multikinase inhibitors being the most promising.

Radiation Therapy

The conventional teaching is that OSA is not sensitive to radiotherapy, although this paradigm is being challenged. Doses as high as 68 Gy may be needed for a meaningful response. Craniofacial OSAs are often treated with radiation when unresectable or are resected with positive margins.[44] Reddy and colleagues reported acceptable local control of unresectable skeletal and pulmonary metastases with biologically equivalent doses of greater than 48 Gy of stereotactic body radiation therapy.[44] Proton therapy has inherent dosimetric advantages. Some early reports suggest a 20%

Table 2
Commonly used grading systems for evaluating histologic response to neoadjuvant chemotherapy

System	Grade Categories	Basis	Threshold for Good Response
Huvos[33]	Grade I: <50% necrosis Grade II: 50%–90% necrosis Grade III: 90%–99% necrosis Grade IV: 100% necrosis	% tumor necrosis only	≥90% necrosis
Salzer-Kuntschik[34]	Grade I: No viable cells Grade II: Single tumor cell or 1 vital cell cluster < 0.5 cm Grade III: Vital tumor < 10% Grade IV: Vital tumor 10% to 50% Grade V: Vital tumor > 50% VI: No response to chemotherapy	% necrosis + residual cellularity	Grade I to III are good responders
Picci[35]	Total response: No viable tumor Good response: ≥90% necrosis Poor response: 60%–89% necrosis	% necrosis only	≥90% necrosis
Chui Prognostic Index[36]	Composite score based on necrosis, mitotic rate, lymphovascular invasion, tumor size/site	Multiple histologic and clinical factors	Higher score = worse prognosis

survivorship rate in pediatric patients with unresectable localized disease, although this is accompanied by significant toxicities.[45] In another study by Cierniek and colleagues, patients with R1 or R2 resection of OS received 68.4 Gy and demonstrated 5 year disease free survival (DFS) and OSA rates of 65% and 67%, respectively.

Carbon ion radiotherapy has shown promising results in OSA. It is also theorized that carbon ions have a Bragg peak similar to protons, but with a greater linear energy transfer, thereby inflicting more DNA damage in tumor cells.[46] Early results from Japan and Europe have been encouraging.[47,48]

Local Recurrence

Factors contributing to local recurrence in OSA include the inability to achieve an adequate surgical margin (intralesional or marginal excision), limb salvage surgery, poor response to chemotherapy, large tumor size, difficult anatomic sites (spine and pelvis), and age of the patient.[49] Local recurrence in OSA should be aggressively treated by surgical resection in the absence of metastatic disease but portends a poor prognosis.

Metastatic Disease

Up to one-third of the patients with OSA present with metastatic disease. Lungs are the most common site for metastasis, while bone is the second most common site. Skip lesions and bony metastasis should be resected at the time of local control surgery. For patients with metastatic disease at diagnosis, metastectomy is performed after the completion of local control surgery. Based on the early reports of noninferiority of thoracoscopic pulmonary metastectomy to open thoracotomy in osteosarcoma, COG is conducting a large randomized control trial to compare open versus thoracoscopic metastectomy in osteosarcoma.[50,51] Relapses are commonly seen 1 to 2 years after the upfront treatment and are rare after 10 years. Long-term survival increases with repeat metastectomy in OSA.

While surgical resection of all known metastatic disease offers best opportunity for survival, the value of systemic cytotoxic chemotherapy at relapse is a matter of debate, but it remains a cornerstone for treatment with curative intent. High-dose ifosfamide can be combined with etoposide and cisplatin, but tolerance may be an issue. Available tyrosine kinase inhibitors include regorafenib, cabozantinib, apatinib, levantinib, and anlotinib.[52] Cabozantinib, in particular, has demonstrated significant antitumor activity in clinical and preclinical studies and is being investigated in combination with frontline therapy,[53] maintenance therapy,[54] and for unresectable residual disease.[55]

Ewing Sarcoma

Epidemiology

Ewing sarcoma is the second most common primary bone tumor in children and adolescents, with an incidence of 3 per 100,000 in patients less than 20 years of age.[56] Its cell of origin is primordial bone marrow-derived mesenchymal stem cells and has a small round cell appearance histologically.[57] The frequently associated fusion gene is EWS-FLI1 as a result of a translocation between chromosomes 22 and 11,[57] seen in about 85% of tumors. The estimated survival rate for patients with localized disease is 70% to 78%.[56,58–60]

Ewing sarcoma is diagnosed most commonly in the second decade of life, with a median age of 15 years. In the long bones, the tumor typically occurs in diaphysis. Ewing sarcoma can also occur in the flat bones, such as the scapula, ribs, and pelvis, as well as within the soft tissues of the trunk or extremities. Most frequently, patients will present with persistent, progressive pain and an associated mass. They may also have systemic complaints such as fever, and lab abnormalities may be present.[61]

Imaging

Ewing sarcoma typically appears as an infiltrative bone lesion with an associated soft tissue mass on radiographs and MRI. MRI of the entire bone with and without gadolinium contrast is imperative to evaluate the soft tissue component of the tumor and proximity to major neurovascular structures, identify extent of marrow involvement in relation to the physis as well as additional skip lesions. It is also critical to plan for biopsy trajectory to maximize viable tumor tissue collection and position in line with incision for planned future resection[61](**Fig. 4**A–C).

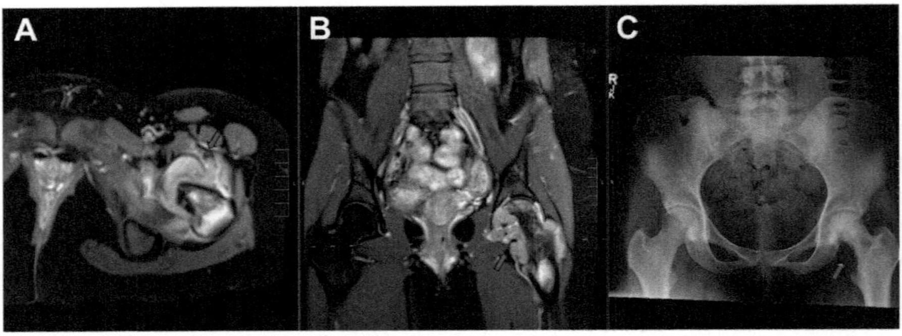

Fig. 4. (*A*) T2 axial image demonstrating Ewing sarcoma of the proximal femur with a soft tissue mass (*blue arrow*). (*B*) T2 coronal image demonstrating Ewing sarcoma of the proximal femur with a soft tissue mass (*blue arrow*). (*C*) Plain radiograph of the pelvis demonstrating a lytic lesion of the left proximal femur and the femoral neck (*red arrow*).

Biopsy

Tissue sampling is of the utmost importance to obtain the correct diagnosis and guide treatment. Similar to osteosarcoma, open or core needle biopsy is considered the gold standard for obtaining an accurate diagnosis in suspected Ewing sarcoma. The COG Bone Tumor Committee recommends obtaining samples from soft tissue component with a 16 gauge needle, collecting 15 to 20 core samples 1.5 to 3 cm in length. When there is not a safely accessible extraosseous component and bone must be sampled, 5 to 7 cores with a 12 or 13 gauge needle is recommended. This approach is typically feasible through a single incision.[28]

Staging

Imaging studies consist of full-length MRI scans of the involved long bone or compartment of the primary site to evaluate for skip lesions. Further evaluation of metastatic disease includes a chest CT and an FDG-PET scan, which has demonstrated superior sensitivity over bone scan.

Routine, bone marrow biopsy and/or aspirate is no longer recommended due to a low incidence of bone metastasis; however, confirmatory bone marrow sample in patients with metastatic pulmonary or bone involvement to determine baseline burden of disease, evaluate treatment response, and communicate prognosis is recommended.[57]

Pathology: Genetic and Molecular Features

Microscopically, Ewing sarcoma is composed of monotonous small round cells with scant cytoplasm, occasionally arranged in a "pseudorosette" formation. The majority of cases demonstrate strong, diffuse membranous staining with CD99. As previously mentioned, EWS-FLI1 is the fusion gene commonly associated with Ewing sarcoma, with approximately 85% to 90% of cases. Less frequently seen is the EWS-ERG fusion in approximately 5% of cases.[62] A retrospective cohort study by Shulman and colleagues investigated the clinical impact of loss of STAG2 protein loss of expression. Their results demonstrated a worse prognosis associated with STAG2 loss of expression, with a 5 year event-free survival rate of 54% in patients with localized disease, compared to 75% in patients who had intact STAG2 expression.[63]

Prognosis

The presence of metastasis is the most significant prognostic factor for outcomes. Several other factors are associated with less favorable prognosis, including older age, larger tumor size, and tumor location in the axial skeleton.[60] A systematic review by Bosma and colleagues concluded that poorer survival rates were reported in tumors with a volume $\geq$ 200 mL or diameter $\geq$ 8 cm, primary site in the pelvis, and histologic response less than 100%.[64]

Treatment

The mainstay of Ewing sarcoma treatment includes a combination of systemic and local therapy. Multiagent chemotherapy is initiated, followed by surgery and/or radiation for local control, with consolidation chemotherapy after surgical resection. Treatment planning requires a multidisciplinary approach.

Chemotherapy

In the United States, the standard chemotherapy regimen for Ewing sarcoma is interval-compressed VDC/IE: vincristine, doxorubicin, and cyclophosphamide alternating with ifosfamide and etoposide every 2 weeks.[61] The addition of vincristine, topotecan, and cyclophosphamide within the standard interval-compressed therapy was not found to have improved EFS or OS in patients with newly diagnosed nonmetastatic Ewing Sarcoma, as demonstrated in the AEWS1031 trial conducted by the COG.[64] The EURO EWING 2012 (EE2012) trial was a randomized controlled trial providing a direct comparison of interval-compressed VDC/IE for induction therapy and the European regimen of vincristine, ifosfamide, doxorubicin, and etoposide (VIDE). Their results favored the COG regimen of VDC/IE, with an EFS of 67% at 3 years compared to 61% in the VIDE group, and an OS of 82% in the VDC/IE group compared to 74% in the VIDE group. They concluded that the VDC/IE regimen should be considered the standard of care, as it was less toxic and more effective.[58]

Radiation

Radiation is an effective form of local control for cases in which close or positive surgical margins are anticipated or achieved, or when there is close proximity and/or displacement of healthy organs.[60] Improvements in MRI and PET scan imaging studies, as well as technical advances such as 3 dimensional conformal radiation therapy, intensity-modulated radiation therapy, and proton beam therapy, have resulted in improved tumor targeting and tissue sparing.[60]

The AEWS1031 trial reported on preoperative radiotherapy for improved local control, with a lower dose and smaller target volume. Eight patients in this cohort received 36 Gy to the tumor with an additional 1 cm margin, with an additional postoperative boost radiation of 19.8 Gy for patients who had an R_2 resection. Low-dose, small-volume preoperative radiotherapy resulted in a high rate of R_0 resection.[65] With the results of their study, there is potential for lower dose and volume protocols in future research.[65]

Surgical Considerations in Osteosarcoma and Ewing Sarcoma

The surgical principles for both sarcomas are identical. The overarching goal for surgical resection is to obtain durable local control by achieving a negative margin (R_0) surgical resection. Limb salvage surgery is the standard of care and remains the first choice for most patients and their families, although amputation may be considered in some cases. The development, timing, and displacement of a pathologic fracture have been shown not to impact local recurrence, despite earlier studies claiming to the contrary, and should not preclude limb salvage.[66,67] Relative contraindications to limb salvage include significant morbidity due to involvement of neurovascular structures, very young age, and infection.[68] The following sections will discuss the recent advances in limb salvage surgery.

Bone sarcomas of the proximal humerus in children younger than 10 years can be reconstructed in several ways. One option is a *vascularized fibular epiphyseal transfer (VFET)*, in which part of the fibula, including the growth plate, is transplanted to replace the resected humerus.[69] This technique allows the reconstruction to grow with the child. In some patients, the transferred fibular head changes shape over time and remodels to more closely resemble the native humeral head.[70]

During harvest of the fibular graft, injury to the *peroneal nerve* can occur. When this happens, it is often temporary and improves with time. Fracture of the fibular graft is also relatively common, but most fractures heal with simple treatments such as casting or bracing rather than additional surgery.[70] Some studies suggest that when a VFET fractures, healing at the junction between the graft and the humerus may actually be reliable.

Another option for reconstruction in children is a *resurfaced allograft–prosthetic composite*, which combines donor bone with a prosthetic joint surface. These constructs preserve native bone and can provide good shoulder motion, particularly when the *axillary nerve* is preserved. Most complications related to this type of reconstruction occur within the first 3 years following surgery.[71]

The most commonly used reconstruction overall is *endoprosthetic reconstruction*, which involves placing a metallic implant to replace the segment of bone removed with the tumor. These implants are fixed within the remaining bone. Most often, this fixation is achieved using *polymethylmethacrylate bone cement*, which anchors the stem of the implant inside the medullary canal.[72] Cementless implants are also increasingly used. These implants rely on bone growing into a specially treated surface of the implant rather than on cement. Their use has increased due to favorable outcomes reported in recent years.[73]

In younger children, especially those undergoing tumor resection in the lower extremities, a *growing endoprosthesis* may be used. This is particularly helpful when the growth plate must be removed as part of the cancer operation. These devices can lengthen over time, helping to reduce future limb-length discrepancy. Traditional growing implants require repeated surgical procedures to lengthen the device. These repeated returns to the operating room increase the risk of wound complications and infection. Newer *magnetically controlled growing endoprostheses* allow noninvasive lengthening and have shown encouraging medium-term results.[74]

In some situations, the tumor involves only part of the bone. When this is the case, it may be possible to preserve a significant portion of the patient's native bone and avoid a full metal replacement. *Geometric resections*, in which only a specific portion of bone is removed, can be reconstructed using *hemicortical allografts*. These techniques have been associated with high rates of healing between the allograft and the host bone. In other cases, the joint surface and a small amount of underlying bone can be preserved, leaving a segmental defect in the shaft of the bone. This defect can be reconstructed using a *segmental (intercalary) allograft*.

Both of these biological reconstruction techniques depend heavily on precise bone cuts. Accuracy is improved through the use of customized *3D-printed cutting guides*, which help surgeons reproduce the planned osteotomies intraoperatively.[75] To improve stability at the graft–host junction, the authors prefer a *telescopic taper technique*, in which the allograft is shaped to fit into a tapered cavity created in the host bone using conical reamers. This method provides strong mechanical fixation.[76]

Reconstruction following *hemipelvectomy* remains controversial. However, acceptable outcomes can be achieved using *customized 3D-printed pelvic implants*. These implants replace large portions of the pelvic bone and are typically fixed to the sacrum. In some cases, fixation is extended to the lower lumbar spine. *Spinopelvic fixation* is preferred over fixation to the sacrum alone, as it better resists motion at the bone–implant interface and is associated with lower rates of implant loosening.[77]

Rotationplasty remains a valid reconstructive option in selected patients. Compared with transfemoral amputation, rotationplasty has been shown to provide better quality of life and less chronic pain, although this does not always translate into superior long-term functional outcomes.[78] Rotationplasty is also an effective salvage option following failed endoprosthetic reconstruction.[79] Based on the study by Alexander and colleagues, the authors routinely perform *targeted muscle reinnervation* in all patients undergoing amputation, as this technique has been shown to significantly reduce phantom limb pain.[80]

Infection is a major postoperative concern. Endoprosthetic reconstruction with a quaternary ammonium compound coating recently received FDA approval.[81] Silver-coated endoprostheses are not yet FDA approved in the USA, but have been extensively used in Europe with some benefit.[82] Recent analysis of PARITY trial data suggests that prolonged use of drains (more than 14 days) is not advised. The same study also did not find any benefit in the routine use of incisional wound VAC.[83]

FUTURE DIRECTIONS AND CONCLUSION

Given the plateauing of the survival rates with OSA and EwS, newer approaches to treatment of relapsed and refractory disease are needed.[85,86] As noted above, the results of trials with multikinase inhibitors are eagerly awaited. Drug sensitivity testing for relapse and refractory disease, mRNA-based lipid nanoparticles, antibody-drug conjugates, and chimeric antigen receptor T-cell therapies are at various stages of development.[87–89] On the surgical front, augmented reality, robotic-assisted sarcoma resections, and progress in surgical navigation are exciting developments.[90,91] Further research must be undertaken to overcome the therapeutic plateau for these common childhood sarcomas.

CLINICS CARE POINTS

- Biopsy of suspected bone sarcomas should be performed in specialist sarcoma referral centers, regardless of the technique, and should emphasize sufficient tissue collection for optimal diagnostic workup.
- Extent of necrosis caused by neoadjuvant therapy remains the most important prognosticator, although progress is being made in noninvasive measurement of the therapeutic response.
- Aggressive metastectomy of oligometastatic disease, whole lung radiation in EWS, and novel therapeutics should be pursued in the setting of advanced disease.

DISCLOSURE

T.J. Scharschmidt: consultant for Stryker Orthopaedics and Onkos Surgical; O. Binitie: consultant for Onkos Surgical; R. Gupta: Nothing to disclose. K. Harrison: Nothing to disclose.

REFERENCES

1. Gatta G, Capocaccia R, Botta L, et al. Burden and centralised treatment in Europe of rare tumours: results of RARECAREnet-a population-based study. Lancet Oncol 2017;18(8):1022–39.
2. Mirabello L, Troisi RJ, Savage SA. Osteosarcoma incidence and survival rates from 1973 to 2004: data from the surveillance, epidemiology, and end results program. Cancer 2009;115(7):1531–43.
3. Wold LE, Unni KK, Sim FH, et al. Osteosarcoma. Atlas of orthopedic pathology. Philadelphia: Saunders; 2008. p. 179.
4. Cole S, Gianferante DM, Zhu B, et al. Osteosarcoma: a surveillance, epidemiology, and end results program-based analysis from 1975 to 2017. Cancer 2022;128(11):2107–18.
5. Patel AJ, Rao VY, Fox BD, et al. Radiation-induced osteosarcomas of the calvarium and skull base. Cancer 2011;117(10):2120–6.
6. Halperin EC, Perez CA, Brady LW. Perez and Brady's principles and practice of radiation oncology. Philadelphia: Lippincott Williams & Wilkins; 2008.
7. Venkatraman S, Weisberg EM, Fishman EK. Radiation-induced osteosarcoma of the chest wall after treatment for unresectable thymoma. Radiol Case Reports 2023;18(10):3716–9.
8. Hansen MF, Seton M, Merchant A. Osteosarcoma in Paget's disease of bone. J Bone Miner Res 2006;21(Suppl 2):P58–63.
9. Mankin HJ, Hornicek FJ. Paget's sarcoma: a historical and outcome review. Clin Orthop Relat Res 2005;438:97–102.
10. Yabut SM, Kenan S, Sissons HA, et al. Malignant transformation of fibrous dysplasia A case report and review of the literature. Clin Orthop Relat Res 1988;228.
11. Saucier E, Bougeard G, Gomez-Mascard A, et al. Li-Fraumeni-associated osteosarcomas: the French experience. Pediatr Blood Cancer 2024;71(12):e31362.
12. Bielack SS, Baumhoer D, Hecker-Nolting S, et al. Osteosarcomas in retinoblastoma-survivors. A report of 28 affected patients from the Cooperative Osteosarcoma Study Group (COSS). EJC Paediatric Oncology 2024;3:100158.
13. Vlachos A, Rosenberg PS, Atsidaftos E, et al. Incidence of neoplasia in Diamond Blackfan anemia: a report from the diamond blackfan anemia registry. Blood 2012;119(16):3815–9.
14. Lee RS, Higgs D, Haddo O, et al. Osteosarcoma associated with diamond-blackfan anaemia: a case of a child receiving growth hormone therapy. Sarcoma 2004;8(1):47–9.
15. Hicks MJ, Roth JR, Kozinetz CA, et al. Clinicopathologic features of osteosarcoma in patients with Rothmund-Thomson syndrome. J Clin Oncol 2007;25(4):370–5.
16. Sandoval C, Dunbar J, Ozkaynak M, et al. Osteosarcoma following growth hormone therapy in recurrent acute lymphoblastic leukemia and rapadilino syndrome. Pediatr Hematol Oncol 2012;29(3):270–1.
17. Ishikawa Y, Miller RW, Machinami R, et al. Atypical osteosarcomas in Werner Syndrome (adult progeria). Jpn J Cancer Res 2000;91(12):1345–9.
18. Nishida Y. Osteosarcoma in the elderly: clinical features and outcome. In: Watanabe H, editor. Osteosarcoma. Tokyo: Springer; 2016. p. 59–71.
19. Yaghmai I. Parosteal osteosarcoma. Bone tumors. Berlin, Heidelberg: Springer; 1977. p. 73–82.
20. Cesari M, Alberghini M, Vanel D, et al. Periosteal osteosarcoma: a single-institution experience. Cancer 2011;117(8):1731–5.

21. Cè M, Cellina M, Ueanukul T, et al. Multimodal imaging of osteosarcoma: from first diagnosis to radiomics. Cancers (Basel) 2025;17(4).
22. Nguyen JC, Baghdadi S, Pogoriler J, et al. Pediatric osteosarcoma: correlation of imaging findings with histopathologic features, treatment, and outcome. Radiographics 2022;42(4):1196–213.
23. Oh C, Bishop MW, Cho SY, et al. F-FDG PET/CT in the management of osteosarcoma. J Nucl Med 2023;64(6):842.
24. Welker JA, Henshaw RM, Jelinek J, et al. The percutaneous needle biopsy is safe and recommended in the diagnosis of musculoskeletal masses: outcomes analysis of 155 patients at a sarcoma referral center. Cancer 2000;89(12):2677–86.
25. Henry L. Jaffe 1896–1979. In: Mostofi SB, editor. Who's who in orthopedics. London: Springer London; 2005. p. 161–3.
26. Khal AA, Aiba H, Righi A, et al. Diagnostic challenges in low-grade central osteosarcoma: a retrospective study. Bone Jt J 2024;106(1):99–106.
27. Barrientos-Ruiz I, Ortiz-Cruz EJ, Serrano-Montilla J, et al. Are biopsy tracts a concern for seeding and local recurrence in sarcomas? Clin Orthop Relat Res 2017;475(2):511–8.
28. Dietz MS, Al-Ibraheemi A, Davis JL, et al. Optimizing ewing sarcoma and osteosarcoma biopsy acquisition: a children's oncology group bone tumor committee consensus statement. J Natl Compr Cancer Netw 2024;23(1).
29. Meyers PA, Schwartz CL, Krailo M, et al. Osteosarcoma: a randomized, prospective trial of the addition of ifosfamide and/or muramyl tripeptide to cisplatin, doxorubicin, and high-dose methotrexate. J Clin Oncol 2005;23(9):2004–11.
30. Nakano K. The future of HER2-Targeted treatment for osteosarcoma: lessons from the negative trastuzumab deruxtecan results. Int J Mol Sci 2023;24(23).
31. Piperno-Neumann S, Le Deley MC, Rédini F, et al. Zoledronate in combination with chemotherapy and surgery to treat osteosarcoma (OS2006): a randomised, multicentre, open-label, phase 3 trial. Lancet Oncol 2016;17(8):1070–80.
32. Lewis IJ, Nooij MA, Whelan J, et al. Improvement in histologic response but not survival in osteosarcoma patients treated with intensified chemotherapy: a randomized phase III trial of the European Osteosarcoma Intergroup. J Natl Cancer Inst 2007;99(2):112–28.
33. Richardson SM, Wurtz LD, Collier CD. Ninety percent or greater tumor necrosis is associated with survival and social determinants of health in patients with osteosarcoma in the national cancer database clinical orthopaedics and related research® 2023;481(3).
34. Salzer-Kuntschik M, Delling G, Beron G, et al. Morphological grades of regression in osteosarcoma after Polychemotherapy—study COSS 80. J Cancer Res Clin Oncol 1983;106(Suppl 1):21–4.
35. Picci P, Bacci G, Campanacci M, et al. Histologic evaluation of necrosis in osteosarcoma induced by chemotherapy regional mapping of viable and nonviable tumor. Cancer 1985;56(7):1515–21.
36. Chui MH, Kandel RA, Wong M, et al. Histopathologic features of prognostic significance in high-grade osteosarcoma. Arch Pathol Lab Med 2016;140(11):1231–42.
37. Parambil BC, Khemani P, Puri A, et al. Outcomes based on histological tumor necrosis and predictive clinical and laboratory parameters for necrosis in children with osteosarcoma treated on a non-high dose methotrexate-based chemotherapy backbone. Pediatr Blood Cancer 2025;72(3):e31471.
38. Bielack SS, Kempf-Bielack B, Delling G, et al. Prognostic factors in high-grade osteosarcoma of the extremities or trunk: an analysis of 1,702 patients treated

on neoadjuvant cooperative osteosarcoma study group protocols. J Clin Oncol 2002;20(3):776–90.
39. Kang J-W, Shin SH, Choi JH, et al. Inter-and intra-observer reliability in histologic evaluation of necrosis rate induced by neo-adjuvant chemotherapy for osteosarcoma. Int J Clin Exp Pathol 2017;10(1):359–67.
40. Ho DJ, Agaram NP, Jean MH, et al. Deep learning-based objective and reproducible osteosarcoma chemotherapy response assessment and outcome prediction. Am J Pathol 2023;193(3):341–9.
41. Marina NM, Smeland S, Bielack SS, et al. Comparison of MAPIE versus MAP in patients with a poor response to preoperative chemotherapy for newly diagnosed high-grade osteosarcoma (EURAMOS-1): an open-label, international, randomised controlled trial. Lancet Oncol 2016;17(10):1396–408.
42. Múdry P, Kýr M, Rohleder O, et al. Improved osteosarcoma survival with addition of mifamurtide to conventional chemotherapy – observational prospective single institution analysis. J Bone Oncol 2021;28:100362.
43. Palmerini E, Meazza C, Tamburini A, et al. Is there a role for mifamurtide in nonmetastatic high-grade osteosarcoma? Results From the Italian Sarcoma Group (ISG/OS-2) and Spanish sarcoma Group (GEIS-33) trials. J Clin Oncol 2025;43(28):3113–22.
44. Reddy S, Upadhyay R, Klamer B, et al. Local control and toxicity outcomes after stereotactic body radiation therapy for metastatic osteosarcoma in pediatric patients. Pediatr Blood Cancer 2025;72(9):e31834.
45. Indelicato DJ, Bradley JA, Spiguel A, et al. Proton therapy for pediatric patients with localized unresectable osteosarcoma. Int J Radiat Oncol Biol Phys 2025; 123(1, Supplement):e169.
46. Brar GS, Schmidt AA, Willams LR, et al. Osteosarcoma: current insights and advances. Explor Target Antitumor Ther 2025;6:1002324.
47. Kamada T, Serizawa I, Tsuji H, et al. Carbon ion radiotherapy for unresectable primary bone sarcoma of the spine. Int J Radiat Oncol Biol Phys 2008;72(1):S106.
48. Seidensaal K, Mattke M, Haufe S, et al. The role of combined ion-beam radiotherapy (CIBRT) with protons and carbon ions in a multimodal treatment strategy of inoperable osteosarcoma. Radiother Oncol 2021;159:8–16.
49. Grimer RJ, Sommerville S, Warnock D, et al. Management and outcome after local recurrence of osteosarcoma. Eur J Cancer 2005;41(4):578–83.
50. Kuo C, Malvar J, Chi Y-Y, et al. Survival outcomes and surgical morbidity based on surgical approach to pulmonary metastasectomy in pediatric, adolescent and young adult patients with osteosarcoma. Cancer Med 2023;12(20):20231–41.
51. Teke ME, Saif A, Sarvestani AL, et al. A phase III, randomized, controlled trial comparing open versus thoracoscopic management of pulmonary metastases in patients with osteosarcoma. Ann Surg Oncol 2022;29(13):7961–3.
52. Assi A, Farhat M, Hachem MCR, et al. Tyrosine kinase inhibitors in osteosarcoma: adapting treatment strategiesa. J Bone Oncol 2023;43:100511.
53. Children's Oncology Group (COG). A study to test the addition of the drug cabozantinib to standard chemotherapy in patients with newly diagnosed osteosarcoma [Internet]. Bethesda (MD): National Library of Medicine (US); 2023. Available at: https://clinicaltrials.gov/study/NCT05691478 (Accessed 1 June 2026).
54. Shah N. CaboMain: a phase 2 study of cabozantinib as a maintenance agent in patients with ultra-high risk pediatric solid tumors. J Clin Oncol 2022;40(16_suppl):TPS10060–.

55. Ipsen Pharma. A phase II, randomized, open-label study to assess the efficacy, safety, and pharmacokinetics (PK) of maintenance cabozantinib (XL184) plus best supportive care (BSC) versus BSC in children, adolescents and young adults (AYA) with unresectable residual osteosarcoma either at diagnosis or at first relapse after standard treatment (CabOSTar). ClinicalTrials.gov. Bethesda (MD): National Library of Medicine (US); 2024. Available at: https://clinicaltrials.gov/study/NCT06341712.
56. Juan Ribelles A, Felix A, Benavent N, et al. Recurrent and refractory ewing sarcoma phase I/II trials: current perspective from the euro-ewing consortium. JCO Precision Oncol 2025;9:e2500377.
57. Eaton BR, Claude L, Indelicato DJ, et al. Ewing sarcoma. Pediatr Blood Cancer 2021;68(Suppl 2):e28355.
58. Brennan B, Kirton L, Marec-Bérard P, et al. Comparison of two chemotherapy regimens in patients with newly diagnosed ewing sarcoma (EE2012): an open-label, randomised, phase 3 trial. Lancet 2022;400(10362):1513–21.
59. Gillani R, Shulman DS, DelRocco NJ, et al. Molecular characterization informs prognosis in patients with localized ewing sarcoma: a report from the Children's Oncology Group. J Clin Oncol 2025;43(35):3750–9.
60. Jamshidi K, Naghizadeh H, Shooroki KK, et al. Optimizing local control in Ewing sarcoma: a critical discussion of radiotherapy and surgical approaches with proposed decision-making algorithm; a narrative review. Radiat Oncol 2025;20(1):165.
61. Callan AK, Alexander JH, Montgomery NI, et al. Contemporary surgical management of osteosarcoma and Ewing sarcoma. Pediatr Blood Cancer 2025;72:e31374.
62. Dehner CA, Lazar AJ, Chrisinger JSA. Updates on WHO classification for small round cell tumors: ewing sarcoma vs. everything else. Hum Pathol 2024;147:101–13.
63. Shulman DS, Chen S, Hall D, et al. Adverse prognostic impact of the loss of STAG2 protein expression in patients with newly diagnosed localised Ewing sarcoma. Br J Cancer 2022;127(12):2220–6.
64. Bosma SE, Ayu O, Fiocco M, et al. Prognostic factors for survival in Ewing sarcoma: a systematic review. Surg Oncol 2018;27(4):603–10.
65. Indelicato DJ, Callan AK, Ahmed SK, et al. Preoperative radiotherapy in patients with localized ewing sarcoma enrolled on AEWS1031: a report from the Children's Oncology Group. Pediatr Blood Cancer 2025;72(8):e31820.
66. Warikoo V, Aron J, Salunke A, et al. Pathological fracture characteristics and their impact on osteosarcoma prognosis: a systematic review. Journal of Orthopaedic Reports 2025;4(3):100502.
67. Gonzalez MR, Bedi A, Karczewski D, et al. Are pathologic fractures in patients with osteosarcoma associated with worse survival outcomes? A systematic review and meta-analysis. Clin Orthop Relat Res 2023;481(12):2433–43.
68. O'Donnell RJ, DuBois SG, Haas-Kogan DA. Sarcomas of bone. In: DeVita VT Jr, Lawrence TS, Rosenberg SA, et al, editors. DeVita, Hellman, and Rosenberg's Cancer: Principles & Practice of Oncology. 11th ed. the Netherlands: Wolters Kluwer; 2019. p. 1450–74.
69. Li J, Tang X, Wang L, et al. Vascularized fibular epiphyseal transfer for biological reconstruction of bone defects following resection in children with proximal humeral sarcoma. BMC Surg 2025;25(1):95.
70. Azoury SC, Shammas RL, Othman S, et al. Outcomes following free fibula physeal transfer for pediatric proximal humerus reconstruction: an international multi-institutional study. Plast Reconstr Surg 2023;151(4):805–13.

71. Costantino E, Hisaki A, Ahmed A, et al. What is the revision-free survival of resurfaced allograft-prosthesis composites for proximal humerus reconstruction in children with bone tumors? Clin Orthop Relat Res 2024;482:979–90.
72. Peng X, Ji W, Yang F, et al. Enhanced clinical outcomes of uncemented prostheses in revision surgery of distal femoral tumor prostheses: a retrospective study. Eur J Med Res 2025;30(1):834.
73. Gong T, Lu M, Sheng H, et al. Survivorship, complications, and functional outcomes of uncemented distal femoral endoprosthesis with short, curved stem for patients with bone tumours. Bone Jt J 2024;106-B(9):1000–7.
74. Li Z, Fan D, Zhao J, et al. Is proximal tibial hemiarthroplasty reconstruction effective in minimizing limb length discrepancy among skeletally immature patients with primary bone sarcomas? Clin Orthop Relat Res 2025;483(11).
75. Gupta R, Martin SP, Sriwastwa A, et al. Musculoskeletal 3D printing. In: Martin SP, Sheikh A, editors. 3D Printing at Hospitals and Medical Centers: A Practical Guide for Medical Professionals. 2nd ed. New York (NY): Springer International Publishing; 2024. p. 105–25.
76. Baleani M, Erani P, Blaise M, et al. Intercalary reconstruction of long bones by massive allograft: Comparison of construct stability ensured by three different host-graft junctions and two types of fixations in a synthetic femur model. Frontiers in Pediatrics. [Original Research] 2022;10–2022.
77. Huang X, Huang D, Lin N, et al. 3D-Printed prosthesis with an articular interface for anatomical acetabular reconstruction after type I + II (+ III) internal hemipelvectomy: clinical outcomes and finite element analysis. J Bone Joint Surg Am 2025;107(2):184–95.
78. Hobusch GM, Hofer C, Döring K, et al. Is rotationplasty still a reasonable reconstruction option for patients with a femoral bone sarcoma? A comparative study of patients with a minimum of 20 years of Follow-up after rotationplasty and lower extremity amputation. Clin Orthop Relat Res 2025;483(10).
79. Hillmann A, Gosheger G, Hoffmann C, et al. Rotationplasty – surgical treatment modality after failed limb salvage procedure. Arch Orthop Trauma Surg 2000; 120(10):555–8.
80. Alexander JH, Jordan SW, West JM, et al. Targeted muscle reinnervation in oncologic amputees: early experience of a novel institutional protocol. J Surg Oncol 2019;120(3):348–58.
81. Onkos Surgical, Inc. De Novo classification request for ELEOS™ and ELEOSx™ limb salvage system. DEN210058. U.S. Food and Drug Administration. 2022. Available at: https://www.accessdata.fda.gov/cdrh_docs/reviews/DEN210058.pdf [1, 2] (Accessed 1 June 2026).
82. Wafa H, Grimer RJ, Reddy K, et al. Retrospective evaluation of the incidence of early periprosthetic infection with silver-treated endoprostheses in high-risk patients. Bone Jt J 2015;97-B(2):252–7.
83. LiBrizzi CL, Sabharwal S, Forsberg JA, et al. Does the use of negative pressure wound therapy and postoperative drains impact the development of surgical site infections?: a PARITY trial secondary analysis. JBJS 2023;105(Suppl 1):34–40.
85. Wood GE, Graves LA, Rubin EM, et al. Bad to the bone: emerging approaches to aggressive bone sarcomas. Am Soc Clin Oncol Educ Book 2023;43:e390306.
86. Goedhart LM, Ho VKY, Ploegmakers JJW, et al. Bone sarcoma follow-up; a nationwide analysis of oncological events after initial treatment. J Bone Oncol 2022;38:100466.
87. Linder-Stragliotto C, Tsagkozis P, Potdar S, et al. Drug sensitivity testing of patient-derived bone sarcomas identifies selective kinase inhibitors for patients

with refractory disease. Clin Transl Oncol 2026. https://doi.org/10.1007/s12094-026-04261-4.
88. Xie L, Xu J, Sun X, et al. ARTEMIS-002: Phase 2 study of HS-20093 in patients with relapsed or refractory osteosarcoma. J Clin Oncol 2024;42:11507.
89. Morya VK, Magar AG, Park SH, Noh KC. Systemic strategies for osteosarcoma: advances and future directions. Discov Oncol 2025;16(1):1367.
90. Vucicevic RS, Castonguay JB, Treviño N, et al. Surgeon perspectives on a virtual reality platform for preoperative planning in complex bone sarcomas. J Orthop 2024;62:43–8.
91. Li Z, Li L, Deng Z, et al. Long-term outcomes of computer navigation-assisted resection for primary pelvic sarcomas. Bone Joint J 2025;107:561–70.

Management of Extracranial Germ Cell Tumors in Pediatric Patients

Brent R. Weil, MD, MPH[a,*], Hatim Thaker, MD[b],
Bryan J. Dicken, MD, MSc[c], Barrie S. Rich, MD[d]

KEYWORDS

• Germ cell tumor • Pediatric • Adolescent • Teratoma • Surgery

KEY POINTS

- Optimal surgical treatment of germ cell tumors (GCTs) of any location involves intact resection of the tumor without rupture or spillage while sparing vital structures whenever possible.
- If upfront surgical resection isn't possible, would require resection of adjacent organs, and/or result in unacceptable morbidity, biopsy and chemotherapy should be pursued.
- Appropriate staging involves both radiographic and intraoperative assessment and is critical for determining appropriate treatment.
- Platinum-based chemotherapy is used for all malignant GCTs with the exception of stage I ovarian or testicular GCTs for which surgical resection alone may be adequate.
- Future efforts will focus on de-escalation of therapy for low-risk tumors, novel treatments for relapsed/refractory GCTs and improving surveillance with serum microRNAs and circulating tumor DNA.

INTRODUCTION

Germ cell tumors (GCTs) are a heterogeneous group of tumors that originate from primordial germ cells. They vary not only in their site of origin, but also in their histology and clinical behavior. GCTs are comprised of both benign and malignant histologies and include seminomatous tumors (seminoma in the testicle, dysgerminoma in the ovary, germinoma in extragonadal sites), nonseminomatous tumors (yolk-sac tumor, choriocarcinoma, embryonal carcinoma), and teratomas (mature and/or immature).

[a] Department of Pediatric Surgery, Boston Children's Hospital, Boston, MA, USA; [b] Department of Urology, Boston Children's Hospital, Boston, MA, USA; [c] Division of Pediatric Surgery, University of Alberta, Stollery Children's Hospital, Edmonton, Alberta, Canada; [d] Division of Pediatric Surgery, Cohen Children's Medical Center, Zucker School of Medicine, Northwell/ Hofstra, NY, USA
* Corresponding author.
E-mail address: brent.weil@childrens.harvard.edu

Surg Oncol Clin N Am 35 (2026) 785–800
https://doi.org/10.1016/j.soc.2026.03.001 **surgonc.theclinics.com**

Abbreviations	
AJCC	American Joint Committee on Cancer
COG	Children's Oncology Group
ENET	embryonic-type neuroectodermal tumor
FSH	follicular stimulating hormone
GCTs	germ cell tumors
HDCT	high-dose chemotherapy
LH	luteinizing hormone
MaGIC	Malignant Germ Cell International Collaborative
OS	overall survival
RPLND	retroperitoneal lymph node dissection
SCT	Sacrococcygeal GCT
TSH	thyroid stimulating hormone

These tumors can arise from within the gonads or at extragonadal sites such as the retroperitoneum, anterior mediastinum, cervical region, or sacrococcygeal region. GCTs can also be intracranial; these tumors are outside the scope of this current work. Further contributing to their heterogeneity, GCTs may occur in childhood, adolescence, or adulthood. Management of these tumors, therefore, may vary depending upon the age at diagnosis, the histology of the tumor, and/or the primary site. This review aims to summarize the fundamentals of pediatric and adolescent extracranial GCTs and review current best practices for optimal treatment.

EPIDEMIOLOGY

Pediatric GCTs are rare, with an estimated incidence of 11.7 and 6.7 per million among males and females, respectively.[1] Although uncommon, GCTs account for approximately 3% of tumors occurring in children aged less than 15, and approximately 14% of tumors among children and young adults aged 15 to 19.[2,3] Mature teratomas of the ovary represent the most common histology. The incidence of malignant GCTs varies based on age, sex, and location. Recent data suggest that the annual incidence of GCTs in the United States, particularly testicular GCTs in adolescent and young adult males, may be rising.[4]

Most GCTs develop in individuals without any known genetic or other predisposing risk factors. A few known conditions associated with elevated risk for development of GCTs have been identified. Males with cryptorchidism or Klinefelter's syndrome are at increased risk for the development of testicular and mediastinal GCTs.[5] Females with Turner's syndrome carry an elevated risk for development of ovarian GCTs.[6] Individuals with gonadal dysgenesis syndromes are also at elevated risk for developing GCTs, particularly gonadoblastoma, in streak gonads.[7] Several cases of GCTs observed to cluster within families have also been reported, suggesting the possibility of additional heritable genetic risk factors.[8] Inherited pathogenic variants in the checkpoint kinase 2 gene may be associated with development of testicular GCTs among some of these families.[9] Testicular microlithiasis is not a risk for development of testicular GCT.[10] Identification of additional genes and environmental risk factors known to be associated with elevated risk for GCT development remains a subject of ongoing research.

CLASSIFICATION

There are several ways of classifying GCTs. Broadly, GCTs can be benign or malignant, and gonadal versus extragonadal, but age and histologic subtype also carry important implications for risk categorization, management, and prognosis. Prepubertal versus postpubertal patients develop different types of GCTs, based on molecular and pathways, and clinically, the site of origin and histologic subtype dictates management. Increased activity and aberrations of the Wnt signaling pathway have been found to drive GCT development, with prognostic implications as well.[11]

Gametes arise from pluripotent primordial germ cells through a step wise maturation process and alterations in this process give rise to GCTs. GCTs are classified into Type I GCTs or Type II GCTs based on the degree of genomic imprinting erasure. Erasure is the epigenetic modification, via DNA methylation, to allow the maternal or paternal allele expression in the gametes. Type I GCTs undergo partial erasure of imprinting and are derived earlier in the primordial germ cell maturation process. These type I teratomas and yolk sac tumors have gain of 1p or loss of 1q mutations and occur in children less than 11 years of age. Thus, prepubertal tumors are typically Type I GCTs. Type II GCTs have full erasure of genomic imprinting and occur later in the germ cell maturation process. These tumors develop in adolescent and adult patients and commonly contain a chromosome 12p gain. Thus, older patients tend to develop Type II GCTs. Isochromosome 12p testing is a specific way to differentiate between prepubertal (benign) and postpubertal (potentially malignant) teratomas.[12–14]

Histologically, GCTs can be classified as teratomas (mature or immature), or malignant GCTs (**Box 1**). Mature teratomas are composed of well-differentiated tissue from ectoderm, endoderm and mesoderm layers, and can therefore contain any tissue type. They typically have benign behavior. However, they are nonresponsive to chemotherapy, so surgical excision is required for treatment.[15]

Immature teratomas, in addition to ectoderm, endoderm, and mesodermal layers, uniquely include immature fetal neuroectodermal tissue as well. Grading is based on the degree of immaturity. These tumors are calcified as grade 1, 2 or 3. Grade 3 tumors (>50% immature neuroepithelium content) have a higher risk of local recurrence and relapse.[16]

Malignant GCTs can be classified as germinomatous or nongerminomatous tumors. Seminoma or dysgerminoma (ie, germinomatous tumors), originating from the testicle and ovary respectively, are rare in children and adolescents and are exquisitely sensitive to chemotherapy and radiation. Nongerminomatous tumors may include yolk sac tumors, embryonal carcinoma, choriocarcinoma, or a mix of several histologic

Box 1
Classification of germ cell tumors

Teratomas
- Mature
- Immature

Malignant GCTs
- *Germinomatous GCTs*
  - Seminoma (testicle)
  - Dysgerminoma (ovary)
  - Germinoma (extra-gonadal)
- *Non-germinomatous GCTs*
  - Yolk sac (endodermal sinus) tumor
  - Choriocarcinoma
  - Embryonal carcinoma
  - Gonadoblastoma

Mixed GCTs
- Different histologies present within the same tumor

subtypes (mixed GCT). While rare, some malignant GCTs may also contain somatic malignancies such as embryonic-type neuroectodermal tumors (ENET) or sarcomas, which will alter risk and management.

ROLE OF TUMOR MARKERS

The 3 standard serum tumor markers for germ cell tumors are alpha fetoprotein (AFP), beta-human chorionic gonadotropin (βHCG,) and lactate dehydrogenase (LDH) (**Table 1**). These are used for diagnosis, risk stratification, and monitoring treatment response or disease progression. Prenatally, AFP is produced by the yolk sac, liver and intestines, with a peak concentration between 12- and 14-week gestation. Postnatally, synthesis of AFP in the liver subsides, and AFP levels normalize to adult AFP values within the first 2 years of life. Therefore, AFP levels for patients with suspected GCT must be interpreted based on age-adjusted values reported by Glowska-Ciemny and colleagues or Wu and colleagues.[17,18]

AFP is elevated in yolk sac tumor and embryonal carcinoma, and the trend of AFP after therapy correlates with clinical outcomes.[19] Traditionally, AFP was not thought to be elevated in teratoma. However, patients with testicular teratoma may have AFP elevation in 20% to 25% of cases.[20] Patients with immature ovarian teratoma with or without microscopic foci of yolk sac tumor can exhibit elevated AFP levels as well. AFP is typically not secreted by pure seminoma or choriocarcinoma.

The half-life of AFP is classically 5 to 7 days, but may be as high as 1 to 1.5 months in children aged less than 2. After surgery, levels should normalize within approximately 1 month (or 4–5 half-lives), assuming there is no residual or metastatic disease.[20] Elevation of AFP can also occur from non-GCT origins, such as hepatocellular carcinoma, lung cancer, pancreatic cancer, gastric adenocarcinoma, hepatoblastoma, cystic fibrosis, congenital heart defects, hypothyroidism, folate deficiencies, or platelet aggregation abnormalities.[21]

βHCG, initially secreted by the embryo and then by the syncytiotrophoblasts of the placenta, is produced by choriocarcinoma. Other germ cell tumors such as pure seminoma, yolk sac tumor, and embryonal carcinoma may produce βHCG, but teratoma never does. Approximately 10% to 15% of seminomas may produce βHCG due to the presence of syncytiotrophoblasts.[22] The half-life is 24 to 36 hours, so this tumor marker should normalize within 1 week after surgery. Since this protein is structurally similar to luteinizing hormone (LH), follicular stimulating hormone (FSH), and thyroid stimulating hormone (TSH), false positive results can occur in the setting of male

Table 1
Serum tumor marker and microRNA levels for pediatric germ cell tumors

Germ Cell Tumors—Type	AFP	β-hCG	LDH	microRNA
Mature teratoma	-	-	-	-
Immature teratoma	+/–	-	+/–	+/–
Seminoma/Dysgerminoma	-	-	+	+
Yolk sac tumor	+	-	-	+
Choriocarcinoma	-	+	-	+
Embryonal carcinoma	+	+	+/–	+

+ usually elevated; ± may be elevated; - usually not elevated; AFP, alpha fetoprotein; β-hCG, beta-human chorionic gonadotropin; LDH, lactate dehydrogenase.

hypogonadism in older patients due to pituitary increase in HCG. Other malignancies such as hepatocellular carcinoma, pancreatic or gastrointestinal tumors, renal and bladder cancers may also exhibit elevated βHCG levels.[23]

LDH is a serum tumor marker with the least specificity for GCT but does reflect the degree of disease burden as it is marker of cell turnover. The half-life is 4 to 5 days, and it can be secreted by all germ cell tumor subtypes, as well as any lymphoproliferative process.[21]

While AFP, βHCG, and LDH are important for risk stratification and monitoring treatment response, combined sensitivity of all 3 markers only ranges from 40% to 60%.[24] MicroRNA has emerged as a new biomarker for GCT and is particularly useful in scenarios where conventional serum tumor markers cannot stratify patient risk or guide decisions. For example, it is well-established that patients with clinical stage I testicular tumors and negative serum tumors markers, who often undergo surveillance only after surgical resection, may still have occult disease[25,26]

MicroRNAs are short, noncoding, single stranded RNA molecules that regulate gene expression, and are present in GCTs across all ages, gender, site of origin, or histologic subtype. Only pure teratoma does not shed microRNA. Through extensive studies in testicular germ cell tumors, miR-371a-3p has emerged as the highest sensitivity (90.1%) and specificity (94%) for verifying GCT diagnosis in a mass with negative markers, detecting low stage patients at risk of relapse, and further defining the risk of harboring viable tumor in patients who have persistent metastatic masses after chemotherapy.[27] The Children's Oncology Group (COG) phase 3 clinical trial AGCT1531 (ClinicalTrials.gov ID NCT03067181) is currently investigating the role of microRNAs for detecting early relapse in pediatric GCT, particularly in patients with negative tumor markers.

STAGING AND RISK GROUPS

Pediatric GCTs are staged according to the COG staging system, which is based on intraoperative findings (**Table 2**).[28] This is distinct from to the staging system often used for adult gonadal tumors in adults such as the International Federation of Gynecology and Obstetrics for ovarian tumors, and the American Joint Committee on Cancer (AJCC) system for testicular tumors.

GCTs are stratified as low-risk, standard-risk, or high-risk based on patient age and tumor stage, according to the international collaboration Malignant Germ Cell International Collaborative (MaGIC). Increased stage, age ≥11 years, and stage III to IV extragonadal tumors or stage IV ovarian tumors all appear to be associated with worse long-term disease free survival.[14] This schema guides treatment recommendations, clarifying who can receive reduced therapy and those that would benefit from intensification of treatment. Completely excised malignant stage I gonadal GCTs are considered low-risk and are treated with surgical resection and standardized surveillance, with chemotherapy administered only in the setting of recurrent disease. Current open trials are underway evaluating this management for extragonadal stage I tumors.

Standard- and high-risk malignant GCTs require treatment with platinum-based chemotherapy. An additional risk stratification for postpubertal testicular GCTs exists based on the International Germ Cell Cancer Collaborative Group classification system and are categorized as good-risk, intermediate-risk, or poor-risk based on age, tumor markers, primary site, and the presence of metastatic disease (**Table 3**).[29]

MEDICAL MANAGEMENT

Platinum-based chemotherapy serves as the backbone for the medical treatment of pediatric and adult patients with GCTs.[30] Bleomycin, etoposide, and cisplatin are

Table 2
Children's Oncology Group staging system for pediatric germ cell tumors

Stage	Testis	Ovary	Extragonadal
I	Complete resection via orchiectomy. Lymph nodes negative.	Limited to ovary (with negative evaluation of peritoneum), no evidence of extraovarian disease	Complete resection at any site with negative margins (including coccygectomy for sacrococcygeal teratomas)
II	Trans-scrotal biopsy performed, microscopic disease in scrotum or cord, failure of tumor markers to normalize	Microscopic residual disease, peritoneal evaluation negative, failure of tumor markers to normalize	Microscopic residual disease with negative lymph nodes, failure of tumor markers to normalize
III	Retroperitoneal lymph node involvement without visceral or extra-abdominal involvement	Lymph node involvement, metastatic nodule, gross residual disease or biopsy only, contiguous visceral involvement (omentum, bladder, and intestine), peritoneal evaluation positive	Lymph node involvement, gross residual disease, biopsy only
IV	Distant metastases	Distant metastases	Distant metastases

Table 3
Proposed Malignant Germ Cell International Collaborative pediatric germ cell tumors risk stratification system

Risk Group	Age (yrs)	Location	Children's Oncology Group Stage	Survival (%)
Low	Any age	Testis	I	100
	Any age	Ovary	I	96
	Any age	Extragonadal	I	93
Standard	<11	Testis	II/III	99
	<11	Testis	IV	96
	≥11	Testis	II/III	93
	≥11	Testis	IV	83
	<11	Ovary	II/III	97
	<11	Ovary	IV	92
	≥11	Ovary	II/III	85
	<11	Extragonadal	II/III	91
	<11	Extragonadal	IV	79
Poor	≥11	Testis	IV	83
	≥11	Extragonadal	III	61
	≥11	Ovary	IV	60
	≥11	Extragonadal	IV	40

Adapted from Frazier AL, Hale JP, Rodriguez-Galindo C, et al. Revised risk classification for pediatric extracranial germ cell tumors based on 25 years of clinical trial data from the United Kingdom and United States. J Clin Oncol 2015;33(2):195–201. https://doi.org/10.1200/JCO.2014.58.3369.

administered as the standard regimen for GCTs in adults. The regimen has been adapted for the treatment of children and adolescents with GCTs by including a reduced dose of bleomycin (administered once per 3-week cycle as opposed to weekly) and is commonly referred to as *PEb*.[31] Due to the pulmonary toxicity of bleomycin and ototoxicity and other toxicities of cisplatin, both adult and pediatric studies have examined the role of alternative agents and dose reduction strategies.[32] Recent experience in children suggests, for instance, that carboplatin may be substituted for cisplatin leading to reduced toxicity while maintaining similar event free and overall survival (OS).[33,34] As such, the *JEb* regimen (carboplatin, etoposide, and bleomycin) is commonly used throughout the world and is presently being evaluated in the context of a multi-institutional trial in the United States.

Recognition that most children with GCTs experience excellent OS has led to an interest in identifying scenarios where chemotherapy may be safely reduced or omitted to minimize associated short-term and long-term toxicities.[14] Studies have shown that COG stage I gonadal GCTs can be successfully treated with surgery alone, with many patients requiring no further therapy, while those experiencing relapse can nearly always be salvaged with chemotherapy.[35,36] Observation following complete surgical staging and resection may be appropriate for children with stage I malignant gonadal GCTs. Otherwise, platinum-based chemotherapy in addition to surgical resection is presently recommended as the initial therapy for intermediate and poor risk GCTs (stage I extragonadal outside of a clinical trial and all stage II–IV).

The role of chemotherapy for immature teratoma (IT) is controversial. Platinum-based chemotherapy has traditionally been administered, with adult studies noting higher rates of relapse among women with grades 2 and 3 ovarian ITs not receiving chemotherapy.[37] For pediatric and adolescents, it has been recognized that outcomes for IT are excellent without chemotherapy and that radiographic response to chemotherapy is limited.[38,39] Routine use of chemotherapy for IT, regardless of grade, has generally fallen out of favor among pediatric practitioners.

Tumors that relapse following or remain refractory to standard chemotherapy are particularly challenging to treat and associated with poor prognosis. High-dose chemotherapy (HDCT) followed by autologous stem cell rescue has emerged as a promising treatment regimen and is now widely employed for pediatric and young adult patients.[40] An international, phase 3 randomized trial comparing outcomes associated with established HDCT treatment regimens is ongoing.

SURGICAL MANAGEMENT

Surgical resection is the mainstay of treatment of malignant GCTs. The primary goal of surgery at any site is complete resection whenever safely feasible. This includes removal of all visible and palpable macroscopic disease while avoiding tumor rupture or spillage. Complete surgical staging, which involves assessment for locoregional spread is paramount. For gonadal sites, there is a strong focus on fertility preservation, discussed in detail in later sections. Importantly, tumor markers must be sent before resection of any mass where GCT is in the differential diagnosis.

Upfront surgical resection is recommended when possible. This allows for accurate staging and dictates the need for any further treatment. Furthermore, it can improve symptoms brought on by the tumor itself. Should a tumor prove to be unresectable at diagnosis, which is more frequently encountered in extragonadal sites, evaluation with tumor markers and biopsy (ie core needle biopsy or surgical biopsy) is recommended. Interpretation of any biopsy should be considered carefully given the possibility of sampling error due to the heterogeneity of these often large tumors that can have mixed histologies, including mature teratoma. For unresectable tumors, neoadjuvant treatment is administered with cisplatin-based chemotherapy. Surgical resection of any residual mass after treatment is recommended.

Ovarian Germ Cell Tumors

Appropriate tumor resection involves complete removal of the involved ovary intact with sparing of the fallopian tube if amenable and without disease involvement. If complete resection of the tumor would require resection of an organ other than the ipsilateral ovary and fallopian tube, a biopsy should be performed, and definitive resection delayed until after neoadjuvant chemotherapy. Bilateral oophorectomy and/or hysterectomy should not be performed at the time of initial surgical resection.

Complete surgical staging is critical to perform and document during resection of malignant ovarian GCT to accurately stage and appropriately treat patients. Any preoperative or intraoperative tumor rupture should be documented as this upstages a tumor. The COG recommendations for surgical staging are listed in **Box 2**.[36] Without performance of each step, there is incomplete knowledge of the extent of disease with potential for inappropriate therapy assignments. It is important to point out that these steps are less aggressive than the adult staging recommendations, have no impact on fertility, and can be performed without additional morbidity or time.[36]

Given the simplicity of COG surgical staging, these steps should be performed during resection of all ovarian masses to ensure all critical data is identified should the mass prove to be malignant GCT. This is especially true since imaging characteristics alone often cannot distinguish benign from malignant ovarian lesions and should not be relied upon to determine the need for accurate surgical staging (**Fig. 1**A–C).[41,42] Additionally, the use of intraoperative frozen section has been shown to be unreliable in the pediatric and adolescent population and therefore should also not be used to influence the need for complete surgical staging.[43,44]

Ovarian sparing techniques can be considered in the setting of negative tumor markers with a low suspicion for malignancy. This is important particularly given the 8% to 10% risk of a metachronous lesion.[45] In the setting of bilateral tumors, upfront resection can be performed if any ovarian tissue can be salvaged while performing complete tumor resection. Bilateral oophorectomy is not advised, and in this case, biopsy and neoadjuvant chemotherapy is recommended.

Testicular Germ Cell Tumors

Testicular GCTs in postpubertal patients should be treated with a radical orchiectomy with high ligation of the spermatic cord at the level of the internal ring through an inguinal incision. Ideally, the ilioinguinal nerve is preserved, and the spermatic cord is ligated

Box 2
Children's Oncology Group guidelines for surgical staging of ovarian germ cell tumors

Surgical Staging for Ovarian GCTs
- Collection of peritoneal fluid or washings for cytology before starting dissection
- Examination of peritoneal surfaces with biopsy of any abnormalities
- Palpate retroperitoneal lymph nodes and biopsy only for abnormal findings (ie, firm or enlarged nodes)
- Inspect omentum and biopsy only for abnormalities
- Palpate/inspect contralateral ovary and biopsy only for abnormalities
- Complete resection of involved ovary intact (no capsule entry on field) with sparing of fallopian tube if not involved

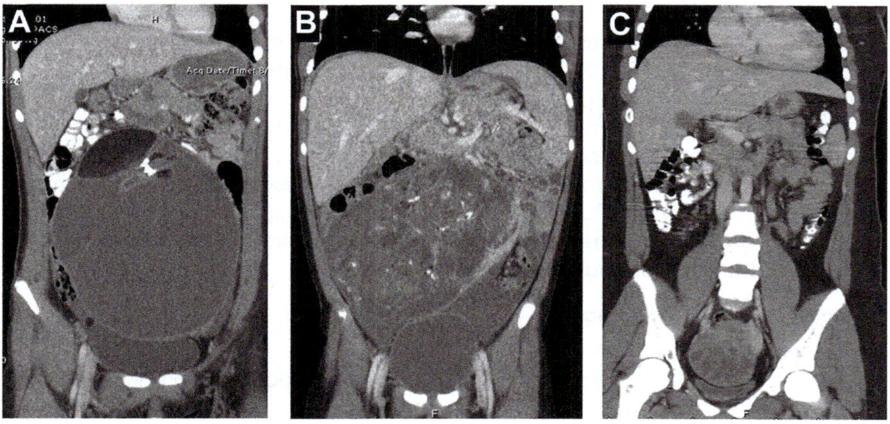

Fig. 1. Coronal CT images of ovarian GCTs. (*A*) Left ovarian MT in a 14-year-old female. The tumor is mostly cystic with solid elements including calcium and fat noted in the most cephalad portion. (*B*) Left ovarian grade 3 IT in a 7-year-old female. The tumor is complex with cystic and solid components including internal fat and calcifications noted. The fluid in the pelvis is worrisome for preoperative rupture. Rupture and diffuse nodularity of the peritoneal cavity was confirmed at laparotomy. Microscopic foci of yolk sac tumor were present throughout the mass on final pathology. (*C*) Right ovarian yolk sac tumor in a 15-year old female. The tumor is complex, also with cystic and solid components.

before manipulation of the testis mass. Preoperative biopsy or intraoperative frozen section while the testis is in situ is not recommended, as this will upstage the tumor. A scrotal incision for orchiectomy is also discouraged as the tumor will be upstaged, and there is a higher risk of local recurrence.[46] However, patients who inadvertently undergo a scrotal orchiectomy can usually be monitored without the need for hemiscrotectomy. In prepubertal males, teratomas with negative tumor markers can potentially be excised with a partial orchiectomy (**Fig. 2**A–E).[47] In contrast, any testicular mass with an elevated AFP, regardless of age, should be treated as potentially malignant and undergo radical orchiectomy.

Surgical management of metastatic testicular cancer is rarely required for prepubertal patients. In postpubertal males, retroperitoneal lymph node dissection (RPLND) may be indicated after orchiectomy for patients with nonseminomatous histology

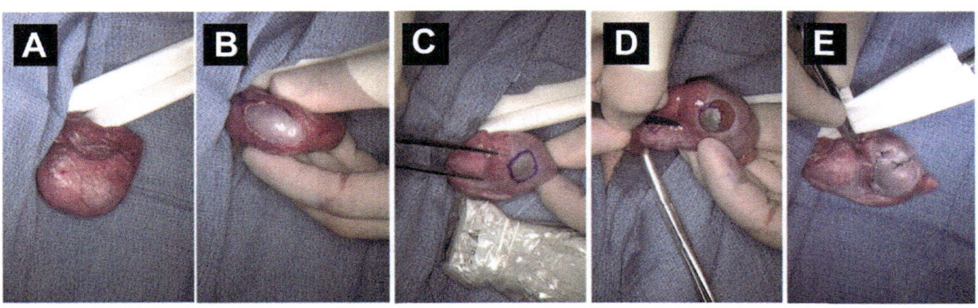

Fig. 2. Steps for performance of a partial orchiectomy. (*A*) Testicle is delivered through an inguinal incision and the spermatic cord is controlled with a vessel loop. (*B*) Tunica vaginalis is incised. (*C*) Tunica albuginea is overlying the tumor with ultrasound guidance. (*D*) Mass is resected with overlying tunica albuginea and seminiferous tubules and sent for frozen section. (*E*) Tunical defect is closed and testicle is replaced into the hemiscrotum.

and AJCC stage 1 or 2 disease with teratoma and somatic type malignancy, stage 1 disease with high-risk features (lymphovascular invasion, embryonal carcinoma predominance) and stage 2A or 2B patients with negative tumor markers. Ongoing trials are evaluating the efficacy of primary RPLND for stage 2A or 2B seminoma, but this is a rare entity in the adolescent and yound adult (AYA) population. Patients with metastatic nonseminomatous retroperitoneal nodal disease are treated with chemotherapy after orchiectomy; postchemotherapy retroperitoneal masses greater than 1 cm warrant RPLND.[48] Presently RPLND in COG protocols is limited to postchemotherapy setting, but the role of prechemotherapy RPLND for pediatric and adolescent GCTs may represent an area of future investigation.

Extragonadal Germ Cell Tumors

Sacrococcygeal germ cell tumors

Sacrococcygeal GCTs (SCTs) presenting in the neonatal period are more likely to be teratomas and predominately external in location. Those occurring later in childhood are associated with an increased risk for malignancy. Optimal surgical treatment for neonatal SCTs involves intact removal of the tumor en bloc with the coccyx while avoiding injury to or resection of adjacent organs, including pelvic floor musculature, so that future bowel, bladder and reproductive function is preserved and optimized.[49,50]

For suspected malignant SCTs, the primary tumor should be assessed with computed tomography (CT) or MRI to determine feasibility of resection and the optimal operative approach. Preoperative imaging should be reviewed, and involvement of the tumor with surrounding structures including neural foramina, the rectum, and/or genitourinary structures assessed. Any suggestion that the tumor cannot be safely separated from vital structures should prompt initial biopsy followed by administration of neoadjuvant chemotherapy in lieu of upfront resection should malignant GCT be confirmed.[34] Provision of neoadjuvant chemotherapy can facilitate eventual, less morbid surgical resection with the expectation for similar OS compared with upfront resection.[28,51] Resection can be performed by a posterior sagittal approach and/or a peritoneal approach based on the degree of internal extension. Should a peritoneal approach be employed for resection, fluid and/or pelvic washings should be sent, and peritoneal surfaces and retroperitoneal lymph nodes assessed to evaluate for disease spread.[28]

Mediastinal germ cell tumors

Primary mediastinal GCTs are commonly large and frequently involve critical structures. As with GCTs at other sites, optimal surgical treatment involves complete resection of the tumor without rupture or spillage while preserving vital structures. The thymus is often involved and should be removed en bloc with the tumor. Large lesions with negative tumor markers and imaging features consistent with MT should be primarily resected. In asymptomatic or minimally symptomatic patients, this can usually be done safely under general anesthesia via lateral thoracotomy, sternotomy, or thoracoscopic approach. Lesions with elevated tumor markers that appear unresectable should be biopsied with chemotherapy administered if malignancy is confirmed.[52] Image-guided, percutaneous core-needle biopsy with multiple cores is preferred. General anesthesia may be contraindicated in patients exhibiting CT or MRI findings of greater than 35 to 50% tracheal compression, peak expiratory flow rates of less than 50% predicted, or those with orthopnea.[53]

Germ cell tumors at other sites

Extracranial GCTs may also arise from the retroperitoneum, vagina, head and neck, and other sites. Cervical GCTs occurring in the neonatal period are often teratomas and require surgical resection for definitive management. Airway compromise is a critical concern and may require immediate postnatal securement of a safe airway and, in some cases, may necessitate in utero or extrapartum interventions. The site of origin for retroperitoneal GCTs may be difficult to determine based on preoperative imaging and the surgeon may need to be prepared for a variety of scenarios at the time of planned surgical resection (**Fig. 3**A–D). Malignant retroperitoneal GCTs may involve vital structures requiring initial biopsy and administration of neoadjuvant chemotherapy. At the time of eventual resection, intraperitoneal fluid and/or washings should be sent for cytology. Retroperitoneal lymph nodes and evidence of peritoneal spread should be assessed, and abnormal-appearing nodes or peritoneal implants should be removed or biopsied. Vaginal GCTs should be managed with the intent for vaginal preservation with neoadjuvant chemotherapy most commonly being given to facilitate a more limited, vaginal-preserving resection.[54]

SURGICAL MANAGEMENT OF METASTATIC, REFRACTORY, AND RECURRENT DISEASE

The role of surgical resection for metastatic disease in GCTs has not been adequately studied, and currently there are no data recommending surgical resection of distant sites of disease. However, there is a role for surgical resection in the setting of recurrent germ cell tumor to the tumor bed. If a recurrent tumor is felt to be resectable, the recommendation is for resection at the time of relapse. If the recurrent disease is felt to be unresectable, and tumor markers are consistent with relapse, then medical therapy is warranted. However, if the mass is unresectable and tumor markers are normal, a surgical biopsy should be strongly considered to rule out somatic malignant

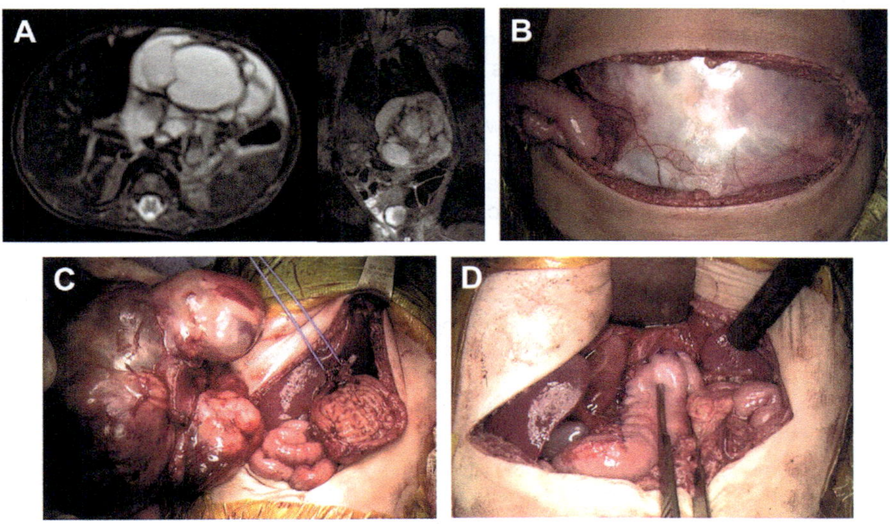

Fig. 3. Newborn infant with abdominal distension, poor oral intake and failure to thrive. (*A*) T2-weighted axial and coronal MR sequences revealing a large intraabdominal mass with mixed cystic and solid (likely fat-containing elements) of uncertain origin. (*B*) Appearance of mass upon transverse laparotomy. (*C*) The mass was firmly adherent to the stomach at the angle of His and was resected along with a small portion of the stomach and gastroesophageal junction. The photo reveals the resected mass on the left, the open stomach and gastric rugae, and a blue vessel loop around the distal esophagus where a nasogastric tube can be seen exiting. (*D*) The gastrotomy repaired primarily and a partial fundoplication performed. Pathology was consistent with mature teratoma.

transformation, growing teratoma syndrome, or a tumor marker negative recurrent tumor. Tissue diagnosis may be critical in these cases.

FUTURE DIRECTIONS

Despite overall excellent outcomes associated with the majority of pediatric GCTs, several challenges remain.[55] These include a need to identify areas where adult and pediatric providers can collaborate to study treatments and outcomes, fostering international collaborations to enroll more patients into clinical trials, improving outcomes for patients with stage III and IV disease, and reducing late effects associated with therapy. To this end, the ongoing COG AGCT 1531 trial is enrolling children and young adults treated at both pediatric and adult centers, and will enroll participants from multiple international centers. A commitment to and means for international collaboration, including establishment of global biobanks, has been further established via the MaGIC consortium.

Additionally, targeted therapies have been evaluated for the treatment of otherwise medically refractory GCTs with some success being reported for tyrosine kinase inhibitors for treatment-refractory GCTs, and cyclin-dependent kinase inhibitors for Rb-expressing, unresectable teratomas.[56,57] Finally, given the limitations associated with the use of tumor markers, promising new methods including measurement of serum microRNA and/or circulating-tumor DNA are either being studied or are already clinically employed for the purposes of better monitoring disease burden, response to therapy and relapse.[24,55]

SUMMARY

In summary, malignant germ cell tumors are a heterogeneous group of tumors. While the fundamentals regarding diagnosis and management pertain to all tumor sites, specific surgical tenets and treatment algorithms should be considered based on site, histology, and age. In this review, we summarize the fundamentals regarding the diagnosis and management for the tumors, the optimal site-specific surgical management, and the controversies that remain. Further work is ongoing and needed to assist in the treatment of refractory/recurrent GCTs.

CLINICS CARE POINTS

- Optimal surgical treatment of germ cell tumors (GCTs) of any location involves intact resection of the tumor without spillage while sparing vital structures whenever possible.
- If upfront surgical resection is not possible and would require resection of adjacent organs, and/or would result in unacceptable morbidity, biopsy and chemotherapy should be pursued as an initial strategy.
- Appropriate GCT staging involves both radiographic and intraoperative assessment and is critical for determining needed treatment.
- Platinum-based chemotherapy is used for all malignant GCTs with the exception of stage I ovarian or testicular GCTs for which a strategy of surgery alone is undertaken.
- Serum tumor markers for germ cell tumors include AFP, βHCG and LDH and are used for diagnosis, risk stratification, and monitoring treatment response or disease progression. Use of serum microRNAs and circulating tumor DNA may complement and enhance the role of traditional serum tumor markers.
- Patient age, tumor stage, and tumor location are critical factors for determining risk and treatment of pediatric GCTs.

DISCLOSURE

All authors have nothing to disclose.

REFERENCES

1. Ries LAG, Smith MA, Gurney JG, et al, editors. Cancer incidence and survival among children and adolescents: united States SEER program 1975-1995. 1999.
2. Shaikh F, Murray MJ, Amatruda JF, et al. Paediatric extracranial germ-cell tumours. Lancet Oncol 2016;17(4):e149–62.
3. Poynter JN, Amatruda JF, Ross JA. Trends in incidence and survival of pediatric and adolescent patients with germ cell tumors in the United States, 1975 to 2006. Cancer 2010;116(20):4882–91.
4. Almeida AA, Wojt A, Metayer C, et al. Racial/ethnic differences in trends of testicular germ cell tumor incidence in the United States, 1992-2021. Cancer 2025; 131(2):e35706.
5. Dieckmann KP, Rübe C, Henke RP. Association of Down's syndrome and testicular cancer. J Urol 1997;157(5):1701–4.
6. Tam YH, Wong YS, Pang KKY, et al. Tumor risk of children with 45,X/46,XY gonadal dysgenesis in relation to their clinical presentations: further insights into the gonadal management. J Pediatr Surg 2016;51(9):1462–6.
7. Dicken BJ, Billmire DF, Krailo M, et al. Gonadal dysgenesis is associated with worse outcomes in patients with ovarian nondysgerminomatous tumors: a report of the Children's Oncology Group AGCT 0132 study. Pediatr Blood Cancer 2018;65(4). https://doi.org/10.1002/pbc.26913.
8. Poynter JN, Richardson M, Roesler M, et al. Family history of cancer in children and adolescents with germ cell tumours: a report from the Children's Oncology Group. Br J Cancer 2018;118(1):121–6.
9. AlDubayan SH, Pyle LC, Gamulin M, et al. Association of inherited pathogenic variants in checkpoint Kinase 2 (CHEK2) with susceptibility to testicular germ cell tumors. JAMA Oncol 2019;5(4):514–22.
10. DeCastro BJ, Peterson AC, Costabile RA. A 5-Year followup study of asymptomatic men with testicular microlithiasis. J Urol 2008;179(4):1420–3.
11. Xu L, Pierce JL, Sanchez A, et al. Integrated genomic analysis reveals aberrations in WNT signaling in germ cell tumors of childhood and adolescence. Nat Commun 2023;14(1):2636.
12. Shah R, Weil BR, Weldon CB, et al. Neonatal malignant disorders: germ cell tumors. Clin Perinatol 2021;48(1):147–65.
13. Pierce JL, Frazier AL, Amatruda JF. Pediatric germ cell tumors: a developmental perspective. Adv Urol 2018;2018:9059382.
14. Frazier AL, Hale JP, Rodriguez-Galindo C, et al. Revised risk classification for pediatric extracranial germ cell tumors based on 25 years of clinical trial data from the United Kingdom and United States. J Clin Oncol 2015;33(2):195–201.
15. Weil BR, Billmire DF. Management of germ cell tumors in pediatric patients. Surg Oncol Clin N Am 2021;30(2):325–38.
16. Pashankar F, Hale JP, Dang H, et al. Is adjuvant chemotherapy indicated in ovarian immature teratomas? A combined data analysis from the malignant germ cell tumor International Collaborative. Cancer 2016;122(2):230–7.
17. Głowska-Ciemny J, Szymanski M, Kuszerska A, et al. Role of alpha-fetoprotein (AFP) in diagnosing childhood cancers and genetic-related chronic diseases. Cancers 2023;15(17):4302.

18. Wu JT, Book L, Sudar K. Serum alpha fetoprotein (AFP) levels in normal infants. Pediatr Res 1981;15(1):50–2.
19. O'Neill AF, Xia C, Krailo MD, et al. α-Fetoprotein as a predictor of outcome for children with germ cell tumors: a report from the malignant germ cell international consortium. Cancer 2019;125(20):3649–56.
20. Montgomery J, Weizer A, Filson C, et al. Role of biochemical markers in testicular cancer: diagnosis, staging, and surveillance. Open Access J Urol 2011;1. https://doi.org/10.2147/OAJU.S15063.
21. Lobo J, Leão R, Jerónimo C, et al. Liquid biopsies in the clinical management of germ cell tumor patients: state-of-the-art and future directions. Int J Mol Sci 2021;22(5):2654.
22. Gilligan TD, Seidenfeld J, Basch EM, et al. American Society of Clinical Oncology Clinical Practice Guideline on uses of serum tumor markers in adult males with germ cell tumors. J Clin Oncol 2010;28(20):3388–404.
23. Stenman UH, Alfthan H, Hotakainen K. Human chorionic gonadotropin in cancer. Clin Biochem 2004;37(7):549–61.
24. Dieckmann KP, Radtke A, Spiekermann M, et al. Serum levels of MicroRNA miR-371a-3p: a sensitive and specific new biomarker for germ cell tumours. Eur Urol 2017;71(2):213–20.
25. Lafin JT, Singla N, Woldu SL, et al. Serum MicroRNA-371a-3p levels predict viable germ cell tumor in chemotherapy-naïve patients undergoing retroperitoneal lymph node dissection. Eur Urol 2020;77(2):290–2.
26. Ghandour RA, Singla N, Bagrodia A. Management of stage II germ cell tumors. Urol Clin North Am 2019;46(3):363–76.
27. Bagrodia A, Daneshmand S, Cheng L, et al. The past and future of biomarkers in testicular germ cell tumors. Société Int D'Urologie J 2020;1(1):77–84.
28. Rescorla F, Billmire D, Stolar C, et al. The effect of cisplatin dose and surgical resection in children with malignant germ cell tumors at the sacrococcygeal region: a pediatric intergroup trial (POG 9049/CCG 8882). J Pediatr Surg 2001;36(1):12–7.
29. Gillessen S, Sauvé N, Collette L, et al. Predicting outcomes in men with metastatic nonseminomatous germ cell tumors (NSGCT): results from the IGCCCG update consortium. J Clin Oncol 2021;39(14):1563–74.
30. Einhorn LH, Donohue J. *Cis* -Diamminedichloroplatinum, vinblastine, and bleomycin combination chemotherapy in disseminated testicular cancer. Ann Intern Med 1977;87(3):293–8.
31. Rogers PC, Olson TA, Cullen JW, et al. Treatment of children and adolescents with stage II testicular and stages I and II ovarian malignant germ cell tumors: a pediatric Intergroup Study—Pediatric Oncology Group 9048 and children's cancer Group 8891. J Clin Oncol 2004;22(17):3563–9.
32. Cushing B, Giller R, Cullen JW, et al. Randomized comparison of combination chemotherapy with etoposide, bleomycin, and either high-dose or standard-dose cisplatin in children and adolescents with high-risk malignant germ cell tumors: a Pediatric Intergroup Study—Pediatric Oncology Group 9049 and children's cancer Group 8882. J Clin Oncol 2004;22(13):2691–700.
33. Mann JR, Raafat F, Robinson K, et al. The United Kingdom children's cancer study group's second germ cell tumor study: Carboplatin, etoposide, and Bleomycin are effective treatment for children with malignant extracranial germ cell tumors, with acceptable toxicity. J Clin Oncol 2000;18(22):3809–18.
34. Frazier AL, Stoneham S, Rodriguez-Galindo C, et al. Comparison of carboplatin versus cisplatin in the treatment of paediatric extracranial malignant germ cell

tumours: a report of the Malignant Germ Cell International Consortium. Eur J Cancer 2018;98:30–7.
35. Rescorla FJ, Ross JH, Billmire DF, et al. Surveillance after initial surgery for stage I pediatric and adolescent boys with malignant testicular germ cell tumors: report from the Children's Oncology Group. J Pediatr Surg 2015;50(6):1000–3.
36. Billmire DF, Cullen JW, Rescorla FJ, et al. Surveillance after initial surgery for pediatric and adolescent girls with stage I ovarian germ cell tumors: report from the Children's Oncology Group. J Clin Oncol 2014;32(5):465–70.
37. Gershenson DM, del Junco G, Silva EG, et al. Immature teratoma of the ovary. Obstet Gynecol 1986;68(5):624–9.
38. Pashankar F, Hale JP, Dang H, et al. Is adjuvant chemotherapy indicated in ovarian immature teratomas? A combined data analysis from the M alignant G erm C ell Tumor International Collaborative. Cancer 2016;122(2):230–7.
39. Marina NM, Cushing B, Giller R, et al. Complete surgical excision is effective treatment for children with immature teratomas with or without malignant elements: a Pediatric Oncology Group/Children's Cancer Group Intergroup Study. J Clin Oncol 1999;17(7):2137–43.
40. Adra N, Abonour R, Althouse SK, et al. High-dose chemotherapy and autologous peripheral-blood stem-cell transplantation for relapsed metastatic germ cell tumors: the Indiana university experience. J Clin Oncol 2017;35(10):1096–102.
41. Billmire D, Dicken B, Rescorla F, et al. Imaging appearance of Nongerminoma Pediatric Ovarian Germ Cell Tumors does not discriminate benign from malignant histology. J Pediatr Adolesc Gynecol 2021;34(3):383–6.
42. Knaus ME, Onwuka AJ, Afrazi A, et al. Multi-institutional review of the preoperative diagnostic accuracy for pediatric ovarian mature cystic teratomas. J Pediatr Adolesc Gynecol 2022;35(4):478–85.
43. Dicken BJ, Billmire DF, Rich B, et al. Utility of frozen section in pediatric and adolescent malignant ovarian nonseminomatous germ cell tumors: a report from the children's oncology group. Gynecol Oncol 2022;166(3):476–80.
44. Gil LA, Lutz CM, Dillon PA, et al. Use and accuracy of intraoperative frozen section analysis for ovarian masses in children and adolescents. J Pediatr Adolesc Gynecol 2022;S1083-3188(22):00295-9.
45. Braungart S, Craigie R, Farrelly P, et al. Ovarian tumors in children: how common are lesion recurrence and metachronous disease? A UK CCLG Surgeons Cancer Group nationwide study. J Pediatr Surg 2020;55(10):2026–9.
46. Capelouto CC, Clark PE, Ransil BJ, et al. A review of scrotal violation in testicular cancer: is adjuvant local therapy necessary? J Urol 1995;153(3 Pt 2):981–5.
47. Shukla AR, Woodard C, Carr MC, et al. Experience with testis sparing surgery for testicular teratoma. J Urol 2004;171(1):161–3.
48. Masterson TA, Cary C. The use of modified templates in early and advanced stage nonseminomatous germ cell tumor. Adv Urol 2018;2018:1–5.
49. Hambraeus M, Hagander L, Stenström P, et al. Long-term outcome of sacrococcygeal teratoma: a controlled cohort study of urinary tract and bowel dysfunction and predictors of poor outcome. J Pediatr 2018;198:131–6.e2.
50. Rescorla FJ. Pediatric germ cell tumors. Semin Pediatr Surg 2012;21(1):51–60.
51. Göbel U, Schneider DT, Calaminus G, et al. Multimodal treatment of malignant sacrococcygeal germ cell tumors: a prospective analysis of 66 patients of the German cooperative protocols MAKEI 83/86 and 89. J Clin Oncol 2001;19(7):1943–50.
52. Schneider DT, Calaminus G, Reinhard H, et al. Primary mediastinal germ cell tumors in children and adolescents: results of the German cooperative protocols MAKEI 83/86, 89, and 96. J Clin Oncol 2000;18(4):832.

53. Shamberger RC, Holzman RS, Griscom NT, et al. Prospective evaluation by computed tomography and pulmonary function tests of children with mediastinal masses. Surgery 1995;118(3):468–71.
54. Vural F, Vural B, Paksoy N. Vaginal teratoma: a case report and review of the literature. J Obstet Gynaecol 2015;35(7):757–8.
55. Fonseca A, Lobo J, Hazard FK, et al. Advancing clinical and translational research in germ cell tumours (GCT): recommendations from the Malignant Germ Cell International Consortium. Br J Cancer 2022;127(9):1577–83.
56. Vaughn DJ, Hwang W, Lal P, et al. Phase 2 trial of the cyclin-dependent kinase 4/6 inhibitor palbociclib in patients with retinoblastoma protein-expressing germ cell tumors. Cancer 2015;121(9):1463–8.
57. Oechsle K, Honecker F, Cheng T, et al. Preclinical and clinical activity of sunitinib in patients with cisplatin-refractory or multiply relapsed germ cell tumors: a Canadian Urologic Oncology Group/German Testicular Cancer Study Group cooperative study. Ann Oncol 2011;22(12):2654–60.

Rare Tumors: Part One

Erica C. Arnold, MD[a], Brian R. Englum, MD, MHS[b],
Emily Christison-Lagay, MD[c], Jennifer H. Aldrink, MD[d,*]

KEYWORDS

- Pediatric thyroid carcinoma • Differentiated thyroid carcinoma • Pediatric melanoma
- Rare tumor • Pediatric

KEY POINTS

- Rare cancers in children, such as differentiated thyroid carcinoma and melanoma, remain challenging to study, and most recommendations are derived from adult guidelines.
- Pediatric thyroid nodules are routinely evaluated using Thyroid Imaging Reporting and Data System (TI-RADS) criteria, with TI-RADS with a modified pediatric size criterion showing superiority to American Thyroid Association and American College of Radiology's TI-RADS for determining nodules indicated for fine needle aspiration.
- Surgical diagnosis and treatment for pediatric patients with melanoma are based on adult guidelines, with considerations for smaller margins or less aggressive therapy in specific cases. Precise classification of histologically indeterminate lesions will be based on molecular analyses.

PEDIATRIC DIFFERENTIATED THYROID CARCINOMA

Introduction

Differentiated thyroid cancer is the most common endocrine malignancy in children and adolescents.[1] Thyroid carcinoma is primarily identified in adolescent patients, with a female predominance of up to 6:1.[1] Over 90% of differentiated thyroid carcinomas (DTCs) are papillary thyroid carcinoma (PTC), while the rest are follicular thyroid carcinomas (FTCs).[1–3]

While most cases of DTC occur spontaneously, certain populations are predisposed to the development of thyroid carcinoma. Patients with a history of radiation exposure of 10 to 30 Gy are at increased risk for DTC by approximately 2% annually, starting 5 years after exposure.[2] Additionally, several syndromes and mutations are

[a] Center for Surgical Outcomes Research, Nationwide Children's Hospital, Columbus, OH, USA; [b] Division of Pediatric Surgery, Department of Surgery, University of Maryland School of Medicine, Baltimore, MD, USA; [c] Division of Pediatric Surgery, Yale School of Medicine, New Haven, CT, USA; [d] Division of Pediatric Surgery, Department of Surgery, Nationwide Children's Hospital, The Ohio State University College of Medicine, Columbus, OH, USA
* Corresponding author. Division of Pediatric Surgery, Nationwide Children's Hospital, FOB Suite 6B, Columbus, OH 43205.
E-mail address: Jennifer.aldrink@nationwidechildrens.org

Surg Oncol Clin N Am 35 (2026) 801–816
https://doi.org/10.1016/j.soc.2026.04.014 surgonc.theclinics.com

Abbreviations	
ACR TI-RADS	American College of Radiology's Thyroid Imaging Reporting and Data System
AJCC	American Joint Committee on Cancer
ATA	American Thyroid Association
CLND	completion lymph node dissection
DTC	differentiated thyroid carcinoma
FNA	fine needle aspiration
FTC	follicular thyroid carcinoma
HR	hazard ratio
PED TI-RADS	Pediatric Thyroid Imaging Reporting and Data System
PTC	papillary thyroid carcinoma
RAI	radioactive iodine ablation
SLNB	sentinel lymph node biopsy
TI-RADS	thyroid imaging reporting and data system
WLE	wide local excision

associated with DTC, including DICER1 syndrome, adenomatous polyposis coli (APC) syndrome (PTC only), Carney complex, Werner syndrome, and PTEN hamartoma syndrome.[1,2,4]

Clinical Presentation

DTC most commonly presents with the detection of a thyroid nodule either by palpation by a practitioner during a routine exam or by the patient/family. Thyroid nodules may present as a mass with or without lymphadenopathy. Most are asymptomatic; less frequently they present with mass-effect symptoms, such as dysphagia, ear/throat pain, or voice alteration.[2] Alternatively, patients with the diffuse sclerosing variant of PTC may present with diffuse enlargement of the thyroid without a discrete mass with ultrasound demonstrating diffuse microcalcifications (**Fig. 1**).[5] Firm, fixed, or large nodules on exam are concerning for malignancy, as are voice changes, which can suggest underlying vocal cord involvement.[1] Thyroid function tests are typically normal.[6]

Evaluation

Patients who present with thyroid nodules should have a thorough history and physical, with attention to family history, cancer predisposition syndromes, and exposure to prior ionizing radiation.[1,6] Laboratory testing should include a thyroid stimulating hormone (TSH), with confirmatory T3/T4 levels for derangements in TSH.[4,6] Ultrasound is the imaging of choice for thyroid evaluation and should include standardized image acquisition, including sweeps of the gland.

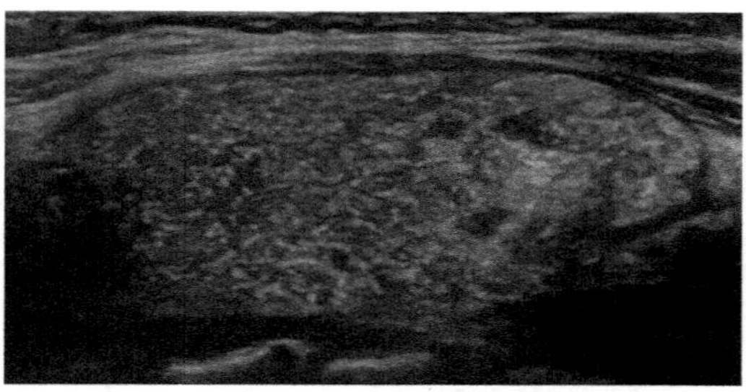

Fig. 1. Ultrasound demonstrating diffusely abnormal thyroid echotexture and innumerable microcalcifications.

Thyroid nodules

Thyroid nodules identified in pediatric patients carry a higher risk of malignancy (20%–25%) compared with adults (5%–15%).[1,2] Based on standardized adult practice, it is common for pediatric thyroid nodules identified on ultrasound to be routinely evaluated using the American College of Radiology's Thyroid Imaging Reporting and Data System (ACR TI-RADS)[7] for risk stratification and determination of the need for fine needle aspiration (FNA) biopsy (**Fig. 2**). This imaging system assesses 5 nodule characteristics: composition, echogenicity, margins, shape, and echogenic foci, with increasing numeric scores as an indication for FNA.[7] In general, nodules with hypoechogenicity, increased nodular vascularity, and microcalcifications are most suspicious for malignancy.[2]

In conjunction with nodule size, TI-RADS can identify nodules at risk for harboring malignancy and those that should undergo FNA. TI-RADS with a modified pediatric size criterion (PED TI-RADS) has been evaluated in multi-institutional pediatric studies and found to miss fewer malignancies and recommend fewer unnecessary FNAs than ACR TI-RADS or the American Thyroid Association (ATA) recommendations.[8] PED TI-RADS recommendations are summarized in **Table 1**.

Thyroid nodules that undergo FNA are evaluated using the Bethesda System for Reporting Thyroid Cytopathology (**Table 2**), which estimates malignancy risk based on cytopathologic features and can be used to guide management.[9] In general, pediatric patients have higher rates of malignancy in each Bethesda category than seen in adults.[3] Patients with Bethesda III (atypia/follicular lesion of undetermined significance) and IV (follicular neoplasm) nodules represent up to 35% of cytology results, with rates of underlying malignancy averaging 28% for Bethesda III and 50% for Bethesda IV lesions, presenting a diagnostic challenge for clinicians.[4] The 2015 ATA guidelines for pediatric thyroid nodules recommend thyroid lobectomy for Bethesda III and IV nodules, with completion thyroidectomy if the surgical pathology

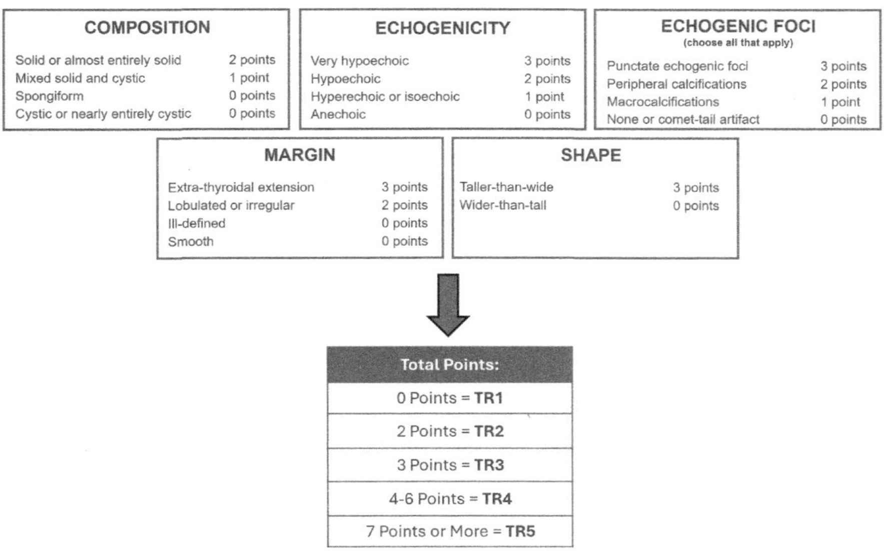

Fig. 2. ACR TI-RADS criteria. (*Data from* Tessler FN, Middleton WD, Grant EG, et al. ACR Thyroid Imaging, Reporting and Data System (TI-RADS): White Paper of the ACR TI-RADS Committee. J Am Coll Radiol 2017;14(5):587–595. https://doi.org/10.1016/j.jacr.2017.01.046.)

Table 1
Recommendations for fine needle aspiration by pediatric and American College of Radiology's Thyroid Imaging Reporting and Data System[7,8]

TI-RADS Score	ACR TI-RADS Recommendations	PED TI-RADS Recommendations
TR1 (Benign)	No FNA recommended	No FNA recommended
TR2 (Not Suspicious)	No FNA recommended	No FNA recommended
TR3 (Mildly Suspicious)	FNA if nodule ≥2.5 cm, Surveillance if nodule ≥1.5 cm	FNA if nodule ≥1.5 cm
TR4 (Moderately Suspicious)	FNA if nodule ≥1.5 cm, Surveillance if nodule ≥1.0 cm	FNA if nodule ≥1.0 cm
TR5 (Highly Suspicious)	FNA if nodule ≥1.0 cm, Surveillance if nodule ≥0.5 cm	FNA for nodule of any size

Data from Tessler FN, Middleton WD, Grant EG, et al. ACR Thyroid Imaging, Reporting and Data System (TI-RADS): White Paper of the ACR TI-RADS Committee. J Am Coll Radiol 2017;14(5):587–595. https://doi.org/10.1016/j.jacr.2017.01.046; and Srivatsa S, Al-Hadidi A, Stanek J, et al. Assessing the Diagnostic Accuracy of TI-RADS in Pediatric Thyroid Nodules: A Multi-institutional Review. J Pediatr Surg 2025;60(1):161924. https://doi.org/10.1016/j.jpedsurg.2024.161924.

demonstrates malignancy.[4] A recent consensus now recommends molecular testing be performed upfront to guide treatment decisions.[3]

Molecular testing

Genetic alterations in pediatric DTC are distinctly different from those of adults. Pediatric DTC molecular changes can be classified into 3 principal tiers: low-risk *RAS*-like mutants (including DICER and NRAS point mutations), intermediate-risk *BRAF*-mutants, and

Table 2
Bethesda classification and management recommendations in pediatric patients[2,3,9]

	Cytopathology	Management Recommendations	Malignancy Risk
Bethesda I	Nondiagnostic	Repeat FNA	1%–5%
Bethesda II	Benign	Ultrasound surveillance if <4 cm, if >4 cm perform lobectomy	0%–10%
Bethesda III	Atypia of undetermined significance or follicular lesion of undetermined significance	Molecular genetic testing: total thyroidectomy for BRAF or fusion mutation, lobectomy if these are absent	0%–44%
Bethesda IV	Follicular neoplasm	Molecular genetic testing: total thyroidectomy for BRAF or fusion mutation, lobectomy if these are absent	60%–71%
Bethesda V	Suspicious for malignancy	Total thyroidectomy ± central neck dissection	70%–86%
Bethesda VI	Malignant	Total thyroidectomy ± central neck dissection	97%–100%

Adapted from Christison-Lagay E, Baertschiger RM. Management of Differentiated Thyroid Carcinoma in Pediatric Patients. Surg Oncol Clin N Am 2021;30(2):235–251. https://doi.org/10.1016/j.soc.2020.11.013.

high-risk kinase, BRAF, and TERT promoter fusions.[10,11] In contrast to adults, where the *BRAF* V600E point mutation is seen in 40% to 60% of PTC diagnoses and associated with invasive disease, *BRAF* V600E is only seen in 20% to 40% of pediatric PTC, and typically in older adolescents.[10,12] There are also mixed data regarding its association with advanced disease, and this risk may differ by age groups, but *BRAF* V600E mutation is overall less aggressive in pediatric patients than in adults.[10,12,13] Finally, kinase fusions are found at a higher rate in pediatric DTC than adults (50% vs 15%) and most commonly involve *RET* and *NTRK* proto-oncogenes.[10,11] These kinase fusions are more common in younger pediatric patients, particularly those less than 10 years of age, and are associated with increased locoregional and distant metastases.[10]

While there have been significant advancements in molecular testing for pediatric DTC in recent years, somatic and germline testing for pediatric DTC is not yet universal.[14]

Burden of Disease

Evaluation for regional and metastatic disease

Advanced disease at presentation is common. As such, ultrasound imaging of both central and lateral cervical nodal basins should be obtained preoperatively to assess for radiographic evidence of lymph node metastases and to assist in surgical planning.[4] Up to 80% of pediatric PTCs may have metastatic spread into the lymph nodes of the central neck, although this spread may be micrometastatic and undetectable by physical exam or ultrasonography. The reported incidence of metastatic spread into the lateral neck varies widely, from approximately 25% to 70%, but is most often reported to be around 30% to 40%.[15,16] In patients with a high suspicion for locally advanced bulky disease, CT with contrast of the neck can be performed to assess the tumor's relation to relevant neurovascular structures.[2] Compared with adults, pediatric DTC patients more often have extrathyroidal extension, larger tumors, and regional nodal disease.[3,17–19]

Staging

Pediatric DTC is staged using the American Joint Committee on Cancer (AJCC) tumor, node, metastasis (TNM) classification system[20,21] and categorized as low-, intermediate-, or high-risk based on the ATA system. The ATA Risk Stratification system (**Table 3**) can be used to guide treatment, postoperative thyroid suppression levels, and surveillance imaging.[3,4,6]

Table 3
American Thyroid Association Risk Stratification of pediatric differentiated thyroid carcinoma[4]

Low-risk	Disease confined to the thyroid Incidentally identified micrometastatic disease in a small number of central (level VI) lymph nodes
Intermediate-risk	Extensive lymph node involvement in the central neck Minimal lymph node involvement in the lateral neck
High-risk	Macroscopic extrathyroidal extension Extensive lymph node involvement in the lateral neck unilaterally or bilaterally Distant metastatic disease

Data from Francis GL, Waguespack SG, Bauer AJ, et al. Management Guidelines for Children with Thyroid Nodules and Differentiated Thyroid Cancer. Thyroid 2015;25(7):716–59. https://doi.org/10.1089/thy.2014.0460.

Treatment

Surgical management of differentiated thyroid carcinoma

Surgical resection is the primary treatment. For many patients with PTC, total thyroidectomy is recommended over thyroid lobectomy.[4] PTC is associated with multifocal disease in up to 65% and bilateral disease in up to 30% of cases,[22,23] and as opposed to lobectomy, total thyroidectomy allows for the subsequent use of radioactive iodine for treatment and imaging, and serum thyroglobulin levels as a screening tool for recurrence.[3,4]

In general, compartment-based dissection for nodal disease is recommended.[3] Central neck dissection (cervical level VI) should be performed for all patients with evidence of central and/or lateral neck nodal metastases preoperatively.[4] The role of prophylactic central neck dissection for clinically negative nodes is contentious, as its risk reduction is modest and the risk of complications in nonexpert hands is high.[4,16] Patients with evidence of lateral compartment nodal disease (cervical levels II–V) should undergo modified radical neck dissection to improve disease-free survival.[3,4,16]

Patients with FTC often present with an indeterminate Bethesda score and undergo thyroid lobectomy, after which pathology reveals the ultimate diagnosis. Thyroid lobectomy is generally sufficient, unless the carcinoma is greater than 4 cm in size, has invasion of 4 or more blood vessels, or has known metastases for which total thyroidectomy is recommended.[4] As FTC spreads hematogenously and rarely presents with nodal metastases, lymphadenectomy is not indicated.[3]

Medical treatment of differentiated thyroid carcinoma

Radioactive iodine ablation (RAI) or ^{131}I is now selectively used based on degree of patient disease. In general, patients with small, localized disease without extensive nodal spread who are deemed low-risk by the ATA guidelines do not require ^{131}I. ^{131}I is recommended for patients with T3 disease or extensive nodal metastases as well as for those with known distant metastases or with low-volume residual unresectable cervical disease.[3,4] Patients with disease at intermediate risk for recurrence should be discussed in a multidisciplinary forum.

Despite excellent survival, less than 20% of DTC pulmonary metastases have complete remission following RAI, but the disease process is often indolent with no (or very slow) progression over decades.[14] Nonetheless, a small fraction of patients present with progressive metastases, highlighting the need for additional therapies.[14,24] An understanding of the molecular characteristics of each tumor is essential to guiding potential targeted therapies. Multitarget and selective tyrosine kinase inhibitors are increasingly prevalent and useful, particularly for patients with progressive or RAI-refractory disease, although not currently standard of care.[6,25] Selpercatinib, a *RET*-inhibitor, is Food and Drug Administration (FDA)-approved for use in pediatric metastatic medullary thyroid cancer and has shown to be effective in patients with *RET*-fused metastatic PTC.[25] Larotrectinib, an *NTRK*-inhibitor, has shown impact in treating a limited number of pediatric *NTRK*-fusion positive DTCs.[26]

Discussion

Complications of treatment

Complications of DTC management include bleeding, infection, nerve injury, hypocalcemia, and RAI complications.

Nerve injury, including recurrent laryngeal nerve (RLN) injury, is uncommon but can significantly impact quality of life. The rate of reported RLN injury in pediatrics varies in the literature from 1% to 23%,[27,28] but a recent 2025 systematic review found a 2%

rate of transient vocal cord palsy and 1% permanent paralysis.[28] Intraoperative RLN monitoring is increasingly used and while it does not replace the need for anatomic identification and preservation of the RLN, it facilitates recognition of a functional neuropraxia or injury and data have demonstrated it is associated with a reduced rate of vocal cord palsy in children.[29,30]

Postoperative hypocalcemia is common following total thyroidectomy as the parathyroid glands have a tenuous blood supply, closely aligned with the thyroid. The parathyroid glands are at greatest risk of devascularization or inadvertent removal with central lymph node dissection.[3] In the case of devascularization, autotransplantation at the time of surgery is recommended, but infrequently performed.[31] Reported postoperative hypocalcemia rates vary widely between 6% and 52%, with rates of permanent hypocalcemia reported between 3% and 8%.[28,32–34] One study found that children who received perioperative calcium and vitamin D supplementation had shorter length of stay and lower odds of postoperative hypocalcemia on multivariable analysis.[35] Another report found that preoperative calcitriol administration in pediatric patients undergoing partial and total thyroidectomy for Graves' disease resulted in fewer intravenous calcium supplementation requirements.[36]

Long term outcomes

Many children with DTC present with disease at intermediate or high risk for recurrence, and overall DTC recurrence is reported to be between 20% and 40%. Factors associated with recurrence include larger tumors, nodal involvement, extrathyroidal extension, lymphovascular invasion, and those with molecular fusions.[3,16,19] Despite this, pediatric DTC is associated with excellent long-term survival. Five-year survival rates approach 100%, even in patients with nodal metastases at 97.1%.[3,18,19,24]

MELANOMA IN CHILDREN AND ADOLESCENTS

Introduction

Melanoma ranks as the fifth most common adult malignancy, with nearly 105,000 estimated new US cases in 2025. Conversely melanoma in children accounts for only 300 to 400 cancer cases per year in the US population less than 20 years of age.[37] The overall incidence of 2.9 per million varies dramatically by age from infancy through adolescence and young adulthood (**Fig. 3**).

Similar to adults, pediatric melanoma is mostly sporadic and related to ultraviolet exposure. While only 1% to 2% of pediatric patients with melanoma are estimated to have germline mutations, 25% are suspected to have a pre-existing risk factor for melanoma,[38] including greater than 100 nevi with diameter greater than 2 mm, dysplastic nevus syndrome, congenital melanocytic nevi, xeroderma pigmentosa, immunodeficiency, prior malignancy, or radiation therapy.[39]

Diagnosis and Work-Up

Evidence suggests that the diagnosis of melanoma is frequently delayed in children, related to low incidence and atypical presentation. Over 60% of children less than 10 year old and 40% of children 11 to 19 year old do not meet traditional adult amelanotic, bleeding or bump, color uniformity, de novo and any diameter, and evolution (ABCDE) criteria for melanoma (asymmetry, border irregularity, color variegation, diameter >6 mm, and evolution). Accordingly some experts propose modified ABCDE criteria that should be included in the consideration of pediatric skin lesions.[40]

Biopsies for concerning skin lesions should follow adult principles.[41] Full thickness biopsies are required to guide further surgery with accurate Breslow depth, and can be

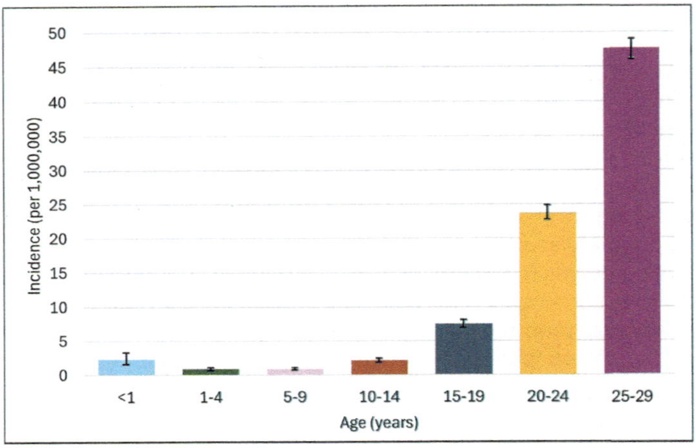

Fig. 3. Melanoma incidence by age (2018–2022 in the United States).

performed via punch, incisional, or excisional surgical biopsy. Shave biopsies should be avoided. Melanoma is staged using the AJCC TNM staging system.[42,43]

Pediatric melanomas are classified as conventional melanoma, melanoma within a congenital nevus, and spitzoid melanoma; however, treatment for these subtypes all follow adult melanoma guidelines. The distinction between atypical Spitz nevus, melanocytic tumors of uncertain malignant potential, and spitzoid melanoma continues to spark debate among dermatopathologists. There is a high rate of reclassification among these entities, with 35% of atypical Spitz nevi later reclassified as spitzoid melanoma,[44] demonstrating the need for specialized dermatopathologist evaluation and the potential for molecular testing to improve diagnostic reliability.[41]

Surgery

Wide local excision

Wide local excision (WLE) is the mainstay of treatment for melanoma, and pediatric melanoma resection follows adult National Comprehensive Cancer Network guidelines.[41] WLE should extend to the muscular fascia, but more aggressive resection involving fascia or muscle do not improve survival or reduce recurrence.[45] Appropriate WLE margins are defined for adults (**Table 4**), and multiple clinical trials have not demonstrated a benefit to margins greater than 2 cm.[46] These guidelines are based on trials excluding children, and retrospective studies indicate lower rates of local recurrence in children compared to adults[47]; therefore, pediatric specialists advocate for considering smaller margins when standard margins significantly impact cosmetic or functional outcomes.[48]

Sentinel lymph node biopsy

Sentinel lymph node biopsy (SLNB) involves injection of a tracing agent (frequently the radiotracer Tc-99) and subsequent lymphoscintigraphy to evaluate all potential nodal basins, as sentinel nodes may be in multiple basins. The radiotracer with or without an intradermal injection of blue dye (ie, methylene blue) or indocyanine green is used to locate one or more sentinel nodes for excision. In 20% of cases, clinically negative nodes will be positive for microscopic metastatic disease identified histologically in an SLN.[49] Compared to adults, children with melanoma have higher rates of lymph node sampling (37% vs 60%) and nodal positivity (23% vs 35%).[50] For patients

Table 4
Surgery recommendations based on Breslow depth

Breslow Depth	WLE Margin	SLNB
Melanoma in situ	0.5–1.0 cm	No
≤1.0 mm	1.0 cm	
<0.8 mm		
Without HRF		No
With HRF[a]		Consider
≥0.8 mm		Consider
>1.0 mm–2.0 mm	1.0–2.0 cm	Yes
>2.0 mm	2.0 cm	Yes

Abbreviation: HRF, high-risk features.
[a] HRF: ulceration, lymphovascular invasion, mitotic rate ≥2 per mm^2.

with clinically negative nodes, pediatric indications for SLNB are based on adult guidelines: (1) No SLNB for lesions less than 0.8 mm in depth without concerning features, (2) consideration of SLNB for lesions between 0.8 and 1.0 mm or less than 0.8 mm with concerning features (ulceration, lymphovascular invasion, or mitotic rate ≥2 per mm^2), and (3) routine SLNB for all lesions ≥1 mm.[41]

SLNB has both prognostic and therapeutic value, with trials of intermediate-thickness (1.2–3.5 mm) melanoma showing that positive SLNB confers a 2.5-fold increased hazard for both recurrence and death.[51] In this study, disease-free survival was improved in the SLNB group for both intermediate and thick melanoma.[51] Pediatric studies have also demonstrated the prognostic utility of SLNB, with 7-year melanoma-specific survival of 89% versus 100% in pediatric patients with melanoma with and without positive SLNB, respectively, but survival benefit has not been shown.[52]

Completion lymph node dissection

The value of completion lymph node dissection (CLND) is nuanced both in adults and children. While SLNB has a low reported rate of complication, with seroma and infection being the most common (6% and 5%), CLND rates for these complications are significantly higher (23% and 16%).[53] Rates of lymphedema are also higher following CLND (24% vs 6% in patients undergoing observation alone).[54] Trials comparing CLND to nodal observation after positive SLNB have failed to demonstrate survival benefit, although nodal recurrence is lower after CLND.[54] Adult guidelines recommend therapeutic lymph node dissection only in those patients with clinically positive nodal disease or positive SLNB that demonstrates high-risk features (extracapsular extension, >3 nodes involved, >2 nodal basins involved, and microsatellite disease of the primary tumor). In a study of 33 children with melanoma undergoing SLNB with a subgroup of 10 children undergoing subsequent CLND, authors found no survival advantage for CLND and suggested avoiding CLND in those without high-risk features (age ≥10 years, ulceration, mitotic activity >5 per mm^2, *TERT* promoter mutation).[55] A large, multicenter review including 252 patients with melanoma compared outcomes for those with a positive SLN who underwent CLND to those who underwent serial nodal ultrasound surveillance, and found no difference in recurrence or death from disease between the 2 groups.[56] Serial nodal ultrasound surveillance should be considered for carefully selected children with a low burden of nodal disease.

Systemic Therapy

Systemic therapy for advanced melanoma has progressed rapidly in recent years, providing neoadjuvant and adjuvant options even in lower stage or resectable disease that are important for the surgeon to understand.[41,57] Once standard therapy for high-risk melanoma, interferon alfa-2b and other cytotoxic agents have been replaced by monoclonal antibody checkpoint inhibitors and targeted therapies for BRAF/MEK inhibition (**Table 5**).[58]

Table 5
Systemic therapies in melanoma

Drug Name	Mechanism of Action/ Target	Current Recommended Uses
Monoclonal antibody checkpoint inhibitors		
Pembrolizumab	PD-1	Resected IIB/C, IIIB–IV *Neoadjuvant*: Resectable IIIB–IV Unresectable/metastatic
Nivolumab	PD-1	Resected IIB/C, IIIB–IV Unresectable/metastatic
Ipilimumab Combined with nivolumab	CTLA-4	Resected IV Unresectable/metastatic
Relatlimab Combined with nivolumab	LAG-3	Unresectable/metastatic
BRAF/MEK inhibitor combination therapies[a]		
Dabrafenib/Trametinib	BRAF inhibitor/MEK inhibitor	Resected IIIB–IV Unresectable/metastatic
Encorafenib/ Binimetinib	BRAF inhibitor/MEK inhibitor	Unresectable/metastatic
Vemurafenib/ Cobimetinib	BRAF inhibitor/MEK inhibitor	Unresectable/metastatic
Other therapies		
Talimogene laherparepvec	Viral oncolytic therapy	Unresectable/Injectable disease refusing preferred therapies
Imatinib	Targeted c-KIT inhibitor	
Interferon alfa-2b	Immunoregulatory cytokine	
Interleukin-2	Immunoregulatory cytokine	
Dacarbazine	Alkylating agent	
Temozolomide	Alkylating agent	
Paclitaxel	Microtubule inhibitor	
Carboplatin	Alkylating agent	

Abbreviations: CTLA-4, cytotoxic T-lymphocyte–associated protein 4; LAG-3, lymphocyte activation gene 3; PD-1, protein death protein 1.
[a] Therapies only available in melanoma with BRAF V600E or K mutation.

Immunotherapy with checkpoint inhibitors is now front-line therapy for melanoma Stage IIB and beyond, although BRAF/MEK inhibitors are also an option in patients with BRAF V600E/K mutations, underscoring the role of molecular testing in advanced disease.[41,57] BRAF/MEK inhibitors can only be recommended in patients with BRAF mutations V600E or K. BRAF mutations occur in 50% of adult melanoma.[59] While pediatric data are sparse, one study demonstrated a BRAF V600E mutation in 87% of pediatric melanoma.[60]

In resected stage IIB/C melanoma, a randomized trial of the monoclonal antibody protein death protein 1 inhibitor nivolumab demonstrated improved recurrence free survival (RFS) compared to placebo at 1 year (89% and 79%, respectively).[61] Pembrolizumab (also a protein death protein 1 inhibitor) showed similar results.

In patients with resected stage IIIA–IV, nivolumab and pembrolizumab are again recommended. Trials demonstrated improved RFS in pembrolizumab versus placebo (hazard ratio [HR]: 0.57)[62] and in nivolumab versus ipilimumab (HR: 0.51).[63] Ipilimumab is a monoclonal antibody inhibiting cytotoxic T-lymphocyte associated protein 4 and demonstrated improved RFS compared to placebo. In resected stage IIIA–IV melanoma with a BRAF mutation, the above agents can be used, but the BRAF/MEK inhibitor combination of dabrafenib and trametinib may also be considered. This therapy showed RFS improvement versus placebo (HR: 0.47),[63] and a meta-analysis showed comparable outcomes among the 3 regimens.[64]

In unresectable stage IV melanoma, a number of other therapies have been studied and can be tailored based on BRAF status (see **Table 5**). Finally, talimogene laherparepvec is a virus based oncolytic therapy that can be considered in patients not eligible for other therapies.[65]

Of special interest to the surgeon, neoadjuvant therapy in clinical and resectable stage IIIB–IV melanoma with pembrolizumab plus adjuvant therapy showed improved 2-year event-free survival over the adjuvant only arm (72% vs 49%), providing a tool for surgeons to consider before resecting these advanced stage lesions.[66]

While pediatric studies have demonstrated safety for several newer agents (NCT02124772),[67] we still lack pediatric efficacy data in melanoma. While adult guidance has been cautiously applied to the pediatric population, some experts have advocated for use of BRAF/MEK targeted inhibitors in pediatric patients with BRAF mutations due to the long-term complications of checkpoint inhibition, with greater than 40% of patients reporting chronic adverse events that persisted greater than 12 weeks after cessation of therapy.[68]

Outcomes

Overall, pediatric melanoma has excellent outcomes, with 5-year survival of 89% to 96%.[69] Pediatric melanoma outcomes vary by stage, with 10-year disease-free survival of 83%, 67%, and 63% stage I, II, and III, respectively.[69] Stage IV with distant metastatic disease is very rare, less than 3% of pediatric cases, and outcomes are unclear. While rates of node-positive disease were higher in children, it did not convey the same mortality risk as adults. In node-positive disease, children had a 6-year survival of 88% compared to 57% in adults.[50] Rates of thick melanoma (>1.5 mm Breslow depth) are higher in pediatric compared to young adult patients, 33% versus 26%; however, 5-year survival in pediatric patients was 92% to 94% regardless of thickness, while young adults had decreased 5-year survival from 97% in thin disease to 82% in thick disease.[70]

Data on recurrence in pediatric melanoma are limited, but reports indicate that a third of recurrences occur 5 years after diagnosis.[71] This highlights the need for long-term follow-up, with proposed regimens that include clinical and ultrasound follow-up every 4 to 6 months for 5 years and then annually.[55]

CLINICS CARE POINTS

- Thyroid nodules should be evaluated using modified pediatric TIRADS scoring, and fine needle aspiration biopsy should follow when appropriate.
- Molecular characterization of indeterminate thyroid nodules should be performed to determine appropriate surgical intervention.
- Children with melanoma may present with varying appearances of the lesion. Currently, adult guidelines are followed for wide local excision, sentinel lymph node biopsy, and completion lymph node dissection versus nodal surveillance. Further study is needed specific to pediatric melanoma.

DISCLOSURE

The authors have nothing to disclose.

REFERENCES

1. Paulson VA, Rudzinski ER, Hawkins DS. Thyroid cancer in the pediatric population. Genes 2019;10(9). https://doi.org/10.3390/genes10090723.
2. Christison-Lagay E, Baertschiger RM. Management of differentiated thyroid carcinoma in pediatric patients. Surg Oncol Clin N Am 2021;30(2):235–51.
3. Christison-Lagay ER, Baertschiger RM, Dinauer C, et al. Pediatric differentiated thyroid carcinoma: an update from the APSA Cancer Committee. J Pediatr Surg 2020;55(11):2273–83.
4. Francis GL, Waguespack SG, Bauer AJ, et al. Management guidelines for children with thyroid nodules and differentiated thyroid cancer. Thyroid 2015;25(7): 716–59.
5. Pillai S, Gopalan V, Smith RA, et al. Diffuse sclerosing variant of papillary thyroid carcinoma–an update of its clinicopathological features and molecular biology. Crit Rev Oncol Hematol 2015;94(1):64–73.
6. Prasad PK, Mahajan P, Hawkins DS, et al. Management of pediatric differentiated thyroid cancer: an overview for the pediatric oncologist. Pediatr Blood Cancer 2020;67(6):e28141.
7. Tessler FN, Middleton WD, Grant EG, et al. ACR Thyroid Imaging, reporting and data System (TI-RADS): white paper of the ACR TI-RADS Committee. J Am Coll Radiol 2017;14(5):587–95.
8. Srivatsa S, Al-Hadidi A, Stanek J, et al. Assessing the diagnostic accuracy of TI-RADS in pediatric thyroid nodules: a multi-institutional review. J Pediatr Surg 2025;60(1):161924.
9. Cibas ES, Ali SZ. The 2017 bethesda system for reporting thyroid cytopathology. Thyroid 2017;27(11):1341–6.
10. Yang AT, Lai ST, Laetsch TW, et al. Molecular landscape and therapeutic strategies in pediatric differentiated thyroid carcinoma. Endocr Rev 2025;46(3): 397–417.
11. Franco AT, Ricarte-Filho JC, Isaza A, et al. Fusion oncogenes are associated with increased metastatic capacity and persistent disease in pediatric thyroid cancers. J Clin Oncol 2022;40(10):1081–90.
12. Geng J, Wang H, Liu Y, et al. Correlation between BRAF (V600E) mutation and clinicopathological features in pediatric papillary thyroid carcinoma. Sci China Life Sci 2017;60(7):729–38.

13. Henke LE, Perkins SM, Pfeifer JD, et al. BRAF V600E mutational status in pediatric thyroid cancer. Pediatr Blood Cancer 2014;61(7):1168–72.
14. Mehrhoff C, Dagalakis U, Bauer AJ, et al. Navigating multidisciplinary care in pediatric thyroid carcinoma: insights from Children's Oncology Group sites. Pediatr Blood Cancer 2025;72(10):e31919.
15. Lin S, Zhong Y, Lin Y, et al. Prediction model for lateral lymph node metastasis of papillary thyroid carcinoma in children and adolescents based on ultrasound imaging and clinical features: a retrospective study. BMC Med Imaging 2024; 24(1):228.
16. Rubinstein JC, Herrick-Reynolds K, Dinauer C, et al. Recurrence and complications in pediatric and adolescent papillary thyroid cancer in a high-volume practice. J Surg Res 2020;249:58–66.
17. Gilja S, Kumar A, Londino AV 3rd, et al. Pathologic characteristics and surgical outcomes of pediatric versus adult well-differentiated thyroid cancer. Otolaryngol Head Neck Surg 2024;171(6):1682–9.
18. Durante C, Haddy N, Baudin E, et al. Long-term outcome of 444 patients with distant metastases from papillary and follicular thyroid carcinoma: benefits and limits of radioiodine therapy. J Clin Endocrinol Metab 2006;91(8):2892–9.
19. Hay ID, Gonzalez-Losada T, Reinalda MS, et al. Long-term outcome in 215 children and adolescents with papillary thyroid cancer treated during 1940 through 2008. World J Surg 2010;34(6):1192–202.
20. Tuttle RM, Haugen B, Perrier ND. Updated American Joint Committee on Cancer/Tumor-Node-Metastasis Staging System for differentiated and anaplastic thyroid cancer (eighth edition): what changed and why? Thyroid 2017;27(6):751–6.
21.. Tuttle RM, Haugen BR, Perrier ND. Differentiated thyroid cancer. In: Amin MB, Edge SB, Greene FL, et al, editors. AJCC cancer staging manual. 8th edition. Cham, Switzerland: Springer International Publishing; 2017. p. 873–90.
22. Jarzab B, Handkiewicz Junak D, Włoch J, et al. Multivariate analysis of prognostic factors for differentiated thyroid carcinoma in children. Eur J Nucl Med 2000; 27(7):833–41.
23. Grigsby PW, Gal-or A, Michalski JM, et al. Childhood and adolescent thyroid carcinoma. Cancer 2002;95(4):724–9.
24. Sugino K, Nagahama M, Kitagawa W, et al. Distant metastasis in pediatric and adolescent differentiated thyroid cancer: clinical outcomes and risk factor analyses. J Clin Endocrinol Metab 2020;105(11). https://doi.org/10.1210/clinem/dgaa545.
25.. Potter SL, Rainusso N, Sher AC, et al. Selpercatinib increases radioactive iodine avidity in RET-fusion pediatric thyroid carcinoma. Pediatrics 2025;156(6): e2024070336. https://doi.org/10.1542/peds.2024-070336.
26. Waguespack SG, Drilon A, Lin JJ, et al. Efficacy and safety of larotrectinib in patients with TRK fusion-positive thyroid carcinoma. Eur J Endocrinol 2022;186(6): 631–43.
27. Olson SL, Ingram ME, Graffy PM, et al. Effect of surgeon volume on pediatric thyroid surgery outcomes: a systematic review. J Pediatr Surg 2022;57(9):208–15.
28. Roy R, Babu A, Song Z, et al. Outcomes in pediatric thyroid surgery across multiple institutions. J Surg Res 2025;312:55–67.
29. Rich BS, Brown EG, Rothstein DH, et al. The utility of intraoperative neuromonitoring in pediatric surgical oncology. J Pediatr Surg 2023;58(9):1708–14.
30. Yeung F, Wong KP, Lang BH, et al. Paediatric thyroidectomy: when and why? A 25-year institutional experience. J Pediatr Surg 2022;57(7):1196–200.

31. Ramos-Gonzalez GJ, Canas JA, Green A, et al. Predictors, trends, and outcomes of parathyroid autotransplantation in pediatric total thyroidectomy. J Surg Res 2025;306:26–32.
32. Wu SY, Chiang YJ, Fisher SB, et al. Risks of hypoparathyroidism after total thyroidectomy in children: a 21-Year experience in a high-volume cancer center. World J Surg 2020;44(2):442–51.
33. Overman RE Jr, Hsieh LB, Menon R, et al. 4-Hour postoperative PTH level predicts hypocalcemia after thyroidectomy in children. J Pediatr Surg 2020;55(7): 1265–9.
34. Nordenström E, Bergenfelz A, Almquist M. Permanent hypoparathyroidism after total thyroidectomy in children: results from a national registry. World J Surg 2018;42(9):2858–63.
35. Banks L, Kelly NA, Onwuka A, et al. Does preoperative calcium and 1, 25 OH vitamin D supplementation impact postoperative hypocalcemia and length of stay following pediatric thyroidectomy? Int J Pediatr Otorhinolaryngol 2024;178: 111895.
36. Breuer CK, Solomon D, Donovan P, et al. Effect of patient age on surgical outcomes for graves' disease: a case-control study of 100 consecutive patients at a high volume thyroid surgical center. Int J Pediatr Endocrinol 2013;2013(1):1.
37. Board PDQPTE. Childhood melanoma treatment (PDQ®): health professional version. *PDQ cancer information summaries*. Bethesda (MD): National Cancer Institute; 2025.
38. Pappo AS. Melanoma in children and adolescents. Eur J Cancer 2003;39(18): 2651–61.
39. Aldrink JH, Polites S, Lautz TB, et al. What's new in pediatric melanoma: an update from the APSA cancer committee. J Pediatr Surg 2020;55(9):1714–21.
40. Cordoro KM, Gupta D, Frieden IJ, et al. Pediatric melanoma: results of a large cohort study and proposal for modified ABCD detection criteria for children. J Am Acad Dermatol 2013;68(6):913–25.
41. NCCN Guidelines Version 2.2025: Melanoma: cutaneous. 2025. Available at: https://www.nccn.org/professionals/physician_gls/pdf/cutaneous_melanoma.pdf.
42. Gershenwald JE, Scolyer RA, Hess KR, et al. Melanoma staging: evidence-based changes in the American Joint Committee on Cancer eighth edition cancer staging manual. CA Cancer J Clin 2017;67(6):472–92.
43. Gershenwald JE, Scolyer RA, Hess KR, et al. Cutaneous melanoma. In: Amin MB, Edge SB, Greene FL, et al, editors. AJCC cancer staging manual. 8th edition. Cham, Switzerland: Springer International Publishing; 2017. p. 563–85.
44. Massi D, Tomasini C, Senetta R, et al. Atypical spitz tumors in patients younger than 18 years. J Am Acad Dermatol 2015;72(1):37–46.
45. Kenady DE, Brown BW, McBride CM. Excision of underlying fascia with a primary malignant melanoma: effect on recurrence and survival rates. Surgery 1982; 92(4):615–8.
46. Thomas JM, Newton-Bishop J, A'Hern R, et al. Excision margins in high-risk malignant melanoma. N Engl J Med 2004;350(8):757–66.
47. Aldrink JH, Selim MA, Diesen DL, et al. Pediatric melanoma: a single-institution experience of 150 patients. J Pediatr Surg 2009;44(8):1514–21.
48. Basta AV, Fritz CD, Chiang Y-J, et al. The impact of surgical margin in wide local excision of pediatric Melanoma–An argument for a more conservative approach. J Pediatr Surg 2025;60(1):161897.
49. Morton DL, Thompson JF, Cochran AJ, et al. Sentinel-node biopsy or nodal observation in melanoma. N Engl J Med 2006;355(13):1307–17.

50. Lautz TB, Fahy AS, Helenowski I, et al. Higher rates of regional disease but improved outcomes in pediatric versus adult melanoma. J Pediatr Surg 2022;57-(10):425–9.
51. Morton DL, Thompson JF, Cochran AJ, et al. Final trial report of sentinel-node biopsy versus nodal observation in melanoma. N Engl J Med 2014;370(7):599–609.
52. Kim J, Sun Z, Gulack BC, et al. Sentinel lymph node biopsy is a prognostic measure in pediatric melanoma. J Pediatr Surg 2016;51(6):986–90.
53. Morton DL, Cochran AJ, Thompson JF, et al. Sentinel node biopsy for early-stage melanoma: accuracy and morbidity in MSLT-I, an international multicenter trial. Ann Surg 2005;242(3):302–11 [discussion: 311–3].
54. Faries MB, Thompson JF, Cochran AJ, et al. Completion dissection or observation for sentinel-node metastasis in melanoma. N Engl J Med 2017;376-(23):2211–22.
55. Sutthatarn P, Davidoff AM, Bahrami A, et al. Regional lymph node evaluation in pediatric conventional melanoma subtype: a single-center 10-year review. Pediatr Surg Int 2024;40(1):68.
56. Scoville SD, Stanek JR, Rinehardt H, et al. Comparison of outcomes between surveillance ultrasound and completion lymph node dissection in children and adolescents with sentinel lymph node-positive cutaneous melanoma. Ann Surg 2024;279(3):536–41.
57. Seth R, Agarwala SS, Messersmith H, et al. Systemic Therapy for melanoma: ASCO guideline update. J Clin Oncol 2023;41(30):4794–820.
58. Kirkwood JM, Manola J, Ibrahim J, et al, Eastern Cooperative Oncology Group. A pooled analysis of eastern cooperative oncology group and intergroup trials of adjuvant high-dose interferon for melanoma. Clin Cancer Res 2004;10(5):1670–7.
59. Ascierto PA, Kirkwood JM, Grob JJ, et al. The role of BRAF V600 mutation in melanoma. J Transl Med 2012;10:85.
60. Lu C, Zhang J, Nagahawatte P, et al. The genomic landscape of childhood and adolescent melanoma. J Invest Dermatol 2015;135(3):816–23.
61. Kirkwood JM, Del Vecchio M, Weber J, et al. Adjuvant nivolumab in resected stage IIB/C melanoma: primary results from the randomized, phase 3 CheckMate 76K trial. Nat Med 2023;29(11):2835–43.
62. Eggermont AMM, Blank CU, Mandala M, et al. Adjuvant pembrolizumab versus placebo in resected stage III melanoma. N Engl J Med 2018;378-(19):1789–801.
63. Long GV, Hauschild A, Santinami M, et al. Adjuvant dabrafenib plus trametinib in stage III BRAF-mutated melanoma. N Engl J Med 2017;377(19):1813–23.
64. Sharma R, Koruth R, Kanters S, et al. Comparative efficacy and safety of dabrafenib in combination with trametinib versus competing adjuvant therapies for high-risk melanoma. J Comp Eff Res 2019;8(16):1349–63.
65. Andtbacka RH, Kaufman HL, Collichio F, et al. Talimogene laherparepvec improves durable response rate in patients with advanced melanoma. J Clin Oncol 2015;33(25):2780–8.
66. Patel SP, Othus M, Chen Y, et al. Neoadjuvant-adjuvant or adjuvant-only pembrolizumab in advanced melanoma. N Engl J Med 2023;388(9):813–23.
67. Geoerger B, Kang HJ, Yalon-Oren M, et al. Pembrolizumab in paediatric patients with advanced melanoma or a PD-L1-positive, advanced, relapsed, or refractory solid tumour or lymphoma (KEYNOTE-051): interim analysis of an open-label, single-arm, phase 1-2 trial. Lancet Oncol 2020;21(1):121–33.

68. Corley EA, Schmitt AM, Furness AJ, et al. The role of systemic therapy in paediatric cutaneous melanoma: a review. Pediatr Med 2023;6:37.
69. Averbook BJ, Lee SJ, Delman KA, et al. Pediatric melanoma: analysis of an international registry. Cancer 2013;119(22):4012–9.
70. Lange JR, Palis BE, Chang DC, et al. Melanoma in children and teenagers: an analysis of patients from the National Cancer Data Base. J Clin Oncol 2007;25-(11):1363–8.
71. Ipenburg NA, Lo SN, Vilain RE, et al. The prognostic value of tumor mitotic rate in children and adolescents with cutaneous melanoma: a retrospective cohort study. J Am Acad Dermatol 2020;82(4):910–9.

Rare Tumors: Part Two

Erica C. Arnold, MD[a], Josélio Rodrigues de Oliveira Filho, MD[b], Danielle B. Cameron, MD, MPH[b], Sara A. Mansfield, MD, MS[c,*]

KEYWORDS

- Adrenocortical carcinoma • Pediatric ACC • Adolescent and young adult
- Pediatric colorectal carcinoma • Rare tumor

KEY POINTS

- Patients who present with signs of excess hormone production should be evaluated for a potential underlying adrenocortical carcinoma.
- The role for minimally invasive surgery and retroperitoneal lymph node dissection in pediatric adrenocortical carcinoma continues to evolve.
- Colorectal cancer in children and adolescents demonstrates distinct biological features compared to typical adult-onset colorectal cancer and is associated with worse prognosis and overall survival.
- Pediatric patients with persistent gastrointestinal symptoms should be evaluated for colorectal cancer to prevent a delay in diagnosis and worse prognosis.

PEDIATRIC ADRENOCORTICAL CARCINOMA

Introduction

Adrenocortical carcinoma (ACC) is rare in children, making up less than .2% of all pediatric malignancies.[1,2] ACC incidence peaks between 0 and 4 years of age, with another smaller bimodal distribution after age 10.[3] There is a 2:1 ratio of females versus males.[3,4] Pediatric ACC is frequently associated with Li-Fraumeni syndrome (*TP53* mutation), which is present in 50% to 80% of cases, and *IGF2* overexpression with Beckwith-Wiedemann syndrome.[5,6] ACC incidence in children is notably higher in Brazil due to the presence of the *TP53* p.R337H mutation.[1,7] Less common associations include multiple endocrine neoplasia (1.4%), hereditary nonpolyposis colorectal cancer (3%), familial adenomatous polyposis (FAP) (<1%), neurofibromatosis 1 (<1%), and Carney complex (<1%).[8]

[a] Center for Surgical Outcomes Research, Nationwide Children's Hospital, Columbus, OH, USA; [b] Division of Pediatric Surgery, Department of Surgery, Harvard Medical School, Massachusetts General Brigham, Boston, MA, USA; [c] Division of Pediatric Surgery, Nationwide Children's Hospital, Department of Surgery, The Ohio State University College of Medicine, Columbus, OH, USA

* Corresponding author. Nationwide Children's Hospital, 700 Children's Drive, Columbus, OH 43205.

E-mail address: Sara.mansfield@nationwidechildrens.org

Surg Oncol Clin N Am 35 (2026) 817–830
https://doi.org/10.1016/j.soc.2026.04.013 **surgonc.theclinics.com**

Abbreviations	
ACC	adrenocortical carcinoma
AYA	adolescent and young adult
COG	Children's Oncology Group
CRC	colorectal cancer
CRS-HIPEC	cytoreductive surgery combined with hyperthermic intraperitoneal chemotherapy
EFO	event-free survival
ENSAT	European Network for the Study of Adrenal Tumors
FAP	familial adenomatous polyposis
MIS	minimally invasive surgery
OS	overall survival
PSORC	Pediatric Surgical Oncology Research Collaborative
RPLND	retroperitoneal lymph node dissection
TME	total mesorectal excision

Table 1
Symptoms and hormone derangements in pediatric adrenocortical carcinoma[1,10]

Excess Hormone Secretion	Frequency of Presentation	Signs/Symptoms	Laboratory Studies
Virilization: Sex steroids/steroid precursors	80%	Precocious puberty Clitoromegaly Pubic hair development Hirsutism Muscle hypertrophy Acne Penis enlargement Voice changes	Elevated DHEA Elevated androstenedione Elevated 17-hydroxyprogesterone Elevated urinary steroid
Cushing Syndrome: Glucocorticoids	15%–40%	Growth failure Weight gain Facial plethora Abdominal striae Muscle weakness Menstrual changes	Suppressed ACTH Elevated salivary cortisol Elevated 24-h urinary cortisol Elevated urinary steroids Elevated salivary cortisol Suppressed ACTH on low-dose dexamethasone suppression test
Feminization: Estrogen	1%–7%	Gynecomastia (males only) Pseudoprecocious puberty in females	Elevated estradiol Elevated urinary steroid
Conn Syndrome: Mineralocorticoids	1%–4%	Hypertension Polyuria Headache	Elevated aldosterone Decreased renin Elevated aldosterone/renin ratio Hypernatremia Hypokalemia

Abbreviations: ACTH, adrenocorticotropic hormone; DHEA, dehydroepiandrosterone.

Clinical Presentation

Pediatric ACCs are functional in up to 95% of cases (compared with 50% in adult ACC) and most commonly present with symptoms of excess hormone production (**Table 1**).[3] Symptoms of hormone excess may differ by age, puberty status, and gender. Children most commonly present with virilization with or without hypercortisolism (~80%), followed by Cushing syndrome (15%–40%).[3,7–9] Around 10% of pediatric ACCs are nonfunctional and usually present in adolescents.[3] Other potential presentations of ACC include abdominal pain, weight loss, or, rarely, an acute abdomen due to tumor rupture.[8,10]

Evaluation

Laboratory testing

In patients presenting with symptoms of excess hormone secretion, a targeted workup and laboratory testing toward the hormones of interest should be performed (see **Table 1**).[1,7,10] Renal function should also be assessed in case of the need for concurrent nephrectomy.

Imaging

Ultrasound may be used for screening, but computed tomography (CT) or MRI adrenal protocol is necessary for definitive diagnosis of an adrenal tumor. Given the high incidence of *TP53* mutations in this population, MRI is often used to limit ionizing radiation.[8,10] Imaging findings concerning for malignancy include size greater than 4 cm, irregular borders, heterogeneous appearance, low lipid content, and the presence of necrosis or calcifications. Additionally, MRI T2 signal of the adrenal tumor twice that of the liver, and CT findings of a tumor density greater than 10 Hounsfield Units and delayed washout of contrast less than 50% after 10 minutes are worrisome for malignancy (**Fig. 1**).[10]

CT chest should be obtained in addition to fluorodeoxyglucose positron emission tomography (FDG-PET) to assess for distant metastases. FDG-PET is also useful for primary tumor assessment, as ACC exhibits higher uptake compared to a benign adrenal adenoma.[10] ACC most commonly metastasizes to the lungs and liver, with the central nervous system and bones being involved less frequently.[8] All patients with a *TP53*

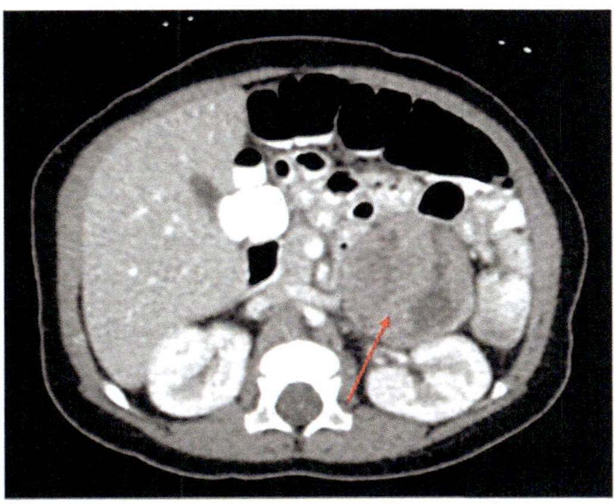

Fig. 1. Left adrenocortical tumor (*red arrow*) on CT abdomen/pelvis with heterogeneous appearance and tumor necrosis.

mutation require an MRI brain to assess for underlying brain malignancy.[11] Localized tumors should not be biopsied to avoid the risk of tumor rupture and seeding.[2,12]

Burden of Disease

Histopathology

The diagnosis of ACC remains challenging. Many histopathologic assessment scales have been developed to differentiate benign adenomas from ACC, including the Weiss and Wienecke classification systems as well as the Five-Item microscopic score and the modified reticulin algorithm (**Table 2**).[13–16] Histopathologic factors that are independently concerning for malignancy include greater than 15 mitoses/20 high-power field and tumor necrosis.[13] Ki-67 index greater than 15% is associated with poorer prognosis.[3,17] Genetic alterations most commonly identified in pediatric ACC are *TP53* mutations, *IGF2* overexpression, *ATRX* variants, and *CTNNB1* variants.[6,17] Combined *TP53* mutation and *ATRX* variants are associated with poor prognosis.[6,7]

Table 2
Histopathologic assessment scales for pediatric adrenocortical carcinoma

Assessment Scale	Criteria Considered	Scoring Determination
Weiss Criteria[14]	High nuclear grade >5 mitosis/50 HPF Abnormal mitoses Clear cells: <25% Diffuse architecture: >33% Tumor necrosis Venous invasion Sinusoid invasion Capsular invasion	*<3 criteria = benign* *3 criteria = indeterminate* *>3 criteria = malignant*
Wieneke Criteria[13,16]	Tumor >400 g Tumor >10.5 cm Tumor extending into periadrenal soft tissue or surrounding organs Vena cava invasion Capsular invasion Venous invasion with vascular venous emboli within the tumor capsule Tumor necrosis >15 mitosis/20 HPF Atypical mitotic features present	*≥4 criteria = malignant*
Modified reticulin algorithm[15]	Reticulin Disruption Tumor necrosis >15 mitoses/20 HPF Venous invasion	*Positive reticulin disruption with ≥1 criteria = malignant*
Five-Item microscopic score[16]	Adrenal capsular invasion Venous invasion Tumor necrosis >15 mitoses/20 HPF Ki-67 >15%	*≤2 criteria = favorable histology* *>2 criteria = unfavorable histology (Used for COG Stage II and III tumors only)*

Abbreviation: HPF, high power field.

Data from Mansfield SA, De Corti F, Aldrink JH, et al. Rare tumors II: Adrenocortical tumors, neuroendocrine tumors of the appendix, pheochromocytoma and paraganglioma, pancreatoblastoma and solid pseudopapillary tumors of the pancreas. Pediatr Blood Cancer. 2025;72 Suppl 2:e31207. https://doi.org/10.1002/pbc.31207.

Staging

There are a variety of staging classification algorithms that exist for ACC, including the European Network for the Study of Adrenal Tumors (ENSAT), Children's Oncology Group (COG), and the Sandrini systems (**Table 3**).[5,9,18,19] The most frequently used is the ENSAT Staging System.

Treatment

Surgical treatment

Given the rarity and limited trial data, pediatric ACC management is derived from that of adults. The mainstay of treatment is surgery with the goal of an R0 resection, either via an abdominal or thoracoabdominal approach.[6,9,10] Inadequate resection is associated with poor outcomes and reduced survival.[2–4,9] Tumor invasion may require en bloc resection of surrounding organs, most frequently nephrectomy. Tumor infiltration of the inferior vena cava (IVC) and/or tumor thrombus extending into the suprahepatic IVC may require intraoperative cardiopulmonary bypass.[1,9] Additionally, perioperative steroid supplementation should be anticipated, as functional tumors often have contralateral adrenal gland suppression.[10,20]

ACC has a high risk of tumor rupture, for which minimally invasive surgery (MIS) has historically been avoided in adults.[21] However, even with open surgery, the rate of

Table 3
Pediatric adrenocortical carcinoma staging classification systems

COG Staging[5]	
I	Entirely resected, small tumor (<200 cm^3 and <100 g) with normal postoperative hormone values
II	Entirely resected, large tumors (≥200 cm^3 and ≥100 g) with normal postoperative hormone values
III	Retroperitoneal lymph node involvement Tumor spillage in otherwise Stage I/II tumors with failure to reach normal hormone levels postoperatively Unresectable, microscopic, or gross residual disease
IV	Distant metastatic disease
ENSAT Staging[9,18]	
I	Tumor ≤ 5 cm, confined to adrenal gland
II	Tumor > 5 cm or gross tumor extension locally without nodal or distant disease
III	Regional lymph node disease or unresectable local tumor extension
IV[a]	Distant metastatic disease
Sandrini Staging[19]	
I	Completed excised tumor <200 cm^3, normal hormone levels postoperatively, no metastases
II	Residual microscopic tumor, tumor >200 cm^3, tumor spillage intraoperatively, or elevated hormone levels postoperatively
III	Gross residual tumor or unresectable tumor
IV	Distant metastatic disease

[a] Modified ENSAT with Stage IVa = 2 involved organs, IVb = 3 involved organs, IVc >3 involved organs.

tumor rupture is around 22%.[9,10] A multi-institutional study through the Pediatric Surgical Oncology Research Collaborative (PSORC) found that for 17 stage I or II lesions resected via MIS, there were no instances of tumor spillage.[9] The tumors resected via MIS approach were generally smaller (4.4 cm vs 9.6 cm, $P<.01$) and did not undergo lymphadenectomy. Importantly, MIS patients had equivalent long-term outcomes as those who underwent open surgery in this very limited sample. These data suggest that MIS may be safe for certain patients with small stage I or II ACC in the appropriate clinical scenarios.[9]

Retroperitoneal lymph node dissection (RPLND) remains controversial. In adults, RPLND has shown oncologic benefit; however, there are limited pediatric data.[22] The COG ARAR0332 protocol demonstrated that for stage 1 disease, primary tumor excision alone can be curative, and for stage II when RPLND was recommended, there was overall poor compliance and low lymph node yield.[5,9] They also found no improvement in event-free survival (EFS) with RPLND in stage ≥II, although this may have been confounded by compliance and yield.[5] A recent PSORC study also found that only 15.9% of patients underwent RPLND, with another 24.6% undergoing some level of lymph node sampling.[9] Similarly, RPLND was not associated with a significant difference in EFS in their cohort.[9] Further research is needed on this topic.

Medical treatment

COG ARAR0332 evaluated the use of combined mitotane/chemotherapy treatment.[5] Stage III and IV patients received 8 cycles of chemotherapy (cisplatin, etoposide, and doxorubicin) and mitotane for 8 months, and potential surgical intervention based on the treatment team's discretion.[5] They identified that stage III patients responded well to chemotherapy and mitotane with a 5-year EFS of 81% and overall survival (OS) of 94.7%.[5] The OS for stage IV disease in ARAR0332 remained poor at 15.6%.[5] German Society for Paediatric Oncology and Haematology (GPOH-97) evaluated the use of vincristine, ifosfamide, adriamycin, carboplatin, and etoposide, with around half of the cohort also receiving mitotane.[23] Those who received mitotane had a significantly better survival than those who received chemotherapy alone.[7,23]

Mitotane is often poorly tolerated as it inhibits steroidogenesis and induces atrophy of the adrenal cortex, which can be associated with endocrine dysfunction and gastrointestinal side effects, as well as speech and motor development delays in children.[1,5,6,8] Mitotane requires blood level monitoring to maintain adequate treatment levels.[6] Adjuvant therapy is indicated for patients with metastatic disease, inadequate surgical resection, and tumor spillage.[1,23] Radiation therapy is not routinely used and should be avoided in those with *TP53* mutations.[1,6]

While immunotherapy is currently being studied in adult ACC, there are limited pediatric data. One pediatric study looking at pembrolizumab, a PD-1 inhibitor, in a variety of solid tumors did show a partial response in 2 of 4 ACC patients included in the study.[24] Further study of targeted therapies and inclusion of pediatric patients is needed.

Discussion

Long-term survival and surveillance

Five-year survival of pediatric ACC patients is around 50% to 70% overall, with those with metastatic disease having 5-year OS less than 20%.[2–4,9] Factors associated with improved survival include stage I disease, smaller tumor size, and age 0 to 3 at diagnosis.[3,4,12] Surveillance imaging and laboratory testing frequency are guided by risk factors.[1]

Future directions

Further research developing targeted therapies and effective treatment regimens for pediatric ACC is critical. Pediatric ACC exhibits different histologic and molecular characteristics than those of adult ACC, highlighting the need for individualized study of pediatric ACC rather than extrapolation of adult ACC data.[9] International data and trial collaboration will be critical for this rare disease.[6]

SUMMARY

Pediatric ACC is rare, with outcomes dependent on the extent of disease. Early diagnosis, younger age, and early stage are associated with improved outcomes. Surgical resection is the mainstay of treatment, with the need for complete tumor resection for the best outcomes. Chemotherapy in conjunction with mitotane is used for advanced disease but is poorly tolerated. Further research is necessary to identify superior treatment regimens for patients with unresectable and metastatic disease to improve survival.

COLORECTAL CANCER IN CHILDREN AND ADOLESCENTS

Introduction

Colorectal cancer (CRC) is exceedingly rare in children and adolescents, with an incidence of roughly 1 to 2 per million per year in individuals under 20 year old.[25] Historically, CRC has been considered a disease affecting adults; however, in recent years, there has been a significant increase in early-onset cases.[26] While early-onset CRC is typically defined in patients younger than 50 years old, adolescent patients represent a unique cohort which should be considered separately.

Pediatric and adolescent CRC often arises sporadically, although there is a subset of patients with underlying genetic cancer predisposition syndromes (eg, FAP or Lynch syndrome). A positive family history of colorectal carcinoma may be identified in about 30% of cases[27] and an underlying genetic tumor risk syndrome can be confirmed in up to 39% of cases.[27,28] There are distinct biological features compared to the typical adult-onset CRC. Pediatric CRCs are more likely to be poorly differentiated, locally advanced at diagnosis and to have mucinous or signet-ring cell histology.[29–31] This more aggressive tumor biology may contribute to the worse outcomes observed in some studies with young patients.[31,32]

Current guidelines for hereditary gastrointestinal cancer recommend germline, mismatch repair deficiency (MMR), and microsatellite instability (MSI) tumor testing for all individuals diagnosed with CRC before age 50, multiple primary malignancies, or a strong family history.[33,34] For surgeons, this information has immediate consequences: patients with FAP, *MUTYH*-associated polyposis, or other adenomatous polyposis syndromes often benefit from subtotal colectomy or proctocolectomy in adolescence or young adulthood, with timing individualized to symptoms and polyp burden, while those with Lynch syndrome should at least be counseled on the option of total colectomy with ileorectal anastomosis given the high lifetime risk of metachronous CRC.[34] However, extensive surgery has not provided a clear survival benefit in patients with Lynch syndrome.[33,35] Identifying a germline mutation also prompts cascade testing and surveillance of at-risk relatives, extending the impact of surgical decision-making beyond the just the patient.

Biology and Histopathology

Pediatric and adolescent CRCs differ markedly from *typical* late-onset adult tumors in both histology and stage at diagnosis.[36] Multiple series have shown that children and adolescents are more likely to be diagnosed with mucinous adenocarcinoma or signet-ring cell carcinoma, with estimates of these *unfavorable* subtypes approaching 40% in some pediatric series, compared with roughly 10% to 15% mucinous and less than 1% signet-ring histology in adult patients.[30,32,37] These tumors are more often poorly differentiated, deeply invasive, and node-positive at presentation.[29,30] Adolescents are more likely to present with peritoneal carcinomatosis,[31] consistent with the known behavior of mucinous and signet-ring cancers.

Presentation and Diagnosis

Children and adolescents with colorectal cancer often present with nonspecific symptoms that overlap with benign gastrointestinal disorders, contributing to diagnostic delays.[37] Abdominal pain, change in bowel habits, rectal bleeding, or weight loss may be initially attributed to more common pediatric conditions (eg, constipation, inflammatory bowel disease, or gastroenteritis).[38] In a population-based analysis of malignant lower gastrointestinal tract tumors in patients less than 20 years, the majority occurred in older adolescents (78.9% age >15 years).[39] In contrast, prepubertal CRC is less frequent, and when it occurs clinicians should have heightened suspicion for an underlying predisposing condition.[38] As a result, the diagnosis of CRC in the young is frequently made at a later stage. In a retrospective analysis of early-onset CRC patients, 70% of those under 25 were diagnosed at stage III or IV, whereas older adults are more commonly diagnosed at stage I or II.[29] The vast majority of patients presented with either locally advanced or metastatic disease.[32,38]

Given this pattern of presentation, thorough evaluation is critical when young patients present with persistent gastrointestinal symptoms. Although CRC is rare in young patients, clinicians should maintain a high index of suspicion given the rise in early-onset cancers and delays in diagnosis can significantly worsen prognosis. Diagnostic workup should include a complete colonoscopic evaluation with biopsy of any suspicious lesions, as well as cross-sectional imaging (eg, abdominal/pelvic MRI or CT) (**Fig. 2**A, B) for staging. Once diagnosed, tumors are staged according to the tumor-node-metastasis (TNM) classification used in adults, which guides subsequent therapy.[40]

Surgical Treatment

Surgical resection remains the cornerstone of curative-intent treatment for colorectal cancer in pediatric, adolescent, and young adult patients.[39] Given the rarity of

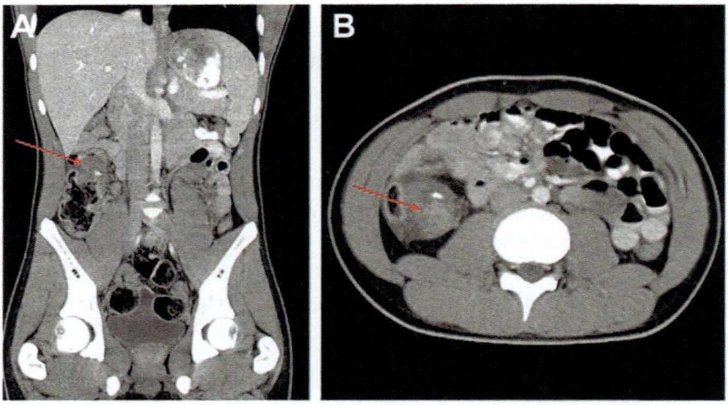

Fig. 2. (*A, B*) CT scan of the abdomen and pelvis demonstrating circumferential thickening of the midascending colon (*red arrow*) with severe luminal stenosis and surrounding inflammation, suggestive of an underlying mass.

adolescent CRC and lack of age-specific data, there are no pediatric or adolescent-specific surgical oncology guidelines for CRC and management therefore follows adult guidelines. In practice, pediatric patients with colon cancer undergo standard oncologic colectomy with en bloc removal of the tumor and regional lymphadenectomy for proper staging.[40] For rectal cancers, total mesorectal excision (TME) is the standard for achieving local disease control, often combined with multimodal therapy. The small pelvis of younger children can make TME technically demanding; thus, these cases are ideally managed by experienced surgical teams in high-volume centers. Minimally invasive approaches, including conventional laparoscopy, and increasingly robotic-assisted techniques may be used in adolescents, mirroring adult CRC practice. In adults, large series and meta-analyses demonstrate that minimally invasive colectomy achieves comparable margin status, lymph node harvest, local recurrence, and long-term survival to open surgery, while reducing blood loss, postoperative pain, and length of stay.[41] Data in pediatric and adolescent patients are limited but reassuring: a series of robotic pediatric oncology procedures showed that these techniques are feasible and safe in older children, with good functional outcomes.[42] Extrapolating from this experience, minimally invasive colectomy or low anterior resection can be considered for adolescents with resectable, nonobstructing tumors when an adequate oncologic resection is achievable and institutional expertise is available. In a multi-institutional analysis of pediatric freestanding centers and pediatric centers within adult institutions, only 82% had adequate lymph node sampling, potentially supporting the role of collaboration between pediatric and adult teams to optimize oncologic staging and outcomes.[32] An open approach remains preferred for bulky T4 lesions, extensive peritoneal metastases requiring cytoreduction, anticipated en bloc multivisceral resections, or in hemodynamically unstable patients.

Multidisciplinary care is essential. While surgical resection of the primary tumor is paramount, most adolescent patients will also require adjuvant chemotherapy, given the high incidence of locally advanced disease at presentation.[30] Common regimens such as FOLFOX, which includes 5-fluorouracil and oxaliplatin or FOLFIRINOX are extrapolated from adult oncology protocols,[40,43] as pediatric-specific clinical trials are lacking, and adolescents are often excluded from active adult based trials. The use of radiation therapy in young CRC patients is more nuanced. Pediatric patients may receive radiation as part of multimodal therapy, although patterns of use may differ from adult practice,[30] which may partly be due to concerns about long-term toxicity in young patients.[44] Nonetheless, for locally advanced rectal carcinoma, neoadjuvant chemoradiation is often considered to improve resectability and local control while weighing the risks and benefits carefully in each case.

In metastatic or recurrent adolescent CRC, aggressive surgical strategies may be indicated. Resection of isolated liver or lung metastases can be pursued if feasible, analogous to adult management. Emerging data also support a role for liver transplantation in carefully selected adults with unresectable liver-limited metastases. The TRANSMET trial demonstrated a significant 5-year OS benefit compared with chemotherapy alone.[45] However, no comparable evidence exists in pediatric or adolescent patients.

Notably, peritoneal carcinomatosis—which is relatively common in adolescents with CRC—has prompted consideration of cytoreductive surgery combined with hyperthermic intraperitoneal chemotherapy (CRS-HIPEC).[46] Although data are limited, CRS-HIPEC has been performed in adolescent CRC patients with peritoneal metastases.[47] In a systematic review of published cases, adolescents who underwent complete cytoreduction and HIPEC for colorectal carcinomatosis achieved disease control in some instances, demonstrating the feasibility of this aggressive approach.[47]

Such interventions are typically considered on a case-by-case basis at specialized centers.

Overall, emphasis should be on the importance of oncologic tumor resection and cytoreduction, when possible, given the poor response of these tumors to systemic therapy.[48]

Multidisciplinary Care Models and Pediatric–Adult Collaboration

Given the rarity and complexity of CRC in children and adolescents, care in specialized centers with robust multidisciplinary infrastructure is essential. Across cancer types, multidisciplinary tumor boards are associated with more accurate staging, increased adherence to evidence-based guidelines, and better coordinated multidisciplinary care.[49] In pediatric oncology, a single-institution study showed that formal multidisciplinary review altered diagnostic interpretation or treatment recommendations in over one-third of children with solid tumors, underscoring the practical impact of these meetings.[50] For pediatric and adolescent and young adult (AYA) CRC specifically, joint conferences that bring together pediatric and adult colorectal surgeons, medical oncologists, radiation oncologists, radiologists, pathologists, and genetic counselors allow integration of high-volume colorectal expertise with pediatric-specific considerations such as growth, treatment tolerance and physiology, fertility, and survivorship. Incorporating genetics into these discussions ensures timely germline testing, cascade screening of at-risk relatives, and appropriate decisions regarding the extent of colectomy in hereditary syndromes. Parallel attention to fertility preservation and long-term surveillance is particularly important for patients who may live for decades after treatment.

Future Directions and Adolescent and Young Adult-specific Programs

AYA patients occupy a space between pediatric and adult oncology, with documented gaps in clinical trial enrollment, survivorship support, and psychosocial care.[51] The rising incidence of AYA CRC and the distinct biology observed in pediatric and adolescent patients underscore the need for prospective, age-focused research efforts.[26,31] Current evidence is largely extrapolated from adult trials, with children and younger AYA patients under-represented or excluded.[33,51] Future priorities include multicenter registries across a broader age continuum that integrate detailed clinicopathologic, germline and somatic profiling, and prospective evaluation of pediatric/AYA-specific surgical and perioperative pathways.[40,42] As immunotherapy and other targeted therapy are increasingly incorporated into management, ensuring access for younger patients will be essential, ideally through harmonized pediatric–adult protocols and shared trial infrastructures.

Dedicated AYA oncology programs aim to bridge this gap by standardizing referral pathways, centralizing multidisciplinary review, and organizing age-specific services such as fertility preservation, psychosocial support, and educational/vocational counseling.[51] For pediatric and AYA CRC specifically, AYA-focused programs and joint pediatric-adult tumor boards could help ensure that patients benefit from high-volume colorectal surgical expertise and access to clinical trials, while also receiving guideline-concordant genetic evaluation and early integration of survivorship and fertility planning. Ultimately, optimizing outcomes will likely require both advances in tumor biology-driven systemic therapies and dedicated combined pediatric–adult CRC clinics, shared tumor boards, and coordinated transition-of-care pathways that address the full spectrum of treatment and survivorship needs.

Outcomes in pediatric and adolescent CRC are likely driven primarily by advanced-stage presentation rather than by an intrinsically worse stage-for-stage prognosis. In a population-based analysis of CRC in patients under 20 years, overall 5-year survival was approximately 40% compared with 60% in adults, a difference largely reflecting later-stage disease at diagnosis.[37] When stage is accounted for, outcomes in young patients with CRC are mixed, sometimes comparable to or better than those of older patients: in a National Cancer Database (NCDB) analysis, stage-specific 5-year survival was higher in patients ≤25 years than in those greater than 25 for stage II (85.6% vs 63.7%) and stage III (60.6% vs 52.9%) disease, with stage IV outcomes similar between groups.[29] Contemporary cohorts of young-onset CRC (20–49 years) similarly demonstrate superior stage-for-stage long-term survival, with 10-year OS of approximately 63% in young-onset versus 42% in late-onset CRC, and cancer-specific survival superior at all stages ($P<.001$).[52] These findings differ from some cohorts in which the survival signal is reversed.[30,31] The apparent divergence may reflect biological differences between truly pediatric CRC and young-onset adult CRC, rather than a genuine contradiction. Additionally, young-onset CRC follows a distinctive pattern of higher early mortality. Landmark analyses show that approximately 63.8% of deaths in young patients occur within 25 months of surgery compared with 42.4% in older patients, yet those who survive beyond this threshold achieve significantly better long-term outcomes.[53] Population-based data indicate a higher cumulative incidence of recurrence at all disease stages with a shorter time to recurrence in early-onset patients, underscoring the need for vigilant postoperative surveillance.[54]

CLINICS CARE POINTS

- Adrenocortical carcinoma can occur at any age and requires a keen index of suspicion in children with excess hormone production.
- Colorectal cancer incidence is increasing in younger patients without known predisposition and warrants a specialized treatment team to optimize outcomes.

DISCLOSURE

The authors have nothing to disclose.

REFERENCES

1. Virgone C, Roganovic J, Vorwerk P, et al. Adrenocortical tumours in children and adolescents: the EXPeRT/PARTNER diagnostic and therapeutic recommendations. Pediatr Blood Cancer 2021;68(Suppl 4):e29025.
2. Cecchetto G, Ganarin A, Bien E, et al. Outcome and prognostic factors in high-risk childhood adrenocortical carcinomas: a report from the European Cooperative Study Group on pediatric Rare Tumors (EXPeRT). Pediatr Blood Cancer 2017;64(6). https://doi.org/10.1002/pbc.26368.
3. Michalkiewicz E, Sandrini R, Figueiredo B, et al. Clinical and outcome characteristics of children with adrenocortical tumors: a report from the International Pediatric Adrenocortical Tumor Registry. J Clin Oncol 2004;22(5):838–45.
4. McAteer JP, Huaco JA, Gow KW. Predictors of survival in pediatric adrenocortical carcinoma: a Surveillance, Epidemiology, and End Results (SEER) program study. J Pediatr Surg 2013;48(5):1025–31.
5. Rodriguez-Galindo C, Krailo MD, Pinto EM, et al. Treatment of pediatric adrenocortical carcinoma with surgery, retroperitoneal lymph Node dissection, and

chemotherapy: the Children's Oncology Group ARAR0332 protocol. J Clin Oncol 2021;39(22):2463–73.

6. Kuhlen M, Schmutz M, Kunstreich M, et al. Targeting pediatric adrenocortical carcinoma: molecular insights and emerging therapeutic strategies. Cancer Treat Rev 2025;136:102942.
7. Pinto EM, Zambetti GP, Rodriguez-Galindo C. Pediatric adrenocortical tumours. Best Pract Res Clin Endocrinol Metab 2020;34(3):101448.
8. Ilanchezhian M, Varghese DG, Glod JW, et al. Pediatric adrenocortical carcinoma. Front Endocrinol 2022;13:961650.
9. Srivatsa S, Aldrink JH, Haque MR, et al. Surgical management and outcomes in pediatric adrenocortical carcinoma: a pediatric surgical oncology research collaborative study. Ann Surg Oncol 2026;33(3):2712–28.
10. Dasiewicz P, Moszczyńska E, Grajkowska W. Adrenal cortical carcinoma: paediatric aspects - literature review. Pediatr Endocrinol Diabetes Metab 2024;30(2): 81–90. Rak kory nadnerczy w populacji pediatrycznej – przegląd literatury.
11. Brondani VB, Fragoso M. Pediatric adrenocortical tumor - review and management update. Curr Opin Endocrinol Diabetes Obes 2020;27(3):177–86.
12. Zambaiti E, Duci M, De Corti F, et al. Clinical prognostic factors in pediatric adrenocortical tumors: a meta-analysis. Pediatr Blood Cancer 2021;68(3):e28836.
13. Wieneke JA, Thompson LD, Heffess CS. Adrenal cortical neoplasms in the pediatric population: a clinicopathologic and immunophenotypic analysis of 83 patients. Am J Surg Pathol 2003;27(7):867–81.
14. Weiss LM, Medeiros LJ, Vickery ALJ. Pathologic features of prognostic significance in adrenocortical carcinoma. Am J Surg Pathol 1989;13(3):202–6.
15. Lopez-Nunez O, Virgone C, Kletskaya IS, et al. Diagnostic utility of a modified reticulin algorithm in pediatric adrenocortical neoplasms. Am J Surg Pathol 2024; 48(3):309–16.
16. Picard C, Orbach D, Carton M, et al. Revisiting the role of the pathological grading in pediatric adrenal cortical tumors: results from a national cohort study with pathological review. Mod Pathol 2019;32(4):546–59.
17. Pinto EM, Rodriguez-Galindo C, Pounds SB, et al. Identification of clinical and biologic correlates associated with outcome in children with adrenocortical tumors without germline TP53 mutations: a St jude adrenocortical tumor registry and Children's Oncology Group Study. J Clin Oncol 2017;35(35):3956–63.
18. Libé R, Borget I, Ronchi CL, et al. Prognostic factors in stage III-IV adrenocortical carcinomas (ACC): an European Network for the Study of Adrenal Tumor (ENSAT) study. Ann Oncol 2015;26(10):2119–25.
19. Sandrini R, Ribeiro RC, DeLacerda L. Childhood adrenocortical tumors. J Clin Endocrinol Metab 1997;82(7):2027–31.
20. Mansfield SA, De Corti F, Aldrink JH, et al. Rare tumors II: adrenocortical tumors, neuroendocrine tumors of the appendix, pheochromocytoma and paraganglioma, pancreatoblastoma and solid pseudopapillary tumors of the pancreas. Pediatr Blood Cancer 2025;72(Suppl 2):e31207.
21. Fassnacht M, Dekkers OM, Else T, et al. European Society of Endocrinology Clinical Practice Guidelines on the management of adrenocortical carcinoma in adults, in collaboration with the European Network for the Study of Adrenal tumors. Eur J Endocrinol 2018;179(4):G1–46.
22. Hendricks A, Müller S, Fassnacht M, et al. Impact of lymphadenectomy on the oncologic outcome of patients with adrenocortical Carcinoma-A systematic review and meta-analysis. Cancers (Basel) 2022;14(2). https://doi.org/10.3390/cancers14020291.

23. Redlich A, Boxberger N, Strugala D, et al. Systemic treatment of adrenocortical carcinoma in children: data from the German GPOH-MET 97 trial. Klin Pädiatr 2012;224(6):366–71.
24. Geoerger B, Kang HJ, Yalon-Oren M, et al. Pembrolizumab in paediatric patients with advanced melanoma or a PD-L1-positive, advanced, relapsed, or refractory solid tumour or lymphoma (KEYNOTE-051): interim analysis of an open-label, single-arm, phase 1-2 trial. Lancet Oncol 2020;21(1):121–33.
25. Wild H, Liebmann A, Maennel L, et al. Colorectal carcinoma in childhood and adolescence: Microsatellite instability correlates with a favorable prognosis. Pediatr Blood Cancer 2025;72(8):e31830.
26. Downham L, Laversanne M, Perdomo S, et al. Increase of early-onset colorectal cancer: a cohort effect. J Natl Cancer Inst 2026;118(4):751–6.
27. Weber ML, Schneider DT, Offenmuller S, et al. Pediatric colorectal carcinoma is associated with excellent outcome in the context of cancer predisposition syndromes. Pediatr Blood Cancer 2016;63(4):611–7.
28. de Voer RM, Diets IJ, van der Post RS, et al. Clinical, pathology, genetic, and molecular features of colorectal tumors in adolescents and adults 25 years or younger. Clin Gastroenterol Hepatol 2021;19(8):1642–51.e8.
29. Akinkuotu AC, Maduekwe UN, Hayes-Jordan A. Surgical outcomes and survival rates of colon cancer in children and young adults. Am J Surg 2021;221(4): 718–24.
30. Poles GC, Clark DE, Mayo SW, et al. Colorectal carcinoma in pediatric patients: a comparison with adult tumors, treatment and outcomes from the National Cancer Database. J Pediatr Surg 2016;51(7):1061–6.
31. Hayes-Jordan AA, Sandler G, Malakorn S, et al. Colon cancer in patients under 25 years old: a different disease? J Am Coll Surg 2020;230(4):648–56.
32. Stetson A, Srivatsa S, Tracy L, et al. Clinical presentation, management, and outcomes of adolescents and young adults with colorectal cancer. J Surg Res 2025; 315:435–42.
33. Cavestro GM, Mannucci A, Balaguer F, et al. Delphi initiative for early-onset colorectal Cancer (DIRECt) International Management Guidelines. Clin Gastroenterol Hepatol 2023;21(3):581–603.e33.
34. Syngal S, Brand RE, Church JM, et al. ACG clinical guideline: genetic testing and management of hereditary gastrointestinal cancer syndromes. Am J Gastroenterol 2015;110(2):223–62 [quiz: 263].
35. Malik SS, Lythgoe MP, McPhail M, et al. Metachronous colorectal cancer following segmental or extended colectomy in Lynch syndrome: a systematic review and meta-analysis. Fam Cancer 2018;17(4):557–64.
36. Busico A, Gasparini P, Rausa E, et al. Molecular profiling of pediatric and young adult colorectal cancer reveals a distinct genomic landscapes and potential therapeutic avenues. Sci Rep 2024;14(1):13138.
37. Sultan I, Rodriguez-Galindo C, El-Taani H, et al. Distinct features of colorectal cancer in children and adolescents: a population-based study of 159 cases. Cancer 2010;116(3):758–65.
38. Saab R, Furman WL. Epidemiology and management options for colorectal cancer in children. Paediatr Drugs 2008;10(3):177–92.
39. Wu P, Deng W, Yan L, et al. Clinicopathologic and prognostic factors for colorectal cancer in children and adolescents: a population-based study. Int J Colorectal Dis 2023;38(1):35.

40. Bergamaschi L, Chiaravalli S, Signoroni S, et al. Management and pharmacotherapy of pediatric colorectal carcinoma: a review. Expert Opin Pharmacother 2023;24(14):1527–35.
41. Leitao MM Jr, Kreaden US, Laudone V, et al. The RECOURSE Study: Long-term oncologic outcomes associated with robotically assisted minimally invasive procedures for endometrial, cervical, colorectal, lung, or prostate cancer: a systematic review and meta-analysis. Ann Surg 2023;277(3):387–96.
42. Vatta F, Gazzaneo M, Bertozzi M, et al. Robotics-Assisted pediatric oncology Surgery-A preliminary single-center report and a systematic review of published studies. Front Pediatr 2021;9:780830.
43. Grothey A, Sobrero AF, Shields AF, et al. Duration of adjuvant chemotherapy for stage III Colon cancer. N Engl J Med 2018;378(13):1177–88.
44. Palmer JD, Tsang DS, Tinkle CL, et al. Late effects of radiation therapy in pediatric patients and survivorship. Pediatr Blood Cancer 2021;68(Suppl 2):e28349.
45. Adam R, Piedvache C, Chiche L, et al. Liver transplantation plus chemotherapy versus chemotherapy alone in patients with permanently unresectable colorectal liver metastases (TransMet): results from a multicentre, open-label, prospective, randomised controlled trial. Lancet 2024;404(10458):1107–18.
46. Vogel JD, Felder SI, Bhama AR, et al. The American Society of Colon and Rectal Surgeons Clinical Practice Guidelines for the management of Colon cancer. Dis Colon Rectum 2022;65(2):148–77.
47. Sorrentino L, Serra F, Cabry F, et al. Peritoneal carcinomatosis from colorectal cancer in the pediatric population: cytoreductive surgery and HIPEC. A systematic review. Eur J Surg Oncol 2021;47(2):211–5.
48. Guana R, Soto Torselli AS, De Leo F, et al. Colorectal adenocarcinoma in children and adolescents: the management of advanced disease. Int J Colorectal Dis 2025;40(1):237.
49. Specchia ML, Frisicale EM, Carini E, et al. The impact of tumor board on cancer care: evidence from an umbrella review. BMC Health Serv Res 2020;20(1):73.
50. Thenappan A, Halaweish I, Mody RJ, et al. Review at a multidisciplinary tumor board impacts critical management decisions of pediatric patients with cancer. Pediatr Blood Cancer 2017;64(2):254–8.
51. Freyer DR, Seibel NL. The clinical trials gap for adolescents and young adults with cancer: recent progress and conceptual framework for continued research. Curr Pediatr Rep 2015;3(2):137–45.
52. Cao AMY, Lonne MLR, Clark DA. Long-term survival outcomes in young-onset colorectal cancer: a population-based cohort study. Colorectal Dis 2025;27(2):e70007.
53. Wang S, Yuan Z, Ni K, et al. Young patients with colorectal cancer have higher early mortality but better long-term survival. Clin Transl Gastroenterol 2022;13-(12):e00543.
54. Nors J, Gotschalck KA, Erichsen R, et al. Risk of recurrence in early-onset versus late-onset non-metastatic colorectal cancer, 2004-2019: a nationwide cohort study. Lancet Reg Health Eur 2024;47:101093.

Surgical Management of Metastatic Pediatric Solid Tumors

Histology-specific Strategies and Multidisciplinary Approaches

Shahab Shaffiey, MD, MSc[a,*], Timothy B. Lautz, MD[b]

KEYWORDS

- Metastasis • Surgical oncology • Fluorescence-guided surgery

KEY POINTS

- Pediatric metastatic cancers differ fundamentally from adult malignancies, with distinct biological drivers and clinical behavior.
- Advances in imaging and diagnostics have markedly improved the detection and management of metastases.
- Complete surgical resection of metastatic lesions (metastasectomy) is a cornerstone of cure in many pediatric solid tumors.
- Multidisciplinary, individualized care is essential for optimizing outcomes and minimizing long-term toxicity.

INTRODUCTION AND BACKGROUND

Pediatric metastatic solid tumors present unique biological and clinical challenges distinct from their adult counterparts, necessitating specialized diagnostic and therapeutic paradigms. A substantial proportion of mortality associated with pediatric solid tumors is directly attributable to metastatic disease itself or to complications arising from its treatment.[1] The management of metastatic disease in children therefore requires a nuanced understanding of tumor biology, age-specific patterns of dissemination, and the complex interplay between systemic therapy, surgery, and radiation.[2,3] This article reviews contemporary approaches to metastatic pediatric solid tumors,

[a] Department of Pediatric and Thoracic Surgery, Nicklaus Children's Hospital, Miami, FL, USA; [b] Department of Surgery, Ann & Robert H Lurie Children's Hospital of Chicago, Northwestern University, Chicago, IL, USA
* Corresponding author. 3200 SW 60th Court, Suite 201, Miami, FL 33155.
E-mail address: Shahab.shaffiey@nicklaushealth.org

Surg Oncol Clin N Am 35 (2026) 831–846
https://doi.org/10.1016/j.soc.2026.05.005 **surgonc.theclinics.com**

Abbreviations	
COG	Children's Oncology Group
CT	computed tomography
ctDNA	circulating tumor DNA
FDG	^{18}F-fluorodeoxyglucose
ICG	indocyanine green
NRSTS	Nonrhabdomyosarcoma soft tissue sarcomas
OS	overall survival
PCNB	percutaneous core-needle biopsy
RMS	rhabdomyosarcoma
SBRT	stereotactic body radiation therapy
WLI	whole-lung irradiation

with particular emphasis on the role of surgery within multidisciplinary, curative-intent treatment strategies.

Over the past several decades, aggressive multimodality therapy has resulted in dramatic improvements in survival for many pediatric cancers. However, these gains have been far less pronounced among patients presenting with metastatic disease at diagnosis or experiencing distant relapse.[4] Metastatic disease remains one of the strongest adverse prognostic factors across pediatric solid tumor histologies. Approximately 10% to 40% of children with solid tumors present with metastatic disease at diagnosis, most commonly involving the lungs.[5] An additional 15% to 20% of patients will subsequently develop distant metastatic disease, again most frequently to the lung.[5] These epidemiologic patterns underscore the central role of pulmonary metastases in pediatric solid tumor management.

The lung is the predominant site of metastatic spread in pediatric solid tumors, accounting for more than 80% of metastatic events in hepatoblastoma and representing the most common initial site of metastasis in osteosarcoma, Ewing sarcoma, and Wilms tumor. Other metastatic sites—including liver, bone, bone marrow, distant lymph nodes, and brain—occur in a histology-dependent fashion and carry varying prognostic and therapeutic implications. Importantly, not all metastatic disease confers equal risk. Prognosis depends on both the site and burden of metastases as well as their responsiveness to systemic therapy, highlighting the need for individualized treatment strategies rather than a uniform approach to all metastatic presentations.[1]

Despite advances in chemotherapy and supportive care, outcomes for children with metastatic disease at diagnosis remain significantly inferior to those with localized tumors. Historically, 5 year survival for metastatic osteosarcoma has remained approximately 20% to 30%, compared with approximately 70% for patients with localized disease. Similarly, metastatic Ewing sarcoma carries an approximate 30% 5 year survival versus approximately 70% for localized disease. Survival for stage IV rhabdomyosarcoma (RMS) remains under 30% in most cooperative group studies, and long-term survival for high-risk neuroblastoma rarely exceeds 40% to 50% despite treatment intensification.[1] Together, these data emphasize metastatic disease as a principal driver of outcome in pediatric oncology and underscore the need for continued therapeutic innovation.

At the same time, outcomes for metastatic pediatric cancer are heterogeneous and strongly influenced by tumor biology and treatment responsiveness. Durable remission is achievable when systemic therapy successfully eradicates micrometastatic disease and local modalities—including surgery—can completely eliminate macroscopic tumor deposits. Improvements in systemic therapy, perioperative care, and surgical technique have transformed several previously lethal metastatic diagnoses into potentially curable conditions. A notable example is metastatic hepatoblastoma, in which children treated on the SIOPEL-4 protocol achieved event-free and overall survival rates of 76% and 83%, respectively, following dose-intensive chemotherapy and complete surgical resection of all disease.[6] These results demonstrate that even traditionally high-risk metastatic disease can be curable in a significant subset of patients with appropriately coordinated multidisciplinary care.

Surgical intervention has, therefore, assumed an increasingly important role in the management of metastatic pediatric solid tumors. In addition to providing diagnostic tissue and enabling molecular characterization, complete surgical resection of metastatic lesions offers a survival advantage in select histologies when all visible disease can be removed.[7–9] Advances in imaging, molecular diagnostics, and multimodal therapeutic strategies have further expanded the feasibility of metastasectomy, particularly for pulmonary disease. However, the burden of therapy for metastatic cancer remains substantial. Children frequently require intensive chemotherapy, complex surgical procedures, and radiation to multiple sites, with attendant risks of acute toxicity and long-term complications including cardiomyopathy, growth disturbance, infertility, and secondary malignancies. This reality has driven modern pediatric oncology protocols toward risk stratification and careful tailoring of treatment intensity to maximize cure while minimizing long-term morbidity. As the surgical management of metastatic disease is reviewed throughout this article, it is within this critical context of balancing aggressive curative-intent therapy against quality of life and long-term health.

DIAGNOSIS AND STAGING OF METASTATIC DISEASE

Accurate diagnosis and staging of metastatic disease in pediatric patients rely on a deliberate combination of advanced imaging modalities and tissue confirmation. Imaging serves as the foundation for detecting metastatic lesions, defining their number, size, and anatomic distribution, and guiding therapeutic planning across multidisciplinary teams. Each imaging technique offers specific advantages and limitations, and optimal staging frequently depends on the complementary use of multiple modalities.

Computed Tomography

Chest computed tomography (CT) remains the gold standard for identifying pulmonary metastases in children. Contemporary multidetector CT scanners can detect lung nodules as small as 1 to 2 mm in diameter, far surpassing the sensitivity of plain radiography and enabling early detection of metastatic disease. CT is similarly employed to evaluate other common metastatic sites depending on tumor histology. However, the high sensitivity of CT comes at the expense of specificity, as benign lesions may be radiographically indistinguishable from metastases, often creating diagnostic uncertainty and challenging decisions regarding intervention. Importantly, CT may underestimate the true burden of metastatic disease. In osteosarcoma, multiple surgical series have demonstrated that the number of pulmonary nodules identified preoperatively underrepresents the actual number of metastatic lesions by approximately 30% to 40%, with very small metastases (<1–2 mm) or lesions obscured by normal anatomic structures escaping detection even on high-quality scans. Despite these limitations, chest CT remains indispensable for staging, surveillance, and operative planning.[10]

MRI

MRI provides superior soft-tissue contrast and avoids ionizing radiation, making it particularly appealing in pediatric populations. Whole-body MRI is increasingly utilized for metastatic evaluation, especially for assessment of bone, marrow, and soft-tissue disease; however, its routine use in pediatric oncology remains limited by variability in protocols and availability. A key limitation of MRI is reduced sensitivity for small pulmonary nodules, and dedicated chest CT remains necessary for reliable detection of lung metastases, particularly for lesions smaller than 5 mm.[11]

Metabolic and Molecular Imaging

PET, most commonly performed as PET/CT or PET/MRI, provides functional imaging of metastatic lesions by identifying metabolically active disease. The most widely used tracer, ^{18}F-fluorodeoxyglucose (FDG), is avid in many high-grade pediatric tumors and can assist in distinguishing viable tumor from necrosis or scar tissue. However, many childhood malignancies are only modestly FDG-avid, and PET sensitivity for small pulmonary nodules is limited, with lesions typically needing to be 7 to 10 mm or larger for reliable detection. As a result, PET complements but does not replace CT for pulmonary staging. Certain tumors require specialized molecular imaging; iodine-123 metaiodobenzylguanidine scanning remains the standard for staging neuroblastoma, where it sensitively detects bone and marrow metastases that may not be apparent on cross-sectional imaging. PET using disease-specific tracers is similarly applied in select histologies and increasingly plays a role in response assessment for metastatic sarcomas and lymphomas.[9,12]

Ultrasound

Ultrasonography is frequently the initial imaging modality for suspected abdominal tumors and may incidentally identify hepatic or retroperitoneal metastases. It is particularly valuable for guiding biopsy of accessible lesions without radiation exposure. However, its limited field of view and operator dependence restrict its utility for comprehensive metastatic surveillance.

Bone Scintigraphy

Technetium-99m bone scintigraphy has largely been supplanted by PET and whole-body MRI but remains in use at some centers to screen for osteoblastic skeletal metastases owing to its sensitivity for osseous turnover. Many contemporary protocols are transitioning away from routine bone scans in favor of cross-sectional or metabolic imaging.

Advanced Imaging Techniques

Emerging technologies such as 3 dimensional volumetric reconstructions, cinematic rendering of CT or MRI data, and patient-specific 3 dimensional printed models are increasingly explored to assist with preoperative planning for complex metastatic resections. While these approaches remain largely investigational, they hold promise for improving surgical precision in selected cases.[13]

Following radiographic identification of suspected metastatic lesions, histologic confirmation is often essential—particularly when metastasis is the initial presentation or when imaging findings are equivocal. Tissue diagnosis prevents misclassification of benign lesions and ensures appropriate risk stratification and treatment planning. Percutaneous core-needle biopsy (PCNB), performed under CT or ultrasound guidance, has become the preferred diagnostic approach for accessible lesions due to its safety, minimally invasive nature, and high diagnostic accuracy, with fewer complications than open biopsy.[14] However, PCNB is less applicable for pulmonary nodules. When tissue confirmation is required for lung lesions, thoracoscopic wedge resection, with or without preoperative localization, is frequently the most straightforward and diagnostically reliable approach. For tumors requiring molecular characterization, the adequacy of biopsy specimens is critical. PCNB reliably yields tissue for histologic diagnosis and key biomarkers, yet comprehensive genomic profiling is successful in only approximately 60% of cases, underscoring the importance of meticulous technique, sufficient sampling, and, when available, real-time pathologic assessment.[15] Surgical biopsy or resection remains appropriate when percutaneous approaches are nondiagnostic, technically infeasible, or unlikely to provide sufficient material for advanced molecular studies.

Molecular profiling of primary and metastatic lesions has become increasingly central to pediatric oncology. Next-generation sequencing is routinely used in relapsed or high-risk tumors to identify potentially actionable alterations, with panel-based testing influencing clinical decision-making in a meaningful subset of patients.[7] While pediatric malignancies harbor fewer targetable mutations than adult cancers, actionable variants are nonetheless identified in select cases and can guide targeted therapy for refractory metastatic disease.[16,17] Despite this, only a small proportion of children ultimately receive matched targeted treatments, reflecting ongoing challenges in translating genomic discoveries into effective therapy.

Liquid biopsy approaches, including circulating tumor DNA (ctDNA), offer a noninvasive method for genomic characterization, dynamic disease monitoring, and early detection of relapse. In Ewing sarcoma, ctDNA assays can detect tumor-specific fusions such as (ewing sarcoma breakpoint region 1 - Friend leukemia virus integration 1 [EWSR1-FLI1]), track disease burden, identify emerging resistance, and in some cases predict relapse before radiographic progression.[18,19] Similar prognostic signal has been reported in RMS, including Children's Oncology Group (COG) intermediate-risk cohorts, and ongoing international trials are incorporating serial ctDNA monitoring to assess real-time treatment response.[20–22]

PRINCIPLES OF SURGICAL MANAGEMENT OF METASTASES

Surgical resection of metastatic disease, or metastasectomy, is a well-established component of therapy for many pediatric solid tumors. Decisions regarding metastasectomy are inherently individualized and depend on tumor histology, anatomic distribution and burden of metastatic disease, response to systemic therapy, and the anticipated morbidity of surgical intervention. Across multiple tumor types, adherence to surgical oncologic principles has been closely associated with improved local control and, in selected settings, meaningful survival benefit.[23] Tumors with limited sensitivity to chemotherapy or radiotherapy are particularly strong candidates for aggressive surgical management, as complete resection of metastatic deposits may represent the most effective modality for durable disease control.[8]

Over decades of practice and retrospective clinical experience, several core principles have emerged to guide the surgical management of pediatric metastatic disease:

1. *Aim for complete resection with negative margins while preserving organ function.* The primary objective of metastasectomy is eradication of all visible disease. Whenever feasible, metastatic lesions should be removed with a rim of normal tissue to ensure oncologic margins, while avoiding unnecessary sacrifice of functional parenchyma that could compromise long-term organ reserve.

2. *Incorporate tumor biology and chemo-radiation sensitivity into patient selection.* Histologic subtype and treatment responsiveness are central determinants of surgical benefit. As a general guiding principle, the less responsive a tumor is to systemic or radiation therapy, the more critical complete surgical resection of metastases becomes.
3. *Neither metastatic number nor short disease-free interval alone contraindicates surgery.* Carefully selected patients with multiple lesions or early recurrence may still benefit from resection when complete clearance is achievable.
4. *Bilateral or multisite metastatic disease can be approached with staged or synchronous resections.* Operative sequencing should be tailored to patient fitness, disease distribution, and systemic therapy integration.

These principles underscore that metastasectomy is rarely performed in isolation but rather as part of a coordinated multimodal treatment plan. While surgery can eradicate macroscopic disease, durable remission generally requires effective systemic therapy to control micrometastatic burden.

Technical Aspects of Pulmonary Metastasectomy

Pulmonary metastasectomy warrants particular emphasis, as lung involvement is the most common metastatic presentation in pediatric solid tumors and frequently determines eligibility for curative-intent therapy. Safe and effective pulmonary metastasectomy requires careful operative planning to maximize completeness of resection while minimizing morbidity. Although open thoracotomy has historically been favored—largely to permit bimanual palpation—minimally invasive approaches and image-guided adjuncts are increasingly incorporated in contemporary practice.[24–26]

Parenchymal-sparing resection

Complete resection with maximal preservation of lung tissue remains a central goal. Wedge resection is preferred for most lesions, with segmentectomy reserved for deep or anatomically constrained nodules.[27] Lobectomy is rarely indicated in children. Parenchymal preservation may be further enhanced using advanced energy devices such as LigaSure (Medtronic, Minneapolis, MN) or bipolar sealing systems, which allow precise excision with controlled sealing of vessels and bronchioles. In selected cases, these techniques may decrease operative time and cumulative lung injury—an important consideration for patients requiring repeated pulmonary resections.

Approach and exposure

Posterolateral muscle-sparing thoracotomy remains a reliable approach for extensive or deep disease and facilitates thorough palpation.[28] Thoracoscopic metastasectomy is appropriate for carefully selected patients with limited, peripheral lesions and has demonstrated outcomes comparable to open approaches in oligometastatic disease.[24,25] The optimal approach continues to be investigated through cooperative group efforts, including the COG randomized trial AOST2031 (NCT05235165), which compares thoracoscopic and open pulmonary metastasectomy in patients with oligometastatic osteosarcoma.[29]

Localization adjuncts

Advances in localization techniques have expanded the feasibility of minimally invasive resection. CT-guided wire or microcoil placement, dye marking with methylene blue or indocyanine green (ICG), and near-infrared fluorescence imaging can assist with identification of small or deep lesions (**Fig. 1**A–D).[30–33] ICG fluorescence-guided surgery has been shown to detect occult nodules within several millimeters

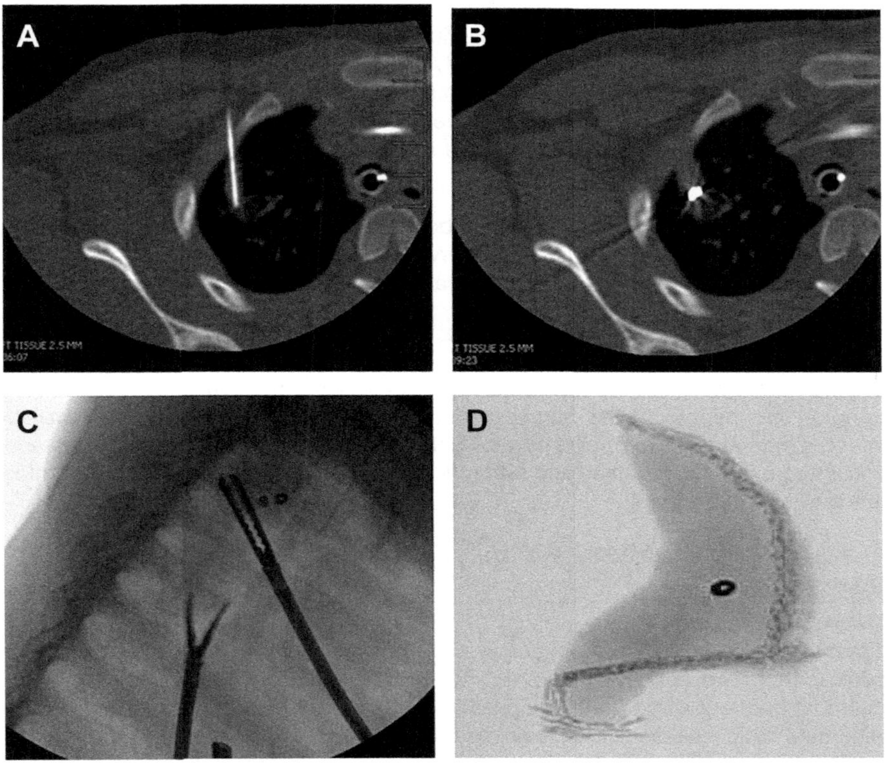

Fig. 1. Workflow for microcoil-based localization of a pulmonary nodule. (*A*) A needle is advanced adjacent to the target lesion under CT guidance, followed by (*B*) deployment of a microcoil. (*C*) In the operating room, fluoroscopy is used to localize the coil in orthogonal views to guide resection. (*D*) Off table fluoroscopy confirms retrieval of the microcoil after resection.

of the pleural surface, although sensitivity declines with depth.[34] Novel tumor-specific fluorophores are under development and hold promise for improving tumor-normal tissue distinction.

Completeness of resection

Across techniques, achievement of an R0 resection remains the strongest predictor of outcome and should guide operative strategy selection.

Surgical Management of Extrapulmonary Metastases

Although the lung predominates as a metastatic site, extrapulmonary metastases to lymph nodes, liver, bone, and brain pose distinct surgical challenges. The overarching objective remains complete resection when safely feasible, integrated within a multidisciplinary strategy.

Lymph node metastases

Surgical assessment of lymph node basins plays a key role in staging and treatment planning. Sentinel lymph node biopsy is indicated in select histologies including RMS and melanoma to avoid understaging cN0 disease.[8] Formal lymphadenectomy may be required in specific tumors such as germ cell or adrenocortical carcinoma.

Liver metastases

Liver involvement is encountered in multiple pediatric solid tumors. In Wilms tumor, hepatic metastases occur in approximately 5% to 10% of metastatic cases.[35] Surgical resection may be curative in select patients but is technically demanding and associated with potential morbidity. Preoperative planning frequently incorporates 3 dimensional imaging to guide parenchymal-sparing strategies.[36]

Bone metastases

Complete surgical excision of isolated bone metastases—particularly in osteosarcoma—is associated with improved survival. Complex reconstructions, including en-bloc spondylectomy or limb-sparing approaches, require meticulous multidisciplinary planning.[37]

Brain metastases

Brain metastases are uncommon but reported in sarcomas, germ cell tumors, renal tumors, and hepatocellular carcinoma. Surgical intervention is typically palliative intent, aimed at symptom relief or local control rather than cure. Maximal safe resection, integrated with radiation and systemic therapy, focuses on preserving neurologic function and quality of life.[38–40]

HISTOLOGY-SPECIFIC CONSIDERATIONS FOR METASTATIC DISEASE

Osteosarcoma

Metastatic pattern

Osteosarcoma is the most common primary malignant bone tumor of childhood and adolescence and spreads predominantly via the hematogenous route. The lung is the most frequent site of metastatic disease. Approximately 20% of patients present with metastatic disease at diagnosis, and an additional approximately 20% to 25% of those initially staged as localized will subsequently develop metastases during the course of treatment, most commonly to the lungs.[41] Extrapulmonary metastases to bone or other visceral organs are less common and usually occur in the setting of progressive or uncontrolled pulmonary disease.[42]

Prognosis

Outcomes for metastatic osteosarcoma remain substantially worse than for localized disease, with reported 5 year overall survival (OS) ranging from approximately 17% to 34%.[43,44] Long-term survival is closely linked to the ability to achieve complete surgical resection of all metastatic sites. Patients who attain complete surgical remission consistently demonstrate superior outcomes compared with those with residual disease. Prognostic factors include metastatic burden, unilateral versus bilateral lung involvement, disease-free interval, and completeness of metastasectomy. Solitary pulmonary lesions confer the most favorable prognosis, whereas increasing numbers of nodules are associated with progressively inferior survival.[45]

Surgery for metastatic disease

Because metastatic osteosarcoma is relatively chemoresistant, complete surgical resection of all detectable metastases is considered standard of care whenever technically feasible. Pulmonary metastasectomy is typically performed after definitive local control of the primary tumor, with the goal of achieving negative margins while preserving lung parenchyma. Bilateral pulmonary disease may be approached with staged or synchronous thoracotomies depending on disease burden and patient fitness. Survival is consistently superior among patients who achieve complete resection compared with those with unresectable or residual metastatic disease.[43,44]

Surgical approach

Open thoracotomy has historically been favored due to the ability to perform bimanual palpation and identify radiographically occult nodules. The clinical impact of this strategy continues to be evaluated. Retrospective series comparing thoracoscopic and open approaches suggest comparable outcomes for carefully selected patients with limited (oligometastatic) pulmonary disease, whereas outcomes appear inferior when thoracoscopy is applied to patients with higher metastatic burden.[44,46] A collaborative multi-institutional analysis similarly demonstrated comparable mortality and pulmonary recurrence rates between video-assisted thoracoscopic surgery and thoracotomy when disease burden was limited.[25] These observations have prompted prospective evaluation through the COG Phase III trial AOST2031 (NCT04890758), which directly compares open thoracotomy and thoracoscopic pulmonary metastasectomy in patients with up to 4 nodules per lung and no extrapulmonary disease.[34,29] When thoracoscopy is employed, accurate preoperative localization of small or deep nodules is essential to ensure completeness of resection.

Repeat metastasectomy and alternative local therapies

Pulmonary relapse following initial metastasectomy occurs in approximately 50% to 70% of patients.[45] Nonetheless, repeat pulmonary metastasectomy can meaningfully prolong survival in carefully selected patients. In a landmark series of more than 170 children and young adults who underwent repeated lung metastasectomies, long-term survival was achieved in nearly one-third of patients, many of whom required more than 1 pulmonary resection.[47] Additional studies confirm improved survival among patients able to undergo repeated complete resections.[48]

When surgical resection is not feasible because of anatomic constraints, comorbidities, or patient preference, stereotactic body radiation therapy (SBRT) or ablative modalities such as radiofrequency ablation may provide local control of isolated pulmonary metastases. In selected patients with oligometastatic disease, SBRT has demonstrated high local control rates with limited toxicity.[49,50] Despite these advances, surgery remains the preferred and most established modality when complete resection can be achieved.

Summary

Control of pulmonary metastatic disease is central to long-term survival in osteosarcoma. Complete metastasectomy—often repeated over time—remains the most effective curative strategy for resectable disease and should be pursued whenever feasible.

Ewing Sarcoma

Metastatic pattern

Ewing sarcoma, including peripheral primitive neuroectodermal tumor, is the second most common primary bone malignancy in children and adolescents and may also arise in soft tissues. Metastatic disease is present at diagnosis in approximately 25% of patients, most commonly involving the lungs, bone, and bone marrow. About half of metastatic patients have pulmonary involvement, frequently in combination with other metastatic sites, while approximately 10% present with isolated lung metastases.[51]

Prognosis

Despite its aggressiveness, Ewing sarcoma is highly sensitive to chemotherapy and radiation therapy. Five-year OS exceeds 70% for localized disease but decreases to approximately 30% for metastatic presentations.[52] Outcomes are more favorable for patients with lung-only metastases, with reported long-term survival of 30% to 50%. Rapid complete response to induction chemotherapy and the use of whole-lung irradiation (WLI) have been associated with improved survival in patients with pulmonary-only disease.[53]

Surgery for metastatic disease

The role of metastasectomy in Ewing sarcoma remains debated given the effectiveness of systemic therapy and radiation. Surgical resection is typically reserved for residual pulmonary lesions after chemotherapy, for diagnostic clarification of indeterminate nodules, or for anatomically favorable extrapulmonary lesions. Contemporary management integrates neoadjuvant chemotherapy, definitive local control of the primary tumor, and treatment of metastatic sites. WLI remains a standard component of therapy for microscopic pulmonary disease, particularly when numerous nodules are present, although select patients with limited lung-only disease and complete surgical clearance may avoid WLI in carefully individualized circumstances.[53]

Summary

Multimodal therapy is essential for metastatic Ewing sarcoma. Chemotherapy and radiation form the backbone of treatment, while metastasectomy may provide additional benefit in selected patients with residual disease.

Rhabdomyosarcoma

Metastatic pattern

Metastatic disease is present at diagnosis in approximately 15% to 20% of children with RMS. The lungs are the most frequent single site of distant spread, followed by bone marrow, bone, and distant lymph nodes. Histologic subtype and fusion status significantly influence metastatic potential, with alveolar and fusion-positive tumors demonstrating a higher propensity for dissemination.[54,55]

Prognosis

Metastatic RMS remains a high-risk category, with 5 year event-free survival generally below 30%. Prognosis varies by site and burden of metastatic disease, with lung-only metastases associated with more favorable outcomes compared with extrapulmonary disease.[56]

Role of pulmonary metastasectomy and radiation

RMS is typically highly responsive to chemotherapy and radiation therapy, limiting the routine role of pulmonary metastasectomy. Surgery is reserved for diagnostic clarification, rare cases of limited persistent disease after systemic therapy, or isolated pulmonary relapse resistant to further chemotherapy. Cooperative Weichteilsarkom Studiengruppe analyses have not demonstrated a clear survival benefit for routine surgical removal of lung metastases, underscoring the dominant role of systemic therapy.[57] WLI is a long-established component of therapy for patients with pulmonary metastases and remains recommended in contemporary high-risk protocols such as COG ARST2031 (NCT04994132).[58]

Summary

Systemic therapy and radiation remain the cornerstones of treatment of metastatic RMS. Metastasectomy plays a selective role, primarily for diagnosis or limited residual or relapsed disease, within a tightly integrated multimodal framework.

Wilms Tumor

Metastatic pattern

Wilms tumor is the most common pediatric renal malignancy. Approximately 10% to 12% of patients present with metastatic disease at diagnosis, with the lungs accounting for the vast majority of metastatic sites. Extrapulmonary metastases are uncommon and usually associated with unfavorable histology or relapse.[59]

Prognosis

Outcomes for metastatic Wilms tumor are generally favorable compared with other stage IV pediatric solid tumors. Modern risk-adapted and response-adapted therapy achieves excellent survival for patients with favorable-histology disease. The COG AREN0533 (NCT00379340) trial established a strategy in which patients with complete radiographic resolution of lung metastases after induction chemotherapy can safely omit WLI, thereby reducing late toxicity without compromising survival.[60]

Role of pulmonary metastasectomy

In contemporary COG protocols, including AREN2331 (NCT06401330), pulmonary metastasectomy functions primarily as a decision-making tool rather than definitive therapy. Resection of a small number of persistent nodules allows determination of residual viable tumor and guides the need for WLI and chemotherapy intensification.[61] This selective approach permits many children to avoid lung radiation while maintaining excellent outcomes.

Summary

Chemotherapy is highly effective for pulmonary metastases in Wilms tumor. Selective, protocol-directed metastasectomy plays a pivotal role in tailoring therapy intensity and minimizing long-term toxicity.

Nonrhabdomyosarcoma Soft Tissue Sarcomas

Metastatic pattern and prognosis

Nonrhabdomyosarcoma soft tissue sarcomas (NRSTS) encompass a heterogeneous group of malignancies with limited chemosensitivity. Metastases are present at diagnosis in approximately 20% to 30% of patients, most commonly to the lungs. Prognosis varies widely by subtype, metastatic burden, and completeness of resection.[62]

Role of metastasectomy

Because systemic therapy is often ineffective, aggressive surgical removal of pulmonary metastases is generally recommended when complete resection is achievable. Open thoracotomy with meticulous palpation is frequently preferred due to the subtle, noncalcified nature of many NRSTS lung metastases. Complete resection offers the best opportunity for long-term survival, whereas incomplete or palliative resections do not confer benefit.[63]

Summary

Surgery remains central to the management of metastatic NRSTS. When technically feasible, metastasectomy should be pursued as part of an aggressive, multidisciplinary approach.

Hepatoblastoma and Hepatocellular Carcinoma

Hepatoblastoma

Metastatic disease is present at diagnosis in approximately 15% to 25% of patients with hepatoblastoma, most commonly to the lungs. Outcomes have improved substantially with modern chemotherapy and aggressive surgical management. Complete resection of all metastatic sites is mandatory prior to liver transplantation and remains a critical prognostic determinant. Pulmonary metastasectomy is indicated for residual lung lesions after chemotherapy and is often facilitated by ICG fluorescence-guided surgery.[64–66]

Hepatocellular carcinoma

Pediatric hepatocellular carcinoma is far less chemosensitive, and outcomes for metastatic disease remain poor. Metastasectomy is rarely curative and is generally reserved for highly selected or palliative situations.

Summary

In hepatoblastoma, complete surgical clearance of metastatic disease is essential for cure and often enables successful liver transplantation. In contrast, metastasectomy in pediatric hepatocellular carcinoma is typically palliative rather than curative.

SUMMARY

Metastatic disease in pediatric solid tumors is biologically heterogeneous, and the role of surgery varies substantially according to tumor histology, patterns of metastatic spread, and responsiveness to systemic therapy. In osteosarcoma, NRSTS, and hepatoblastoma, repeated complete metastasectomy—most commonly targeting pulmonary disease—can transform an otherwise lethal clinical scenario into one associated with meaningful long-term outcomes, including durable remission and extended survival in carefully selected patients. By contrast, in Ewing sarcoma, RMS, and Wilms tumor, systemic therapy and radiation remain the primary drivers of outcome, with metastasectomy employed selectively for diagnostic clarification, confirmation of treatment response, or risk-adapted therapeutic decision-making within contemporary protocolized frameworks.

Across these disease entities, advances in cross-sectional and functional imaging, molecular profiling, and emerging technologies such as ctDNA and fluorescence-guided surgery are refining staging accuracy and operative planning. At the same time, improvements in perioperative care, parenchymal-sparing surgical techniques, and enhanced recovery pathways have reduced treatment-related morbidity and broadened the feasibility of metastasis-directed intervention.

Ultimately, decisions regarding metastasectomy must be made within a robust multidisciplinary framework that integrates pediatric surgical oncologists, medical oncologists, radiation oncologists, radiologists, pathologists, and transplant teams when appropriate. The overarching goal is not simply short-term radiographic clearance, but durable oncologic control achieved with preservation of organ function and minimization of long-term toxicity. As cooperative group trials mature and novel systemic, targeted, and image-guided therapies continue to evolve, pediatric surgical oncologists will remain central in tailoring metastasis-directed strategies that optimize meaningful outcomes while safeguarding the future health and quality of life of children with cancer.

CLINICS CARE POINTS

- Complete resection of all visible metastatic diseases is a key determinant of long-term survival in many pediatric solid tumors, particularly when systemic therapies have limited efficacy.
- Radiographic resolution of metastases does not always indicate complete tumor clearance; viable microscopic disease may persist, underscoring the importance of surgical assessment in selected cases.

- Surgical approach to pulmonary metastases should balance oncologic clearance with parenchymal preservation.
- Multidisciplinary decision-making is essential in metastatic disease management, integrating surgical, medical, and radiation oncology perspectives to tailor therapy based on response and risk.
- Advanced localization tools, such as fluorescence-guided imaging or CT-guided markers, can enhance completeness of resection, particularly for small or deep-seated pulmonary lesions.

DISCLOSURE

S. Shaffiey—None; T.B. Lautz—Research support from On Target Laboratories, United States and consulting income from Stryker Endoscopy.

REFERENCES

1. Perkins SM, Shinohara ET, DeWees T, et al. Outcome for children with metastatic solid tumors over the last four decades. PLoS One 2014;9(7):e100396.
2. Gow KW, Lautz TB, Malek MM, et al. Children's Oncology Group's 2023 blueprint for research: surgery. Pediatr Blood Cancer 2024;71(3):e30766.
3. Pio L, Sarnacki S. Innovative approaches in pediatric surgical oncology. Front Pediatr 2022;10:989822.
4. Liu S, Yin W, Lin Y, et al. Metastatic patterns and prognosis in children with solid tumors. World J Surg Oncol 2023;21:117.
5. Heaton TE, Davidoff AM. Surgical treatment of pulmonary metastases in pediatric solid tumors. Semin Pediatr Surg 2016;25:308–16.
6. Zsiros J, Brugieres L, Brock P, et al. Dose-dense cisplatin-based chemotherapy and surgery for children with high-risk hepatoblastoma (SIOPEL-4). Lancet Oncol 2013;14(9):834–42.
7. Surrey LF, MacFarland SP, Chang F, et al. Clinical utility of next-generation sequencing in pediatric tumors. Genome Med 2019;11(1):32.
8. Croteau NJ, Heaton TE. Pulmonary metastasectomy in pediatric solid tumors. Children (Basel) 2019;6(1):6.
9. Phelps HM, Lovvorn HN 3rd. Minimally invasive surgery in pediatric surgical oncology. Children (Basel) 2018;5(12):158.
10. Duczkowski M, Duczkowska A, Olwert A, et al. Predictors of pulmonary metastases on chest computed tomography in children and adolescents with osteosarcoma - tips for qualifying patients for thoracotomy. BMC Pediatr 2024;24(1):382.
11. de Oliveira AD, de Souza GHY, Guimarães CPBF, et al. Evaluation of whole-body MRI with diffusion-weighted sequences in the staging of pediatric cancer patients. PLoS One 2020;15(8):e0238166.
12. Uslu L, Donig J, Link MP, et al. Value of 18F-FDG PET and PET/CT for evaluation of pediatric malignancies. J Nucl Med 2015;56(2):274–86.
13. Fusco JC, Abdelhafeez AH, Krauel L, et al. Imaging adjuvants in pediatric surgical oncology. Pediatr Blood Cancer 2025;72(Suppl 2):e31241.
14. Teke M, Rich BS, Walther A, et al. A comparison of commonly utilized diagnostic biopsy techniques for pediatric patients with cancer: a systematic review. J Pediatr Surg 2025;60:162038.
15. Overman RE, Kartal TT, Cunningham AJ, et al. Optimization of percutaneous biopsy for diagnosis and pretreatment risk assesment of neuroblastoma. Pediatr Blood Cancer 2020;67:e28258.

16. Bertacca I, Pegoraro F, Tondo A, et al. Targeted treatment of solid tumors in pediatric precision oncology. Front Oncol 2023;13:1176790.
17. Katz L, Ben-Arush M, Blanche E, et al. The clinical utility of next-generation sequencing in childhood and adolescent/young adult solid tumors: a systematic review and meta-analysis. Cancers (Basel) 2025;17(8):1292.
18. Abbou SD, Shulman DS, DuBois SG, et al. Assessment of circulating tumor DNA in pediatric solid tumors: the promise of liquid biopsies. Pediatr Blood Cancer 2019;66:e27777.
19. Krumbholzl M, Eiblwiesert J, Ranft A, et al. Quantification of translocation-specific ctDNA provides an integrating parameter for early assessment of treatment response and risk stratification in Ewing sarcoma. Clin Cancer Res 2021;27-(21):5922–30.
20. Shulman DS, Klega K, Imamovic-Tuco A, et al. Detection of circulating tumour DNA is associated with inferior outcomes in Ewing sarcoma and osteosarcoma: a report from the Children's Oncology Group. Br J Cancer 2018;119:615–21.
21. Abbou S, Klega K, Tsuji J, et al. Circulating tumor DNA is prognostic in intermediate-risk rhabdomyosarcoma: a report from the Children's Oncology Group. J Clin Oncol 2023;41:2382–93.
22. Lak NSM, van Zogchel LMJ, Zappeij-Kannegieter L, et al. Cell-free DNA as a diagnostic and prognostic biomarker in pediatric rhabdomyosarcoma. JCO Precis Onc 2023;7:e2200286.
23. de Campos Vieira Abib S, Chui CH, Cox S, et al. International society of paediatric surgical oncology surgical practice guidelines. Ecancermedicalscience 2022; 16:1356.
24. Kuo C, Malvar J, Chi YY, et al. Survival outcomes and surgical morbidity based on surgical approach to pulmonary metastasectomy in pediatric, adolescent and young adult patients with osteosarcoma. Cancer Med 2023;12(18):18862–74.
25. Lautz TB, Farooqui Z, Jenkins T, et al. Thoracoscopy vs thoracotomy for the management of metastatic osteosarcoma: a pediatric surgical oncology research collaborative study. Int J Cancer 2020;148:1164–71.
26. Türk İ, Çetin M, Sari N, et al. Impact of pulmonary metastasectomy timing and nodule characteristics on survival outcomes in patients with pediatric sarcoma. Turk J Med Sci 2025;55:1151–60.
27. Grapatsas K, Papaporfyriou A, Leivaditis V, et al. Lung metastatectomy: can laser-assisted surgery make a difference? Curr Oncol 2022;29(10):6968–81.
28. Chen L, Liu Z, Stein JE, et al. Intercostal nerve cryoablation is associated with reduced opioid use in pediatric oncology patients. J Surg Res 2023;283:851–7.
29. Teke ME, Saif A, Sarvestani AL, et al. Phase III trial of thoracoscopic vs open pulmonary metastasectomy in osteosarcoma (AOST2031). Ann Surg Oncol 2022;29: 7961–3.
30. Morgan KM, Anderson KT, Johnston ME, et al. Interhospital variability in localization techniques for small pulmonary nodules in children: A pediatric surgical oncology research collaborative study. J Pediatr Surg 2022;57(6):1013–7.
31. Rodrigues JCL, Pierre AF, Hanneman K, et al. CT-guided microcoil pulmonary nodule localization prior to video-assisted thoracoscopic surgery: diagnostic utility and recurrence-free survival. Radiology 2019;291(1):214–22.
32. Morgan KM, Crowley JJ, Many BT, et al. Microcoil localization as an effective adjunct to thoracoscopic resection of pulmonary nodules in children. J Pediatr Surg 2021;56:1172–6.

33. Goldstein SD, Heaton TE, Bondoc A, et al. Evolving applications of fluorescence guided surgery in pediatric surgical oncology: a practical guide for surgeons. J Pediatr Surg 2021;56:1999–2008.
34. Simons DC, van Schalkwijk LHM, van de Sande MAJ, et al. Fluorescence-guided surgery in pediatric oncology: current practice and future directions. Cancers (Basel) 2025;18(1):149.
35. Ehrlich PF, Ferrer F, Ritchey ML, et al. Hepatic metastases at diagnosis in patients with Wilms tumor is not an independent adverse prognostic factor for stage IV Wilms tumor: a report from the Children's Oncology Group/National Wilms Tumor Study Group. Ann Surg 2009;250:484–7.
36. Ryan ML, Wang S, Pandya SR, et al. Integrating artificial intelligence into the visualization and modeling of three-dimensional anatomy in pediatric surgical patients. J Pediatr Surg 2024;59:161764.
37. Kumta SM, Cheng JC, Li CK, et al. Scope and limitations of limb-sparing surgery in childhood sarcomas. J Pediatr Orthop 2002;22:244–9.
38. Gauthier N, Weiser A, Kroiss S, et al. Central nervous system metastases from pediatric solid tumors: a single-institution study. World Neurosurg 2026;207:124786.
39. Jaju A, Li Y, Dahmoush H, et al. Imaging of pediatric brain tumors: a COG Diagnostic Imaging Committee/SPR Oncology Committee/ASPNR White Paper. Pediatr Blood Cancer 2023;70:e30147.
40. Tsang DS, Vargo JA, Goddard K, et al. Palliative radiation therapy for children with cancer. Ped Blood Cancer 2021;68:e28292.
41. Mettmann V, Blattmann C, Friedel G, et al. Primary multi-systemic metastases in osteosarcoma: presentation, treatment, and survival of 83 patients of the Cooperative Osteosarcoma Study Group. Cancers 2024;16:110.
42. Tang J, Guo Y, Lu H, et al. Prognostic nomogram for overall survival in pediatric osteosarcoma with pulmonary metastases: a SEER database analysis. Front Pediatr 2025;13:1574034.
43. Daw NC, Chou AJ, Jaffe N, et al. Recurrent osteosarcoma with a single pulmonary metastasis: a multi-institutional review. Br J Cancer 2015;11(2):278–82.
44. Ferrari S, Briccoli A, Mercuri M, et al. Postrelapse survival in osteosarcoma of the extremities: prognostic factors for long-term survival. J Clin Oncol 2003;21:710–5.
45. Mettmann VL, Baumhoer D, Bielacki SS, et al. Solitary pulmonary metastases at first recurrence of osteosarcoma: presentation, treatment, and survival of 219 patients of the Cooperative Osteosarcoma Study Group. Cancer Med 2023;12: 18399–410.
46. Riccipetitoni G, Bertozzi M, Gazzaneo M, et al. The role of video-assisted thoracoscopic surgery in pediatric oncology: single-center experience and review of the literature. Front Pediatr 2021;9:721914.
47. Pastorino U, Gasparini M, Valente M, et al. Primary childhood osteosarcoma: the role of salvage surgery. Ann Oncol 1992;3:43–8.
48. Briccoli A, Rocca M, Salone M, et al. Resection of recurrent pulmonary metastases in patient with osteosarcoma. Cancer 2005;104:1721–5.
49. Gutkin PM, Gore E, Charlson J, et al. Stereotactic body radiotherapy for metastatic sarcoma to the lung: adding to the arsenal of local therapy. Radiat Oncol 2023; 18:42.
50. Reddy S, Upadhyay R, Klamer B, et al. Local control and toxicity outcomes after stereotactic body radiation therapy for metastatic osteosarcoma in pediatric patients. Pediatr Blood Cancer 2025;72:e31541.
51. Ye C, Dai M, Zhang B. Risk factors for metastasis at initial diagnosis with Ewing sarcoma. Front Oncol 2019;9:1043.

52. Lawlor ER, Sorensen PH. Twenty years on: what we know about ewing sarcoma and the path forward? Cancer Cell 2015;27:265–71.
53. Reiter AJ, Huang L, Craig BT, et al. Survival outcomes in pediatric patients with metastatic Ewing sarcoma who achieve a rapid complete response of pulmonary metastases. Pediatr Blood Cancer 2024;71:e31065.
54. Oberlin O, Rey A, Lyden E, et al. Prognostic factors in metastatic rhabdomyosarcomas: results of a pooled analysis from United States and European cooperative groups. J Clin Oncol 2008;26:2384–9.
55. Vasquez JC, Lou LY, Hiniker SM, et al. Rhabdomyosarcoma with isolated lung metastases: a report from the Soft Tissue Sarcoma Committee of the Children's Oncology Group. Pediatr Blood Cancer 2023;70:e30361.
56. Mercolini F, Sparber-Sauer M, Mascarenhas L, et al. Single-site metastatic rhabdomyosarcoma: an INSTRuCT pooled analysis. Eur J Cancer 2025;229:115793.
57. Dantonello TM, Winkler P, Boelling T, et al. Embryonal rhabdomyosarcoma with metastases confined to the lungs: report from the CWS Study Group. Pediatr Blood Cancer 2011;56:725–32.
58. Haduong JH, Heske CM, Allen-Rhoades W, et al. An update on rhabdomyosarcoma risk stratification and the rationale for current and future Children's Oncology Group clinical trials. Pediatr Blood Cancer 2022;69:e29511.
59. Pater L, Melchior P, Rube C, et al. Wilms tumor. Pediatr Blood Cancer 2021;e28257.
60. Dix DB, Seibel NL, Chi YY, et al. Treatment of stage IV favorable histology Wilms tumor with lung metastases: a report from the Children's Oncology Group AREN0533 study. J Clin Oncol 2018;36:1564–70.
61. Children's Oncology Group. AREN2331: treatment of favorable-histology Wilms tumor with pulmonary metastases. ClinicalTrials.gov Identifier: NCT05134107.
62. Hawkins DS, Spunt SL, Skapek SX, et al. Children's Oncology Group 2013 blueprint for research: soft tissue sarcoms. Pediatr Blood Cancer 2013;60:1005–8.
63. Polites SF, Rhee DS, Seitz G, et al. Contemporary surgical management of pediatric non-rhabdomyosarcoma soft tissue sarcoma. Pediatr Blood Cancer 2024;71:e31289.
64. Honda M, Uchida K, Irie T, et al. Recent advances in surgical strategies and liver transplantation for hepatoblastoma. Cancer Med 2023;12:1585–97.
65. Riehle KJ, Vasudevan SA, Bondoc A, et al. Surgical management of liver tumors. Pediatr Blood Cancer 2025;72(2):e31289.
65. Lake CM, Bondoc AJ, Dasgupta R, et al. Indocyanine green is a sensitive adjunct in the identification and surgical management of local and metastatic hepatoblastoma. Cancer Med 2021;10:4322–30.

Minimally Invasive Surgery and New Technologies in Pediatric Oncology

Lucas Krauel, MD, PhD, FEBPS[a], Stefano Avanzini, MD[b], Thomas Blanc, MD, PhD, FEAPU[c,d], Andrew Davidoff, MD[e,*]

KEYWORDS

- Minimally invasive surgery • Robotics • Pediatric surgical oncology
- Three-dimensional (3D) surgical planning • Image-guided surgery

KEY POINTS

- Minimally invasive surgery (MIS) is increasingly applied in pediatric oncology, offering reduced morbidity and faster recovery while maintaining oncologic safety in carefully selected cases.
- Robotic surgery expands the potential of MIS in children, providing enhanced dexterity, precision, and visualization, although cost and access remain limiting factors.
- Three-dimensional surgical planning transforms conventional imaging into patient-specific models, enhancing surgical precision, training, and communication with families.
- Artificial intelligence is emerging as a driver of automated workflows, risk prediction, and decision support in pediatric surgical oncology.
- Children benefit uniquely from these innovations due to smaller anatomy, frequent tumors with complex vascular involvement, and the need to improve family-centered communication and understanding.

INTRODUCTION

Minimally invasive surgery (MIS) has become a cornerstone in many areas of pediatric surgery, with proven benefits including reduced postoperative pain, shorter hospitalization, faster return to normal activity, and improved cosmesis. In pediatric surgical oncology, however, the application of MIS has historically been limited by concerns

[a] Pediatric Surgery Department, SJD Barcelona Children's Hospital, Universitat de Barcelona, Barcelona, Spain; [b] Pediatric Surgery Department, IRCCS Istituto Giannina Gaslini, Genova, Italy; [c] Department of Paediatric Urology, Paediatric Surgery & Transplantation, Hôpital Necker-Enfants Malades, Assistance Publique-Hôpitaux de Paris, Paris, France; [d] Université Paris Cité, Paris, France; [e] Department of Surgery, St. Jude Children's Research Hospital, Memphis, TN, USA

* Corresponding author. Pediatric Surgery Department, SJD Barcelona Children's Hospital, Passeig de Sant Joan de Déu, 2, 08950 Barcelona, Spain.

E-mail address: Andrew.Davidoff@STJUDE.ORG

Surg Oncol Clin N Am 35 (2026) 847–865
https://doi.org/10.1016/j.soc.2026.04.017 surgonc.theclinics.com
1055-3207/26/

Abbreviations	
3D	3-dimensional
AI	artificial intelligence
CT	computed tomography
ICG	indocyanine green
IDRF	image-defined risk factor
MIS	minimally invasive surgery
RAS	robotic-assisted surgery
RPLNS	retroperitoneal lymph node sampling
VR/AR	virtual and augmented reality

about compromising oncologic principles, the technical challenges posed by small anatomy, and the lack of robust data compared to adult series.

Over the past 2 decades, advances in technology, perioperative care, and collaborative research have led to a gradual expansion of indications for MIS in children with solid tumors. In particular, neuroblastoma, Wilms tumor, and ovarian tumors, in selected patients, have been explored as candidates for MIS approaches.[1,2]

Differences between pediatric and adult oncology remain important. Children present unique tumor biology, higher survival rates, and a greater emphasis on preserving long-term quality of life. Therefore, any innovation in surgical technique must be balanced against strict oncologic safety standards and multidisciplinary treatment strategies.

The rapid adoption of adjunctive technologies such as 3-dimensional (3D) surgical planning, virtual and augmented reality (VR/AR), intraoperative image guidance, and the integration of artificial intelligence (AI) has opened new possibilities to enhance precision and safety. These tools are particularly valuable in pediatric oncology, where tumors often encase major vessels and critical organs in very small anatomic spaces.[3–5]

This article reviews the current landscape of MIS in pediatric oncology, highlights emerging technologies, and discusses how these innovations may shape the future of surgical oncology in children.

CURRENT LANDSCAPE OF MINIMALLY INVASIVE SURGERY IN PEDIATRIC ONCOLOGY

Indications and Procedures

Initially, MIS in pediatric oncology was largely confined to diagnostic purposes: obtaining tumor biopsies, staging procedures, and evaluation of resectability.[6] Over time, its scope expanded to therapeutic resections in selected tumors. The role of MIS is highly dependent on tumor histology. For example, adrenal and neuroblastic tumors without major vascular encasement (L1 tumors) are often amenable to laparoscopic or thoracoscopic removal, whereas adrenocortical carcinomas generally require open resection due to their friability and the necessity for R0 excision.[7] Similarly, thoracoscopic removal of posterior mediastinal neuroblastomas without image-defined risk factors (IDRFs) offers a clear advantage in terms of cosmesis and musculoskeletal preservation, avoiding the morbidity of thoracotomy.[8]

Outcomes: Then versus now

Long-term oncologic outcomes remain the cornerstone of evaluating MIS in pediatric oncology. Large institutional studies have demonstrated the feasibility and safety of MIS when oncologic principles are respected.[9] Early reports emphasized diagnostic procedures, while more recent data document successful therapeutic resections with acceptable rates of complication and recurrence. Importantly, survival outcomes in MIS have been shown to be equivalent to open approaches in carefully selected patients.[10] Furthermore, MIS facilitates faster recovery and shorter hospital stays, both crucial in pediatric oncology where timely resumption of systemic therapy is often important.

Pediatric versus Adult Differences

Translating MIS techniques from adult to pediatric oncology is not straightforward. Children differ in tumor biology, body size, and tolerance to pneumoperitoneum or single-lung ventilation. Instrumentation designed for adults is often poorly suited to small pediatric patients, where the margin for technical error is extremely narrow. Moreover, certain pediatric tumors—such as neuroblastoma—do not always require complete microscopic clearance, unlike their adult counterparts (eg, adrenocortical carcinoma), which profoundly affects surgical decision-making.[7] Thus, while MIS adoption has been rapid in adult oncology, its uptake in pediatrics has been more deliberate and nuanced.

MINIMALLY INVASIVE SURGERY IN SPECIFIC PEDIATRIC TUMORS

Neuroblastoma

Neuroblastoma is one of the most frequent pediatric solid tumors for which MIS has been increasingly applied. Tumors located in the adrenal gland or posterior mediastinum are often suited to laparoscopic or thoracoscopic resection, provided that IDRFs such as major vascular encasement are absent. For L1 tumors, MIS offers excellent visualization and reduced morbidity. In contrast, L2 tumors encasing vessels still represent a challenge, and many surgeons prefer open approaches. However, recent papers have demonstrated the feasibility of neuroblastic tumor resection with selected IDRF.[11] Recent experiences have shown that even piecemeal resection of neuroblastomas is oncologically accepted, as this allows macroscopic vessel clearance from the tumor.[8]

Renal Tumors

Wilms tumor remains the most frequent pediatric renal tumor. The established standard is open nephrectomy with lymph node sampling, due to the importance of avoiding tumor spillage. Nevertheless, laparoscopic nephrectomy has been explored in highly selected patients, particularly in the context of the International Society of Pediatric Oncology approach, where neoadjuvant chemotherapy reduces tumor volume. When other types of renal tumors are suspected (ie, clear cell sarcoma or rhabdoid tumors), a strict adherence to R0 resection is recommended, making MIS less frequently used. Partial nephrectomy via MIS is rare in children, due to the risk of tumor spillage, but has been attempted in patients with predisposition syndromes and with small, favorably located tumors.[10] There is yet no follow up on these patient populations to determine long-term outcomes.

Sarcomas

Rhabdomyosarcomas in the retroperitoneum or bladder region can occasionally be resected using MIS, typically after neoadjuvant chemotherapy. The MIS approach allows precise dissection and can reduce morbidity by preserving pelvic nerves. Retroperitoneal lymph node sampling (RPLNS) in paratesticular rhabdomyosarcoma has also been performed laparoscopically, with the potential advantages of reduced postoperative discomfort, shorter hospital stay, and improved preservation of nerve function. More recently, robotic-assisted RPLNS has been introduced, offering enhanced dexterity, 3D visualization, and refined nerve-sparing capabilities. The integration of indocyanine green (ICG) fluorescence imaging with robotic near-infrared technology may further facilitate lymphatic mapping and anatomic identification during dissection. Sentinel node evaluation may help identify involved nodes in pediatric paratesticular rhabdomyosarcoma; however, current evidence is limited and it should not be used as a substitute for template-based retroperitoneal nodal sampling. Cooperative-group consensus recommends that adequate surgical nodal staging includes sampling from the retroperitoneal template with retrieval of at least 7 nodes even if a sentinel node is identified. Therefore, sentinel techniques should be considered complementary and investigational rather than substitutive to standard retroperitoneal nodal evaluation.[12]

Ovarian Tumors

MIS plays a central role in the management of pediatric ovarian masses. For benign lesions, ovarian-sparing surgery is the standard, and laparoscopic excision offers excellent cosmetic and functional outcomes. For malignant ovarian tumors, however, the goal is complete removal of the affected ovary with or without the fallopian tube, depending on involvement. While MIS can facilitate inspection of the contralateral ovary and staging biopsies, large tumors often require a small laparotomy for intact specimen removal as well as adequate staging.[12] In this context, regardless of whether a minimally invasive or open approach is adopted, the paramount objective remains a complete and oncologically sound surgical staging. Accurate peritoneal inspection, appropriate sampling of peritoneal fluid or washings, omental assessment, and thorough evaluation of lymph nodes—when indicated—are essential to ensure correct risk stratification and to guide adjuvant therapy. The choice of surgical access should therefore be dictated not by technical preference alone, but by the ability to achieve comprehensive staging without compromise.

Pulmonary Metastases

Thoracoscopy is commonly used in the evaluation and management of pulmonary nodules in children with cancer. Its role in therapeutic metastasectomy remains debated, particularly in osteosarcoma, where complete clearance of lung disease is essential for cure. The lack of tactile sensation in thoracoscopy raises concerns about missing small nodules, and in these cases, thoracotomy may still be preferred. However, thoracoscopic resection of solitary nodules is considered safe and beneficial, minimizing postoperative morbidity while preserving oncologic outcomes (Children's Oncology Group, AOST2031; NCT05235165).

ROBOTIC SURGERY IN PEDIATRIC ONCOLOGY

Robotic-assisted surgery (RAS) represents the most recent and perhaps the most promising development in pediatric surgical oncology. The integration of robotics into pediatric practice has gradually evolved from urologic procedures and gastrointestinal surgery to oncologic resections, where precision, visualization, and delicate dissection are paramount.

Technical Advantages

Robotic systems such as the Intuitive da Vinci surgical system provide a stable 3D high-definition visualization with up to 10-fold magnification, wristed instruments with 7 degrees of freedom, tremor filtration, and motion scaling. These features markedly enhance precision and ergonomics, allowing surgeons to perform complex dissections, vascular control, and intracorporeal suturing in anatomically confined regions.

Such advantages are especially valuable in the mediastinum, retroperitoneum, and pelvis, where rigid laparoscopic instruments and 2-dimensional visualization can limit exposure and maneuverability. The robotic interface also enables dual-console teaching, facilitating safe training in complex pediatric procedures.

Indications for Robotic-Assisted Tumor Surgery

Robotic surgery should be considered in selected pediatric patients when it provides clear technical or functional advantages without compromising oncologic safety. Indications depend on tumor location, size, relation to vital structures, and surgeon experience (**Table 1**).

Tumor-specific Indications

Neuroblastoma

The most frequent indication for robotic or laparoscopic oncologic surgery in children is resection of a neuroblastoma. Ideal candidates are those with localized or intermediate-risk tumors (INRGSS L1–L2) with limited vascular contact. RAS facilitates safe dissection around the renal hilum, celiac trunk, and aorta, with improved exposure of the posterior retroperitoneum (**Fig. 1**). Studies by Blanc and colleagues[13] and Aldrink and colleagues[14] confirm feasibility in children greater than 10 kg, with low conversion.

Adrenal Tumors

Both benign (ganglioneuromas) and malignant (neuroblastoma, adrenocortical carcinoma) adrenal lesions can be approached robotically when confined and without vascular invasion. The robotic approach provides superior dexterity for adrenal vein control and preservation of adjacent structures. Special caution and expertise are required in cases of adrenocortical carcinoma because of the friable nature of the tumor and the oncologic consequences of spill of malignant tumor cells.

Table 1
Indications for robotic-assisted tumor surgery over standard laparoscopy/thoracoscopy

Category	Indication
Tumor characteristics	Well-circumscribed tumors with clear radiological planes, where en bloc resection can be achieved without capsule violation.
Tumor size	Lesions $\leq$ 6–8 cm in maximum diameter, or with a tumor-to-abdominal cavity ratio permitting safe manipulation and extraction.
Vascular involvement	Tumors with limited vascular involvement, avoiding direct encasement of major vessels. Encased renal vessels and iliac vessels can be managed in RAS in selected neuroblastic tumors.
Response to therapy	Lesions responsive to neoadjuvant therapy, resulting in reduced size and vascular adherence.
Anatomic location	Tumors in confined but accessible spaces where the robotic platform offers ergonomic and visualization benefits—notably the mediastinum, adrenal bed, retroperitoneum, and deep pelvis.
Technical complexity	Procedures requiring fine dissection and reconstruction, such as nephron-sparing surgery, vascular or ureteral reconstruction, and thoracic resections adjacent to the spine or diaphragm.

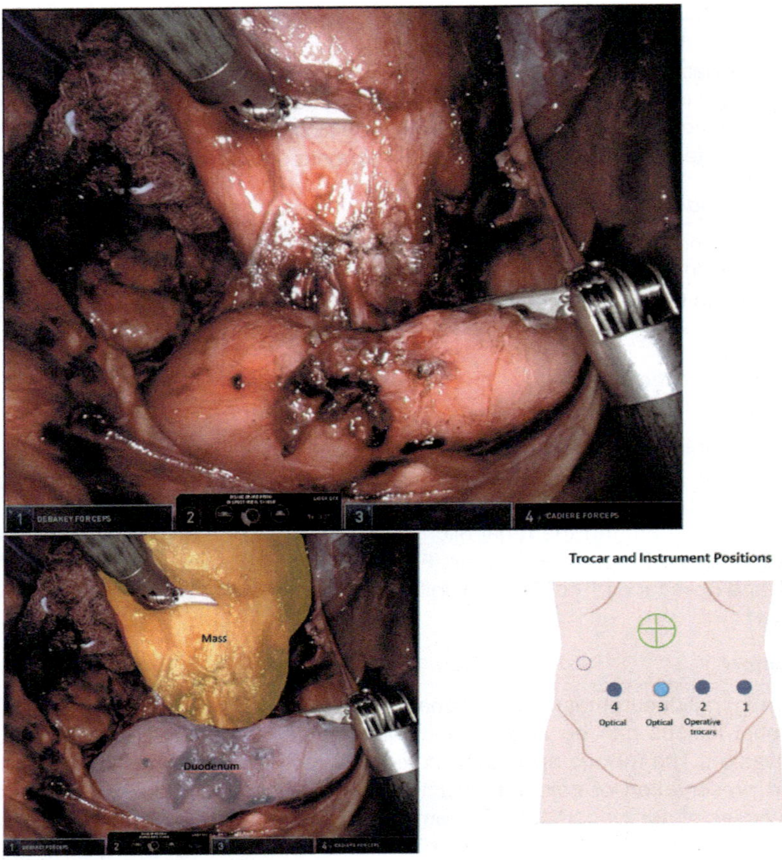

Fig. 1. Robot-assisted laparoscopy for the resection of a right retroperitoneal neuroblastoma. The image shows the tumor and the duodenum in close contact and trocar positioning.

Renal Tumors

Selected cases of Wilms tumor following neoadjuvant chemotherapy—characterized by a small residual mass, absence of venous thrombus, no midline crossing, and no infiltration of extrarenal structures—have been safely resected robotically. Robotic assistance is also advantageous for nephron-sparing surgery in bilateral or syndromic cases (eg, Beckwith–Wiedemann syndrome), allowing meticulous parenchymal reconstruction. Lymph node sampling can be performed with robotic assistance, as recommended by current guidelines (**Fig. 2**).

Thoracic and mediastinal tumors

Posterior mediastinal neurogenic tumors and selected anterior mediastinal masses represent favorable indications for minimally invasive and robotic approaches. In older children and adolescents, the robotic platform may reduce the need for rib spreading, thereby potentially decreasing postoperative pain and improving recovery. The enhanced 3D visualization and articulated instruments provide superior dexterity

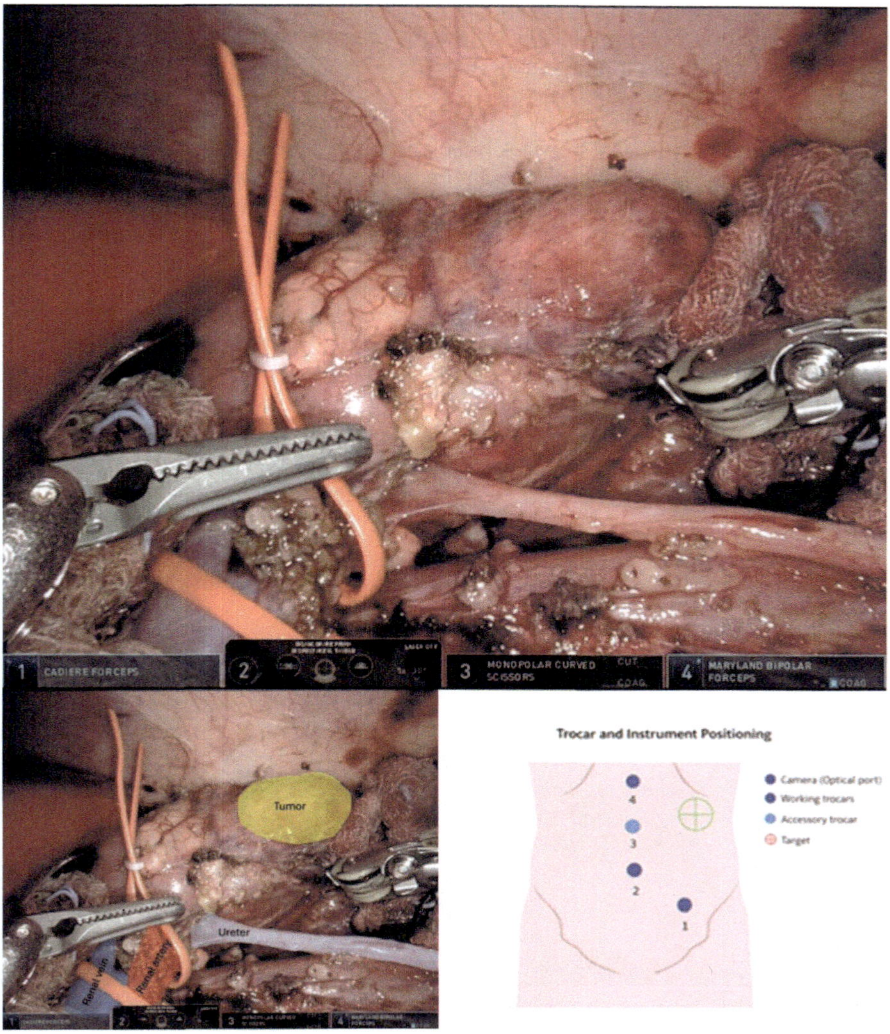

Fig. 2. Robot-assisted laparoscopy for the resection of a left lower pole Wilms tumor using a nephron-sparing technique. The image highlights vascular isolation of the renal pedicle, the left ureter, and the lower renal pole as well as trocar positioning.

and angulation, which is particularly advantageous when dissecting around fixed bony structures such as the ribs and spine, and when operating in close proximity to the sympathetic chain or major vascular structures. However, this approach also has limitations. In smaller children with narrow intercostal spaces, the need to accommodate 8-mm ports may represent a technical constraint and can limit applicability. Furthermore, although robotic precision theoretically facilitates careful dissection near the sympathetic chain, there is currently no clear published evidence demonstrating a reduced incidence of complications—such as Horner's syndrome—compared with open surgery. From a technical standpoint, patient positioning typically involves lateral decubitus, with the ipsilateral upper limb elevated above the head to optimize intercostal exposure. In many cases, complete lung exclusion or single-lung ventilation is not mandatory, particularly for smaller posterior mediastinal lesions, which may simplify anesthetic management (**Fig. 3**).

Pelvic and ovarian tumors

Ovarian masses may benefit from a robotic approach due to enhanced visualization of reproductive organs and pelvic vasculature. Robotic instrumentation allows delicate tissue handling and facilitates fertility-preserving surgery when applicable. In malignant ovarian tumors, the risk of intraperitoneal spillage warrants special consideration and case-by-case discussion in a multidisciplinary context.

Sarcomas

Certain localized soft tissue sarcomas, particularly in the retroperitoneum or pelvis, may be considered for robotic excision if surrounded by a clear capsule and not invading major vessels or bone.

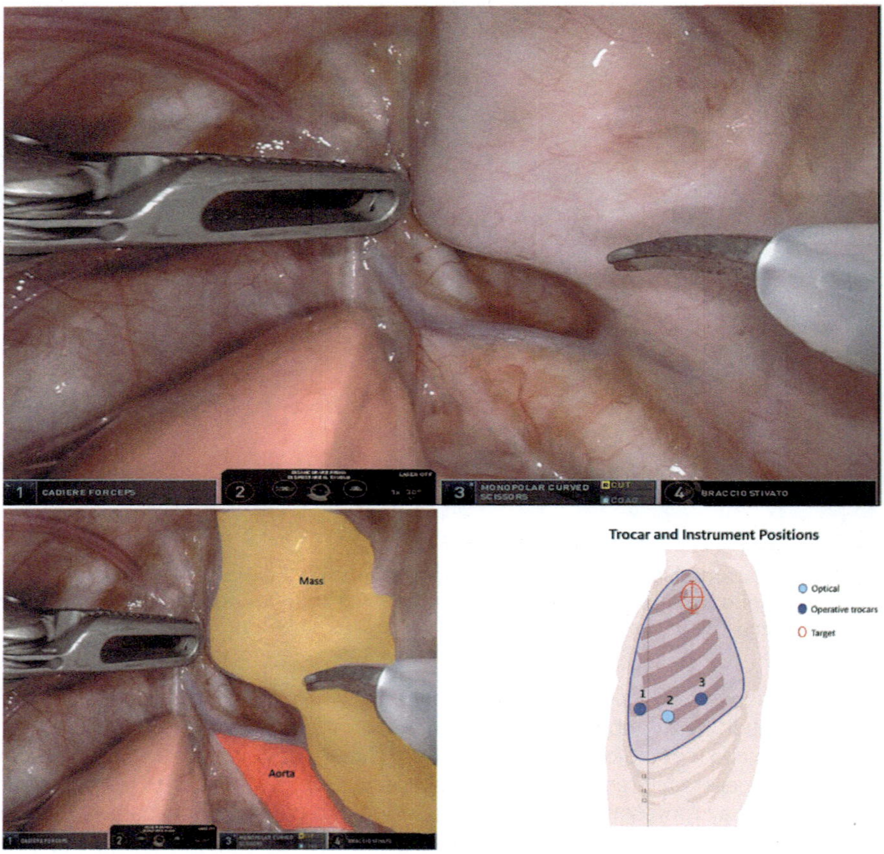

Fig. 3. Robot-assisted thoracoscopy for the resection of a mediastinal neuroblastoma located at the left thoracic apex, in close contact with the aortic arch and the supra-aortic vessels. Trocar positioning. Of note, single-lung ventilation is often not required for this type of procedure.

Contraindications to the Robotic Approach

Robotic resection should be avoided when it might compromise oncologic principles or patient safety. Contraindications can be absolute or relative (**Table 2**).

Patient Selection and Preoperative Planning

Patient selection remains the cornerstone of successful robotic oncologic surgery. Candidates should be evaluated by a multidisciplinary tumor board including pediatric surgeons, oncologists, radiologists, and anesthesiologists.

Contrast-enhanced cross-sectional imaging with magnetic resonance or computed tomography (CT) is essential to define tumor boundaries, vascular relationships, and potential invasion.

3D reconstruction and virtual surgical planning can facilitate port placement and predict safe dissection planes.

Neoadjuvant chemotherapy often downsizes the tumor, transforming borderline cases into suitable candidates for robotic resection; however, this approach must be weighed with late effects of these drugs.

The operative approach (transperitoneal, retroperitoneal, or transthoracic) and patient positioning must be tailored to tumor location, with clear planning for specimen retrieval in a protective bag to prevent spillage. The use of extended-length robotic ports in selected pediatric cases allows the remote center to be positioned more or completely externally relative to the body wall, increasing the working distance between ports. This technical adjustment can reduce external arm collisions and improve internal triangulation, thereby expanding the range of motion and maneuverability—particularly in patients with limited abdominal domain.

Table 2
Contraindications to the robotic approach

Category	Contraindication
Absolute	Tumor rupture risk due to fragile capsule or cystic degeneration.
	Vascular encasement of major structures (aorta, vena cava, and mesenteric vessels) that precludes safe dissection.
	Extensive local invasion into adjacent organs or diaphragm where en bloc resection cannot be safely achieved robotically.
	Uncontrolled coagulopathy or cardiorespiratory instability incompatible with pneumoperitoneum, pneumothorax, or single-lung ventilation.
	Absence of institutional surgical expertise in robotic pediatric oncology.
Relative	Large tumors (>8–10 cm) occupying more than one-third of the abdominal cavity, where manipulation risks capsule rupture.
	Extensive adhesions from previous surgery or infection.
	Inability to achieve R0 margins due to tumor size or location when a margin-negative resection is required
	Very small children (<10 kg), where limited abdominal space restricts port placement and maneuverability.
	Tumors crossing multiple compartments (eg, thoracoabdominal neuroblastoma) that may require combined open access.
	Requirement for complex vascular reconstruction, which remains technically challenging robotically in infants.

Intraoperative Considerations

Key principles during robotic tumor resection include:

Maintaining oncologic principles: minimal direct tumor grasping, avoidance of capsule violation, and achieving en bloc resection when required.

Use of vessel-sealing devices under direct vision or Hem-o-lok vessel occlusion clips, and readiness for conversion if vascular control becomes unsafe.

Adequate lymph node sampling as indicated by tumor type **Fig. 4**.

Specimen extraction is performed in a protected endoscopic bag, either through a minilaparotomy (Pfannenstiel incision) or via an enlarged port site, avoiding morcellation.

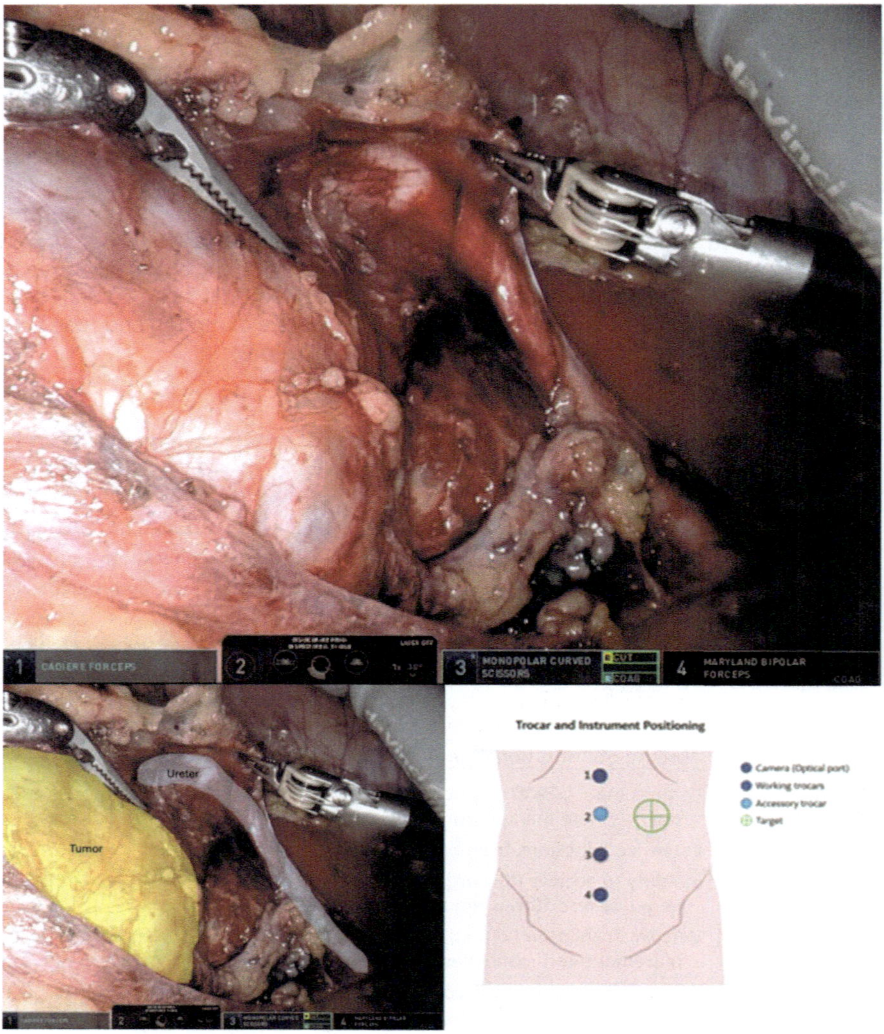

Fig. 4. Robot-assisted laparoscopy for RPLNS in a testicular germ cell tumor. The image shows the left ureter and a large lymph node conglomerate and trocar positioning.

Outcomes and Oncologic Safety

Contemporary evidence supports the safety and efficacy of robotic surgery when applied under appropriate indications. Blanc and colleagues[13] reported a nationwide study of 100 robotic tumor resections, with no intraoperative ruptures, 8% conversions, and excellent short-term outcomes. Aldrink and colleagues[14] reported complete resection in all 39 cases, with a median hospital stay of 1.5 days and no major complications. Many other smaller institutional reports confirm low blood loss, shorter recovery, and improved cosmesis compared with open surgery. Oncologic adequacy—in terms of margin status, local recurrence, and survival—appears comparable to open procedures in properly selected cases, although long-term data remain limited.

THREE-DIMENSIONAL SURGICAL PLANNING AND SIMULATION

3D technologies have transformed the way surgeons conceptualize and prepare for complex oncologic procedures in children. Conventional 2-dimensional imaging provides essential diagnostic information, but often falls short in conveying the true spatial relationships between tumors and surrounding critical structures. By converting radiologic data into interactive, patient-specific models, 3D surgical planning enables a more accurate understanding of anatomy and pathology, facilitating safer and more precise surgical strategies. These tools extend beyond static visualization: they can be printed into physical 3D prototypes, explored in immersive virtual or augmented reality environments, and even integrated into simulation platforms for operative planning and, potentially, rehearsal.[4,5,15]

In pediatric surgical oncology, where tumors frequently involve delicate anatomic regions and organ preservation is of paramount importance, 3D planning holds particular promise. The ability to anticipate technical challenges, test different surgical approaches, and communicate plans within the multidisciplinary team—and even with patients and families—represents a paradigm shift toward precision surgery. Moreover, the rapid evolution of AI, segmentation algorithms, and advanced visualization systems continues to lower barriers of cost and time, making these technologies increasingly feasible in routine clinical practice.[16,17]

Workflow and Technologies

The workflow of 3D surgical planning begins with acquisition of high-resolution imaging, most commonly contrast-enhanced CT or MRI, which provide the necessary detail to capture tumor extent and its relationship with adjacent structures. The next critical step is segmentation, the digital process of isolating and labeling relevant anatomy from raw imaging data. By delineating tumors, vessels, and organs of interest, segmentation transforms conventional scans into distinct 3D objects that form the foundation of patient-specific models. This process can be performed manually, slice by slice, refined with semiautomatic tools, or increasingly accelerated by AI-based algorithms designed to reduce time and user variability[4,16]

Once segmentation is complete, the data can be processed into various outputs. Virtual reconstructions allow surgeons to rotate, magnify, or render structures transparent, improving appreciation of complex spatial relationships. Physical 3D-printed models provide tactile prototypes that can be examined preoperatively, sterilized for intraoperative reference, or even used in training and education (**Fig. 5**).[5,18]

Emerging platforms in VR/AR enable interactive manipulation of anatomy, rehearsal of different surgical approaches, and real-time team communication in an immersive environment. Mixed reality headsets, for instance, allow surgeons to overlay

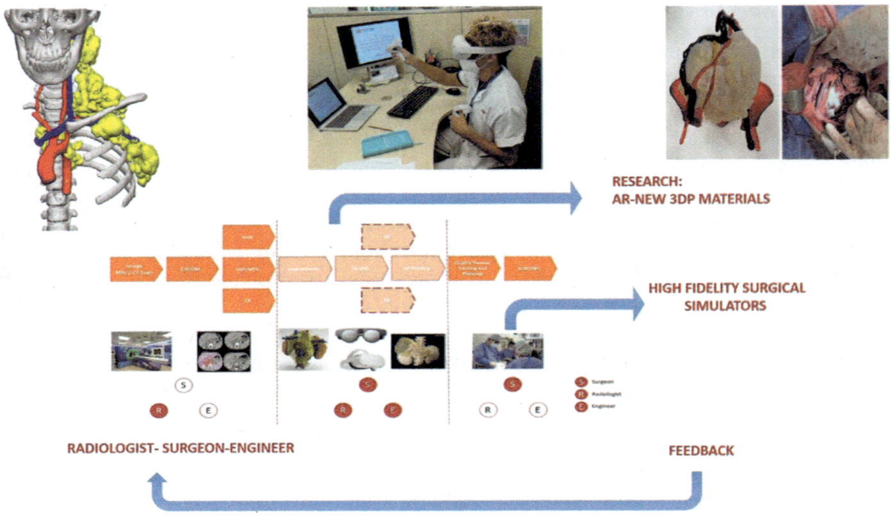

Fig. 5. Integrated workflow for 3D surgical planning and simulation. Process from image acquisition and segmentation to virtual/printed models, high-fidelity simulators, and AR applications, developed through continuous collaboration among radiologists, surgeons, and engineers.

patient-specific anatomy onto the operative field, bridging the gap between planning and execution (**Fig. 6**A-C).

The successful application of these technologies requires multidisciplinary collaboration between radiologists, biomedical engineers, and surgeons to ensure accuracy, clinical relevance, and usability. Advances in material science and sterilization protocols have also enabled safe intraoperative use of models, further strengthening their role as practical tools in surgical oncology.[19] Together, these technologies constitute a flexible and scalable workflow that can be adapted to different institutional resources, ultimately supporting safer resections, greater organ preservation, and more precise operative strategies in pediatric patients.

Clinical Applications

Physical 3D prototypes and virtual models have been successfully applied in complex pediatric oncologic scenarios, providing surgeons with an opportunity to rehearse procedures in advance, anticipate risks, and refine operative strategies.[3,5] **Fig. 7**.

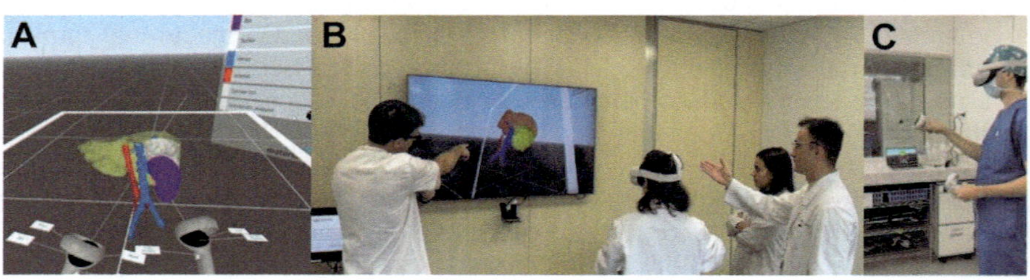

Fig. 6. Use of virtual surgical planning across clinical contexts. (*A*) Virtual 3D visualization of the tumor and surrounding anatomy. (*B*) Interactive teaching session with residents and fellows. (*C*) Preoperative visualization in the operating room to support surgical decision-making.

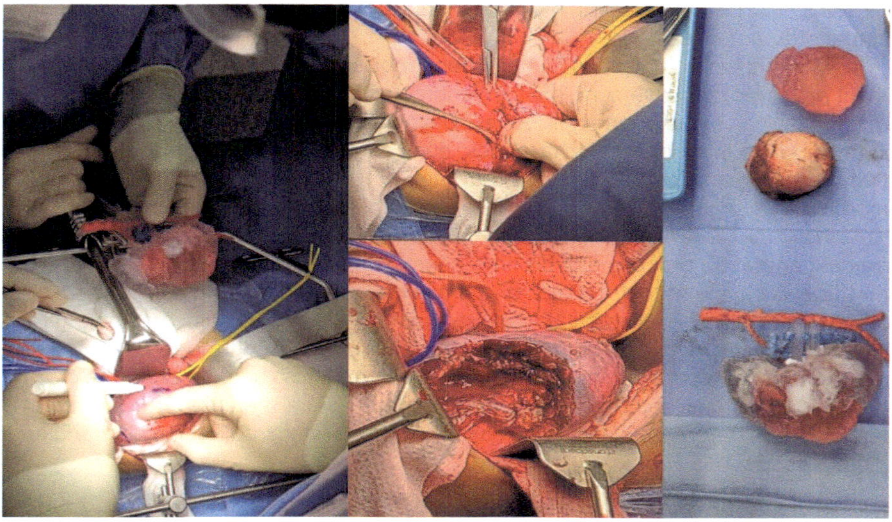

Fig. 7. Different aspects of nephron-sparing surgery using 3D-printed models for surgical guidance.

A Delphi-based expert consensus[20] included 3D modeling among the techniques that may be considered in this setting, although without providing outcome-based validation. Increasingly, 3D planning is being integrated into virtual and augmented reality platforms, broadening opportunities for rehearsal, simulation, and intraoperative guidance.[21] Beyond their role in operative preparation, 3D models have emerged as versatile instruments across several domains of pediatric surgical oncology. In clinical practice, they provide surgeons with tangible or virtual references that improve spatial understanding, aid intraoperative navigation, and support safer resections. In teaching and training, they allow residents and fellows to practice surgical steps, test alternative approaches, and rehearse complex resections in a controlled environment, thereby accelerating the learning curve for challenging oncologic procedures.

3D models also strengthen multidisciplinary communication. By offering a shared visual language, they facilitate discussion among surgeons, oncologists, radiologists, anesthesiologists, and radiation oncologists, ensuring that operative planning is seamlessly integrated into the broader treatment strategy. Finally, they play a unique role in family-centered care. Parents often find conventional imaging difficult to interpret, but physical or virtual 3D models provide an intuitive explanation of their child's condition and the proposed intervention. This enhances understanding, reduces anxiety, and builds trust in the treatment plan.[22]

Impact on outcomes

While randomized data remain limited, a growing body of evidence suggests that 3D surgical planning has a measurable impact on clinical outcomes in pediatric oncology. Early series indicate that its use may shorten operative time, decrease intraoperative complications, and improve the likelihood of achieving complete resections with negative margins.[3,23] In renal tumors, consensus statements highlight the value of 3D models for assessing the feasibility of nephron-sparing procedures, particularly in bilateral or centrally located lesions where preserving renal function is critical.

Similarly, in abdominal and thoracic tumors, 3D reconstructions provide enhanced clarity of tumor–vessel.[23,24]

In neuroblastoma, 3D planning has been reported to improve preoperative assessment of vascular encasement, enabling more accurate stratification of cases for minimally invasive versus open approaches. Beyond resection feasibility, models also aid in anticipating intraoperative challenges, such as vascular control or organ mobilization, reducing unexpected findings that may otherwise prolong surgery or increase morbidity.

At the same time, current limitations must be acknowledged. The segmentation and model generation process can be time-consuming, and results may vary depending on the experience of the operator or the availability of semiautomated and AI-based tools. Costs, although steadily decreasing, remain a barrier in some settings, particularly for centers without in-house engineering support. Furthermore, most published data come from feasibility and proof-of-concept studies, underscoring the need for larger, prospective, multicenter trials to validate clinical benefits and assess cost-effectiveness before 3D planning can be fully incorporated into routine pediatric oncologic practice.

Pediatric-specific insights

Compared to adults, pediatric patients benefit uniquely from 3D surgical planning and simulation. The smaller anatomic scale of children amplifies the challenges of surgical precision, as millimetric differences in dissection can have significant consequences for organ function and long-term outcomes. Pediatric tumors also frequently present with intimate vascular or visceral relationships, such as encasement of major vessels or extension into critical anatomic compartments, where clear spatial understanding is paramount. In these scenarios, 3D planning provides a level of anatomic detail and clarity that is especially advantageous, supporting safer resections and more confident organ-preserving strategies.

Another pediatric-specific dimension is the role of 3D models in family education and engagement. Parents of children with cancer often struggle to interpret conventional CT or MRI images, yet their role in decision-making is central. Physical or virtual 3D models provide an intuitive tool to explain the tumor, its relationship to surrounding organs, and the rationale for the proposed operation. Families consistently report that such models improve comprehension, reduce anxiety, and strengthen trust in the care team. This aligns closely with the principles of family-centered care, which are particularly emphasized in pediatrics.[25]

Finally, 3D planning resonates with the educational needs of pediatric oncology teams, where training opportunities may be limited by the relative rarity of specific tumor types. Patient-specific models and simulations provide a reproducible way to expose trainees to anatomically complex cases, accelerating the learning curve without compromising patient safety.

INTRAOPERATIVE NAVIGATION AND IMAGE-GUIDED TECHNIQUES

Intraoperative navigation in pediatric surgical oncology has evolved considerably, moving from conventional ultrasound-based guidance to a broad spectrum of advanced molecular and imaging technologies. Among these, fluorescence-guided surgery (FGS) has gained particular attention. ICG is currently the most widely used fluorescent tracer in children, owing to its safety profile and established use in hepatobiliary surgery. In oncology, ICG has been applied to aid in intraoperative identification of tumor margins, sentinel lymph node mapping, and detection of small or otherwise occult metastases.[26] The main limitation of ICG remains its shallow penetration depth (<1 cm), which restricts visualization to superficial or exposed lesions. To overcome this, next-generation targeted fluorophores are in active development, such as conjugates directed against tumor-specific markers like GD2, which promise enhanced sensitivity and specificity for pediatric tumors[27–29]

Early clinical experience with other targeted agents, such as the folate-receptor–directed fluorophore pafolacianine, has shown feasibility in young patients undergoing pulmonary metastasectomy for osteosarcoma, improving real-time detection of metastatic nodules beyond white-light inspection and illustrating the potential of molecular FGS to enhance surgical accuracy in pediatric solid tumors.[30]

Radioguided surgery represents another complementary technique. In neuroblastoma, the use of metaiodobenzylguanidine, a norepinephrine analog selectively taken up by neuroblastoma cells, has enabled intraoperative localization of both primary tumors and metastatic deposits, extending detection capabilities deeper into tissues where fluorescence guidance is limited. Building on this, hybrid dual-labeled agents that combine fluorescent and radiotracer properties are currently under investigation, offering the possibility of multimodal guidance with improved accuracy.[31]

Advances in intraoperative navigation, although experimental in this setting, also include the integration of segmented 3D imaging into the surgical field. By overlaying patient-specific reconstructions onto the anatomy in real time, surgeons can visualize tumor–organ–vessel relationships directly during resection, effectively merging preoperative planning with intraoperative decision-making.[21,24]

Taken together, these innovations mark a shift toward more precise, biology-driven intraoperative navigation in pediatric surgical oncology. While many remain at early stages of clinical translation, the combination of fluorescence, radioguided techniques, and image overlay holds great promise for improving tumor localization, achieving complete resections, and ultimately advancing outcomes for children with cancer.

VIRTUAL REALITY, ARTIFICIAL INTELLIGENCE, AND SMART SURGICAL PLATFORMS

VR and AR are becoming increasingly integrated into pediatric surgical oncology. VR platforms enable immersive rehearsal of operations using patient-specific imaging data, allowing surgeons to explore anatomy, plan dissection strategies, and practice technical maneuvers in a risk-free environment. AR applications, in turn, overlay segmented models directly onto the patient in the operating room, providing real-time visual guidance during resection and effectively merging planning with execution.

AI is emerging as a key enabler of these technologies. Machine learning algorithms are increasingly applied to automate image segmentation, substantially reducing the time and variability associated with manual workflows. AI also holds promise for predicting surgical complexity, anticipating intraoperative risks, and supporting real-time decision-making by integrating imaging, operative, and physiologic data.

Looking ahead, the development of smart surgical platforms that combine robotics, AI, and connected devices—represents a major frontier. These platforms are designed not only to assist with visualization but also to actively enhance precision and safety and store data for further learning.

CURRENT GAPS AND RESEARCH OPPORTUNITIES

Despite encouraging results, several gaps remain in the evidence base for MIS and robotic surgery in pediatric oncology. Randomized controlled trials are scarce, largely due to the rarity of pediatric solid tumors and challenges in accrual. Most available data are retrospective, single-center, and heterogeneous in terms of case selection.

Another limitation is the lack of standardized criteria for selecting patients for MIS versus open surgery. While IDRFs and size provide guidance, their predictive value for MIS feasibility remains imperfect.[7]

FUTURE PERSPECTIVES AND RECOMMENDATIONS

The trajectory of pediatric oncologic surgery clearly points toward broader integration of MIS and robotic technologies. As experience accumulates, indications are likely to expand, particularly in the context of adrenal, thoracic, and pelvic tumors. While the robotic approach offers unparalleled precision, it remains limited by the size of instruments (8 mm), port spacing requirements, cost, and the lack of haptic feedback. The development of pediatric-specific robotic systems with 5 mm instruments, shorter arms, and improved force feedback will likely expand its indications. Training also remains crucial: structured curricula, dual-console mentorship, and multicenter registries are needed to ensure safety and consistency. The incorporation of AI-based planning, augmented reality, and fluorescence navigation represents the next frontier in robotic pediatric oncology. Collaborative registries and multi-institutional studies will be essential to generate high-quality evidence and refine guidelines.

SUMMARY

MIS has secured an important role in pediatric oncology, evolving from a diagnostic adjunct to a therapeutic option for selected tumors. Robotic-assisted techniques promise to overcome many of the limitations of conventional laparoscopy, offering enhanced dexterity and visualization for complex resections. While evidence is growing, cautious case selection and strict adherence to oncologic principles remain critical. Future integration of robotics, advanced imaging, and collaborative research will continue to shape the landscape of pediatric oncologic surgery.

CLINICS CARE POINTS

- Reserve minimally invasive surgery (MIS) for tumors without image-defined risk factors (IDRFs); L1 neuroblastic tumors and well-circumscribed lesions with clear radiologic planes are the most reliable candidates for laparoscopic or thoracoscopic resection.
- Confirm absence of major vascular encasement (aorta, vena cava, celiac trunk, SMA) on cross-sectional imaging before planning an MIS or robotic approach; encasement of these vessels is an absolute contraindication.
- Use neoadjuvant chemotherapy strategically: tumor downsizing and reduced vascular adherence can convert borderline lesions into candidates for MIS or robotic resection.
- Do not pursue MIS when R0 margins cannot be assured.
- Adrenocortical carcinoma, clear cell sarcoma, and rhabdoid tumors require open resection because of capsule fragility and the imperative to avoid spillage.
- Avoid tumor rupture at all costs in Wilms tumor; given its impact on staging and the need for intensified therapy, open nephrectomy remains the standard, with laparoscopy reserved for highly selected post-chemotherapy cases (small residual mass, no venous thrombus, no midline crossing).
- Always extract specimens in a protective endoscopic retrieval bag through a mini-laparotomy or enlarged port site; never morcellate oncologic specimens.
- In children under 10 kg, anticipate that limited working space and interport distances under 7 cm will compromise robotic instrument triangulation; weigh this against the benefits before committing to a robotic approach.

- Maintain readiness to convert to open surgery whenever vascular control becomes unsafe; conversion is a sign of sound judgment, not failure. Reported robotic conversion rates remain low (around 8%).
- Adhere to oncologic discipline intraoperatively: no direct tumor grasping, no capsule violation, and en bloc resection within intact planes.
- Recognize the depth limitation of indocyanine green (ICG) fluorescence (penetration under 1 cm); it is best suited to superficial or exposed lesions and sentinel node mapping, not deep-seated disease.
- Consider radioguided (MIBG) localization for small, deep, or relapsed MIBG-avid neuroblastoma lesions where fluorescence guidance is insufficient.
- In thoracoscopic metastasectomy, account for the loss of tactile feedback; small or deep pulmonary nodules may be missed, and thoracotomy may still be preferred when complete clearance is essential, as in osteosarcoma.
- During posterior mediastinal resections, dissect carefully along the sympathetic chain to avoid Horner's syndrome; single-lung ventilation is often unnecessary for apical lesions.
- Validate any 3D-printed model intended for intraoperative use against approved sterilization protocols, and verify segmentation accuracy with the radiology team, as model fidelity depends on operator experience and imaging quality.
- Route every candidate through a multidisciplinary tumor board (surgery, oncology, radiology, anesthesiology) before selecting a minimally invasive or robotic approach, and do not attempt these resections without institutional expertise in pediatric robotic oncology.

REFERENCES

1. Blanc T, Meignan P, Vinit N, et al. Robotic surgery in pediatric oncology: lessons learned from the first 100 tumors—A nationwide experience. Ann Surg Oncol 2022;29(2):1315–26.
2. Pachl M, Lautz TB, Aldrink JH, et al. Minimally invasive and robotic-assisted approaches applied to pediatric surgical oncology. Pediatr Blood Cancer 2025;72-(Suppl 2):e31162.
3. Krauel L, Fenollosa F, Riaza L, et al. Use of 3D prototypes for complex surgical oncologic cases. World J Surg 2016;40(4):889–94.
4. Valls-Esteve A, Adell-Gómez N, Pasten A, et al. Exploring the potential of three-dimensional imaging, printing, and modeling in pediatric surgical oncology: a new era of precision surgery. Children (Basel) 2023;10(5):832.
5. Fusco JC, Abdelhafeez AH, Krauel L, et al. Imaging adjuvants in pediatric surgical oncology. Pediatr Blood Cancer 2025;72(Suppl 2):e31241.
6. Spurbeck WW, Davidoff AM, Lobe TE, et al. Minimally invasive surgery in pediatric cancer patients. Ann Surg Oncol 2004;11(3):340–3.
7. Cecchetto G, Riccipetitoni G, Inserra A, et al, Italian Group of Pediatric Surgical Oncology. Minimally-invasive surgery in paediatric oncology: proposal of recommendations. Pediatr Med e Chir 2010;32(5):197–201.
8. Gurria JP, Malek MM, Heaton TE, et al. Minimally invasive surgery for abdominal and thoracic neuroblastic tumors: a systematic review by the APSA Cancer Committee. J Pediatr Surg 2020;55(11):2260–72.
9. Abdelhafeez A, Davidoff AM, Lautz TB, et al. Twenty years of minimally invasive procedures in pediatric oncology: St. Jude update. J Pediatr Surg 2018.
10. Malek MM, Behr CA, Aldrink JH, et al. Minimally invasive surgery for pediatric renal tumors: a systematic review by the APSA Cancer Committee. J Pediatr Surg 2020;55(11):2251–9.

11. Irtan S, Brisse HJ, Minard-Colin V, et al. Minimally invasive surgery of neuroblastic tumors in children: indications depend on anatomical location and image-defined risk factors. Pediatr Blood Cancer 2015;62(2):257–61. Epub 2014 Oct 4. PMID: 25284263.
12. Wijnen MWHA, Davidoff AM. Minimally invasive techniques in pediatric surgical oncology. Surg Oncol Clin N Am 2021;30(2):417–30.
13. Blanc T, Meignan P, Vinit N, et al. Robotic Surgery in Pediatric Oncology: nationwide experience. Ann Surg Oncol 2021.
14. Svetanoff WJ, Carter M, Diefenbach KA, et al. Robotic-assisted pediatric thoracic and abdominal tumor resection: an initial multi-center review. J Pediatr Surg 2024;59(8):1619–25.
15. Valls-Esteve A, Tejo-Otero A, Adell-Gómez N, et al. Advanced strategies for the fabrication of multi-material anatomical models of complex pediatric oncologic cases. Bioengineering (Basel) 2023;11(1):31.
16. Lozano-Montoya J, Jimenez-Pastor A, Fuster-Matanzo A, et al. ABAR stratification in neuroblastoma patients through machine learning in the multicenter P cohort. Front Oncol 2025;15:1528836.
17. Ryan ML, Wang S, Pandya SR. PSRIAII the V and M of TDA in PS patients. J Pediatr Surg 2024. https://doi.org/10.1016/j.jpedsurg.2024.07.014. Epub 2024 Jul 15. PMID: 39095281.
18. Krauel L, Valls-Esteve A, Tejo-Otero A, et al. 3D-Printing in surgery: beyond bone structures. A review. Ann 3D Print Med 2021;4:100039.
19. Valls-Esteve A, Lustig-Gainza P, Adell-Gomez N, et al. A state-of-the-art guide about the effects of sterilization processes on 3D-printed materials for surgical planning and medical applications: a comparative study. Int J Bioprint 2023;9(5).
20. Fitski M, Bökkerink GMJ, Davidoff AM, et al. Nephron-sparing surgery for patients with Wilms tumor: a surgical Delphi study consensus statement. Pediatr Blood Cancer 2025;72(4):e31636.
21. de Groot NT, van der Zee JM, Bökkerink GMJ, et al. Introducing holographic surgical navigation in pediatric wilms' tumor. Bioengineering (Basel) 2025;12(8):896.
22. Robertson DJ, Abramson ZR, Davidoff AM, et al. Virtual reality applications in pediatric surgery. Semin Pediatr Surg 2024;33(1):151387.
23. Simons DC, Buser MAD, Fitski M, et al. Multi-modal 3-Dimensional visualization of pediatric neuroblastoma: aiding surgical planning beyond anatomical information. J Pediatr Surg 2024;59(8):1662–71.
24. Spijkerboer KGP, Fitski M, Siepel FJ, et al. Augmented reality-guided localization of a chest wall tumor in a pediatric patient. Eur J Cancer 2022;170:103–5. PMID: 35598357.
25. Abramson ZR, Robertson DJ, Shah NR, et al. Modern imaging guidelines for 3-D modeling of pediatric solid tumors: a new era of surgical oncology operative planning. Children 2025;12:1622.
26. Pio L, Wijnen MHWA, Giuliani S, et al. Identification of pediatric tumors intraoperatively using indocyanine green (ICG). Ann Surg Oncol 2023;30(12):7789–98.
27. Privitera L, Waterhouse DJ, Preziosi A, et al. Shortwave infrared imaging enables high-contrast fluorescence-guided surgery in neuroblastoma. Cancer Res 2023;83(12):2077–89. PMID: 36934744.
28. Wellens LM, Deken MM, Sier CFM, et al. Anti-GD2-IRDye800CW as a targeted probe for fluorescence-guided surgery in neuroblastoma. Sci Rep 2020;10:17667.

29. Rosenblum LT, Sever RE, Gilbert R, et al. Dual-labeled anti-GD2 targeted probe for intraoperative molecular imaging of neuroblastoma. J Transl Med 2024;22(1): 940. PMID: 39407274; PMCID: PMC11476241.
30. Lehane A, Polites SF, Dodd A, et al. Let it glow: intraoperative visualization of pulmonary metastases using pafolacianine, a next-generation fluorescent agent, for young adults undergoing pulmonary metastasectomy. Pediatr Blood Cancer 2024;71(11):e31293.
31. Krauel L, Pasten A, Gorostegui M, et al. Use of radioguided surgery for small and difficult-to-locate relapsed MIBG (+) high-risk neuroblastoma lesions. Cancers (Basel) 2024;16(19):3348.

Image-Guided and Fluorescence-Guided Surgery in Pediatric Oncology

Current State of the Art

Alida F.W. van der Steeg, MD, PhD, MBA[a,*], Marcus M. Malek, MD[b], Joseph C. Fusco, MD, MPH[c]

KEYWORDS

- Pediatric surgical oncology • Image-guided surgery • Fluorescence-guided surgery
- Precision surgery • Multimodal imaging

KEY POINTS

- Pediatric tumors pose distinct surgical challenges requiring high precision and organ preservation.
- Image-guided surgery improves anatomic orientation through navigation, tracking, and 3-dimensional modeling.
- Fluorescence-guided surgery enables real-time visualization of tumors and lymphatics using nontargeted and targeted tracers.
- Integrated, artificial intelligence-supported multimodal guidance represents the future of personalized pediatric cancer surgery.

INTRODUCTION

Adherence to the fundamental principles of surgical oncology, achieving complete resection with negative margins, accurate staging through lymph node assessment, and avoidance of injury to vital structures, all pose unique challenges in pediatric surgical oncology. These challenges arise from the distinctive biological and anatomic features of pediatric tumors, as well as the smaller body size and greater vulnerability of children to treatment-related morbidity.[1,2]

[a] Princess Máxima Center for Pediatric Oncology, Heidelberglaan, Utrecht, the Netherlands; [b] Division of Pediatric General and Thoracic Surgery, UPMC Children's Hospital of Pittsburgh, Pittsburgh, PA, USA; [c] Department of Pediatric Surgery, Monroe Carrel Jr Children's Hospital at Vanderbilt, Nashville, TN, USA

* Corresponding author. Princess Máxima Center for pediatric oncology, Heidelberglaan 25, 3584 CS, Utrecht, the Netherlands.
E-mail address: a.f.w.vandersteeg@prinsesmaximacentrum.nl

Surg Oncol Clin N Am 35 (2026) 867–883
https://doi.org/10.1016/j.soc.2026.05.003 **surgonc.theclinics.com**
1055-3207/26/

Abbreviations	
CAIX	vascular endothelial growth factor
EGFR	epidermal growth factor receptor
EM	Electromagnetic
EPR	enhanced permeability and retention
FGS	fluorescence-guided surgery
HMD	head-mounted display
ICG	indocyanine green
IGS	image-guided surgery
IOUS	intraoperative ultrasound
NIR	near-infrared

Pediatric solid tumors differ fundamentally from their adult counterparts in both origin and behavior. Whereas adult malignancies are predominantly epithelial in nature, many pediatric cancers derive from embryonal or mesenchymal lineages, such as Wilms tumor, hepatoblastoma, rhabdomyosarcoma, and osteosarcoma.[3] Consequently, their growth patterns are often infiltrative but less predictable, and they may intimately involve developing organs and critical vascular or neural structures. This biological heterogeneity complicates intraoperative decision-making, as the surgeon must balance maximal tumor clearance with preservation of organ function and growth potential.

While the surgical outcome in pediatric oncology is significantly influenced by the surgeon's experience, the availability of specialized perioperative imaging tools may also impact results.[4,5] Despite advances in multimodal treatment, surgical resection remains the cornerstone of cure for most pediatric solid malignancies. Incomplete resection can lead to local recurrence or necessitate intensification of adjuvant therapies, both of which may increase late effects. Conversely, overly aggressive resections may compromise function, especially in organs such as the kidney, liver, or extremities, where long-term sequelae can impact quality of life and development.[6,7] Hence, precision and selectivity during surgery are crucial, underscoring the need for technologies that enhance intraoperative visualization and orientation.

Intraoperative decision-making traditionally relies on visual inspection and tactile feedback. However, both are limited in differentiating viable tumor tissue from adjacent healthy parenchyma, particularly after neoadjuvant chemotherapy, which can alter tissue texture and color. These limitations have driven the emergence of intraoperative image-guided technologies, designed to integrate preoperative imaging, real-time tracking, and intraoperative visualization to assist the surgeon in achieving precise tumor localization and margin assessment.[8,9]

Within this domain, 2 technological paradigms have emerged:

1. Image-guided surgery (IGS), which provides *navigation and localization* based on preoperative or intraoperative imaging; and
2. Fluorescence-guided surgery (FGS), which enhances *visualization and tissue discrimination* through optical contrast agents.

These modalities are complementary. IGS helps orient the surgeon spatially within the operative field, enabling accurate correlation between imaging and anatomy. FGS, on the other hand, augments tissue differentiation in real time, allowing visualization of tumor boundaries, sentinel lymph nodes, and vital structures such as vessels and ureters. Both are now entering widespread clinical use in pediatric surgical oncology, supported by increasing evidence of safety and utility.[10,11]

Given the smaller anatomy of pediatric patients, higher susceptibility to radiation exposure, and need for organ preservation, the clinical implementation of IGS and FGS in children poses unique technical and ethical considerations distinct from adult oncology. This review summarizes the current state in image-guided and fluorescence-guided surgery for pediatric solid tumors, focusing on clinical applications, limitations, and future perspectives.

IMAGE-GUIDED SURGERY

Principles and Workflow

IGS aims to translate preoperative imaging data into intraoperative navigation information, allowing the surgeon to locate anatomic landmarks and tumor boundaries with millimetric precision. The general workflow involves (1) acquisition of high-resolution preoperative imaging (MRI or computed tomography [CT]), (2) segmentation and 3-dimensional (3D) modeling of relevant structures, (3) registration of the virtual model with the intraoperative anatomy, and (4) real-time tracking of surgical instruments relative to this registered dataset.[12]

In pediatric oncology, the application of IGS is particularly valuable because of the frequent need to operate in confined spaces (eg, retroperitoneum or hepatic hilum) and the high priority of organ preservation. Furthermore, the complex deformability of pediatric tissues, especially in soft-tissue tumors after neoadjuvant chemotherapy, makes intraoperative orientation challenging. In pediatric oncologic resections, where millimeters often delineate critical vascular, biliary, or collecting system structures, navigation systems must achieve sub–2 mm target registration error to be clinically meaningful. Recent validation studies in pediatric renal and hepatic surgery have demonstrated that navigation-assisted workflows can reliably reach this accuracy threshold near the hilum and major vessels, underscoring the feasibility and clinical value of high-fidelity image guidance in children.[13]

While IGS technologies have become well-established in adult neurosurgery and orthopedic oncology, their adoption in pediatric soft-tissue surgery is more recent and remains under clinical evaluation[9,14] The following sections outline the key components and technologies of IGS, with emphasis on their clinical translation and relevance in pediatric surgical oncology. As pediatric soft tissues deform substantially during respiration, mobilization, and tumor manipulation, registration accuracy degrades rapidly once surgery begins, highlighting the need for navigation systems that can adapt to real-time anatomic change.

Segmentation and 3-Dimensional Modeling

Accurate segmentation of preoperative imaging is the foundation of any navigation system. Advanced software allows the isolation of tumor volume, vessels, collecting systems, and surrounding organs, generating a 3D model that can be manipulated interactively. These 3D reconstructions offer an intuitive understanding of spatial relationships that is not achievable from two-dimensional imaging alone.[15,16]

In the pediatric setting, segmentation can be particularly complex due to smaller anatomic dimensions, less distinct tissue contrast, and variability in imaging protocols across centers.[17] Semiautomated and artificial intelligence (AI)-assisted segmentation tools are increasingly used to improve reproducibility and reduce manual workload.[18] Once segmented, the 3D model is exported to navigation platforms or even 3D-printed for preoperative planning and surgical simulation. Several centers have demonstrated the educational and operative value of 3D-printed models in Wilms tumor and hepatoblastoma resections.[19,20]

Clinically, 3D models have been shown to aid in defining resection planes and assessing the feasibility of nephron-sparing or parenchyma-sparing approaches. In complex renal tumors, for instance, surgeons can preoperatively evaluate the relationship between the tumor and the renal vasculature, thereby reducing operative time and blood loss.[21] Similarly, in hepatoblastoma, 3D models can help identify the optimal transection plane, balancing oncologic radicality with maximal preservation of functional parenchyma.[22,23]

Optical Tracking Systems

Optical tracking systems use infrared cameras to detect reflective markers placed on surgical instruments or patient reference frames (**Fig. 1**A, B). These markers provide real-time position data, enabling the surgeon to visualize instrument trajectories related to the preoperative 3D model displayed on a monitor.[24,25]

This technique offers submillimetric accuracy under ideal conditions but requires an unobstructed line of sight between the cameras and the markers. Pediatric cases can be challenging in this respect because smaller operative fields and additional personnel around the table can intermittently block the view of markers. Moreover, intraoperative organ motion and deformation (eg, due to respiration, manipulation, or resection) can reduce accuracy unless periodic re-registration is performed.[26] In pediatric cases, optical tracking accuracy can also be compromised by drape shifts or subtle patient repositioning, both of which alter the spatial relationship between the reference frame and the surgical field, underscoring the need for frequent verification or reregistration during navigation.

Integration with intraoperative ultrasound (IOUS) is particularly promising. By registering the IOUS images with the preoperative dataset, surgeons can compensate for tissue deformation and update the navigation model in real time.[27,28]

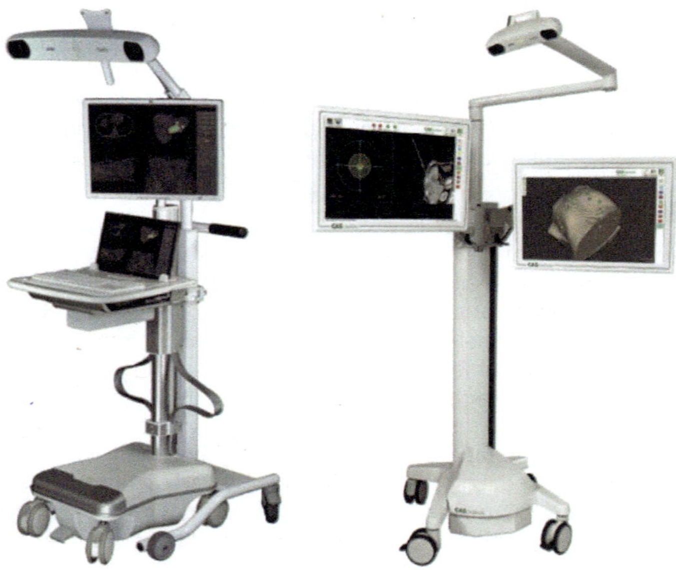

Fig. 1. Image-guided liver surgery systems using optical tracking.

Electromagnetic Tracking Systems

Electromagnetic (EM) tracking systems use low-intensity magnetic fields generated by a field emitter to detect the position and orientation of miniature sensors embedded in surgical instruments (**Fig. 2**). Unlike optical systems, EM tracking does not require a direct line of sight, which is a major advantage in small or deep operative fields.[29]

The flexibility and minimal hardware footprint of EM systems make them attractive for pediatric use, where the surgical field is crowded and delicate. However, EM tracking is more susceptible to distortions from metallic instruments and equipment in the operating room.[30]

Clinically, EM tracking has shown potential in localizing deep intrahepatic or intrathoracic lesions, particularly when combined with IOUS. This *sensorized ultrasound* approach enables precise correlation between the ultrasound probe's position and the 3D preoperative model, allowing the surgeon to *see beyond* the immediate field of view.[31] In adult liver surgery, IOUS has been used to verify resection margins in real time and confirm complete tumor removal before transection of the parenchyma.[32]

In renal surgery, EM navigation may assist in delineating the renal hilum and detecting accessory vessels, reducing the risk of inadvertent vascular injury. Emerging work on miniaturized EM sensors—small enough to be integrated directly into laparoscopic instruments or embedded within ultrasound probes—offers a promising next step toward extending navigation accuracy into minimally invasive pediatric procedures.

Tumor Localization and Hybrid Navigation

An emerging trend in IGS is the combination of navigation technologies with intraoperative imaging modalities, such as cone-beam CT, MRI, or fluorescence. These *hybrid navigation* systems enable intraoperative updates of the image dataset, thereby maintaining accuracy despite anatomic shifts.[33,34]

For instance, intraoperative MRI or ultrasound can be used intraoperatively to reregister navigation data after major tissue mobilization or resection. Although this increases time under anesthesia, its use in children can be justified for highly complex cases where achieving negative margins is critical. Integration of IGS with FGS,

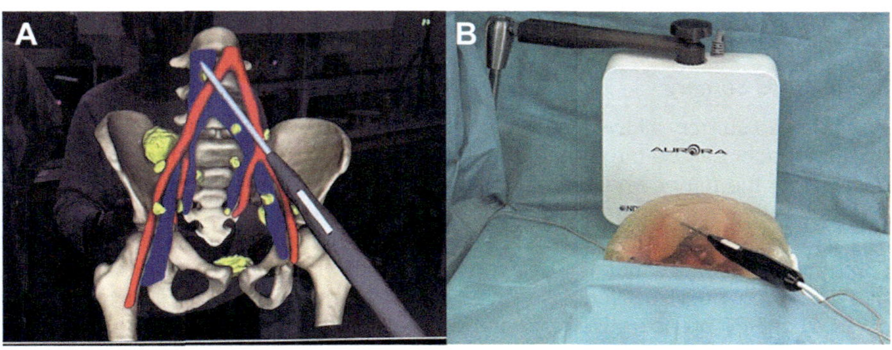

Fig. 2. (*A, B*) Right image shows a phantom of the abdominal cavity with the retroperitoneal vessels visible and the navigation pointer connected to a sensor placed in the abdominal cavity. The left image shows the corresponding 3D image with the pointer near the vena cava. The white box is the electro-magnetic field generator necessary for the navigation. This generator can also be placed underneath the operating table.

discussed later in this review, offers an attractive solution to visualize anatomic and functional information simultaneously.

In sentinel node mapping or metastasectomy, navigation can assist in identifying lymphatic drainage patterns or locate deep-seated lesions that are difficult to palpate. Combining navigation with near-infrared (NIR) fluorescence tracers, for example, allows for dual-modality localization of lesions and sentinel nodes.[35] The integration of navigation data with intraoperative ultrasound and fluorescence imaging represents an early form of multimodal data fusion, a foundational step toward creating real-time *digital twin* surgical environments that continuously reflect evolving anatomy during pediatric tumor resection.

Holographic Projection and Head-Mounted Devices

Recent advances in augmented reality (AR) include head-mounted displays (HMDs) such as the Microsoft HoloLens or the Apple Vision systems overlay the reconstructed anatomy onto the patient's body, providing intuitive spatial orientation without the need to divert attention to a separate monitor.[36] To distinguish current capabilities from future potential, it may be helpful to note that most holographic systems presently provide static visualization, whereas true deformable holographic navigation will require dynamic updates driven by real-time tracking or biomechanical modeling to account for intraoperative organ shift and deformation.

In pediatric oncology, holographic projection is still in early development but holds great potential. Pilot studies have demonstrated its utility in preoperative planning and intraoperative visualization of complex tumor relationships, such as chest wall tumors and retroperitoneal masses.[16,37–39] Surgeons can interact with the hologram via gestures or voice commands, rotating or slicing the model to explore different planes.

Clinically, this can enhance understanding of tumor-vessel interfaces and guide dissection, especially when critical structures are obscured from direct view. Moreover, because holographic overlays are based on preoperative imaging, they can be used in combination with optical or EM tracking for dynamic alignment.

Although technical limitations—such as registration drift, latency, and limited depth perception—still restrict clinical adoption, the rapid pace of hardware and software improvement suggests that intraoperative AR may soon become a valuable adjunct in pediatric surgical oncology (**Fig. 3**).

Radioguided Surgery

Radioguided surgery allows real time intraoperative detection of tumor tissue. In brief, the radiotracer can be targeted to the tumor (given intravenously) or directly injected adjacent to the tumor where it may highlight the tumor itself or be taken up by local lymphatics where it will drain to and highlight the sentinel node. Radioguided surgery (RGS) has been in use for decades to guide sentinel lymph node biopsy, most commonly for breast cancer or melanoma.[40,41] Following tracer administration, the tumor can then be visualized using single-photon emission computed tomography (SPECT) or PET preoperatively or can be detected intraoperatively using a handheld gamma probe. While the gamma probe does not provide a visual aid, it does help orient the surgeon to tumor or lymph node location and can be detected through several cm of tissue.[42] This is a distinct advantage of RGS when compared with fluorescence-guided surgery, where lesions deep to skin or an organ surface can be difficult to detect.[43,44]

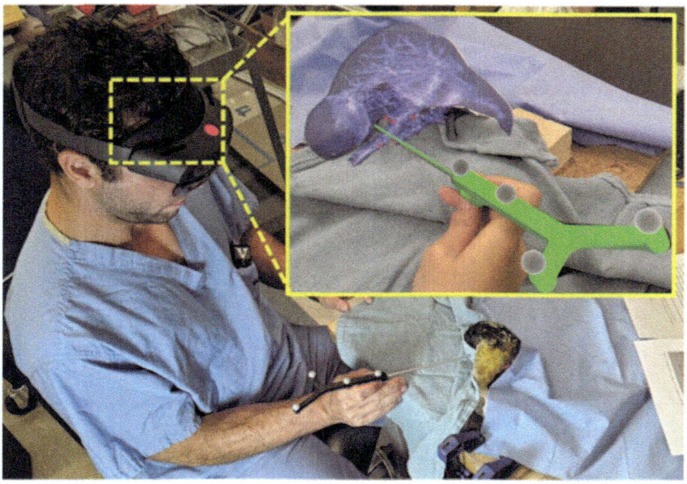

Fig. 3. Bench-top workflow demonstrating mixed reality (MR) visualization using a head-mounted display. A patient-specific 3D hologram (*purple*) derived from preoperative cross-sectional imaging is coregistered to a physical organ model. Optical tracking markers (*green* instrument with reflective spheres) enable spatial alignment and interaction with the hologram, illustrating point-based registration and real-time manipulation.

FLUORESCENCE-GUIDED SURGERY

Principles and Rationale

FGS enhances intraoperative visualization by converting molecular or anatomic information into optical signals detectable in real time (**Fig. 4**). A fluorescent agent is administered preoperatively or intraoperatively and becomes selectively enriched in specific tissues either through physiologic mechanisms (nontargeted tracers; blood or lymphatic flow) or molecular recognition (targeted tracers; tumor antigen or tumor microenvironment). When illuminated with light of a specific excitation wavelength, the fluorophore emits light of a longer wavelength that can be seen in the visual spectrum, or in the case of near-infrared (NIR) fluorophores, captured by dedicated open surgery cameras or integrated into endoscopic cameras.[45–47]

This technique offers several advantages particularly relevant to pediatric oncology. Pediatric tumors are often smaller, more deformable, and more intimately associated with vital structures than those in adults. The ability to visualize tumor margins, sentinel nodes, or critical anatomy in real time can therefore increase surgical precision and reduce postoperative morbidity. Moreover, because FGS provides functional (agent must get to the lesion) rather than merely structural information, it complements the anatomic guidance offered by image-guided surgery.

Fluorescence imaging is typically performed in the NIR spectrum (700–900 nm), which penetrates tissues up to several millimeters while minimizing background autofluorescence and light scattering. This wavelength range allows real-time imaging even through overlying tissue, making it suitable for minimally invasive pediatric procedures.[47]

Nontargeted Fluorescent Agents

Indocyanine green

Indocyanine green (ICG) is the most widely used fluorescent dye in pediatric surgery (**Table 1**). It is a water-soluble tricarbocyanine molecule that binds to

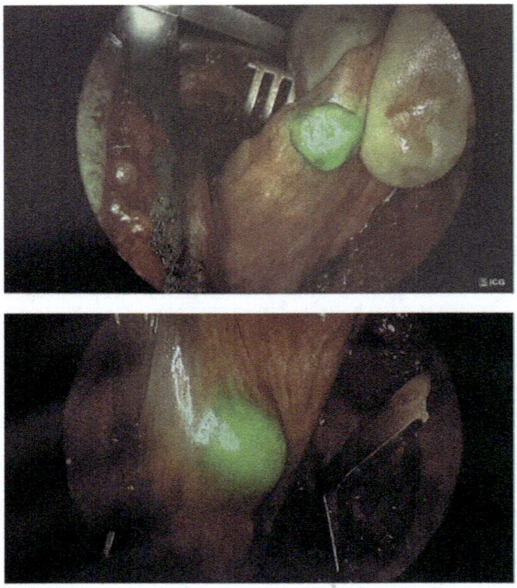

Fig. 4. Intraoperative findings in a child with a large intraabdominal Burkitt's lymphoma and associated pleural effusion. The patient underwent video-assisted thoracoscopic surgery (VATS) for pleural fluid drainage and chest tube placement, followed by diagnostic laparoscopy with tissue biopsy and peritoneal fluid sampling. This case demonstrates the combined use of minimally invasive approaches to reduce morbidity and expedite return to chemotherapy.

plasma proteins and is rapidly excreted by the liver into bile. Its excitation and emission peaks (approximately 805 and 835 nm, respectively) make it ideal for NIR imaging.[48]

Clinical applications in pediatric oncology include:

- *Tumor detection and margin assessment:* ICG accumulates passively in tumor tissue via the enhanced permeability and retention (EPR) effect, although this mechanism is less consistent in pediatric tumors than in adult solid malignancies.[49] Nevertheless, small clinical series have demonstrated

Table 1
Recommended indocyanine green administration protocols for common pediatric surgical oncology applications, including hepatoblastoma resection, pulmonary metastasectomy, and lymphatic mapping

Indication	Dose	Timing	Route
Hepatoblastoma surgery	0.5–1.0 mg/kg	24–72 h preoperatively	Intravenous
Pulmonary metastasectomy	0.5–4.0 mg/kg	24 h preoperatively	Intravenous
Lymphatic mapping	0.5–1.0 mg/kg	Immediately preoperatively	Intralesional
Primary osteosarcoma surgery	1.0 mg/kg	3 h preoperatively	Intravenous

Standard dosing is 0.5 to 1.0 mg/kg, with timing and route adjusted according to operative indication to optimize tumor fluorescence, lesion localization, or lymphatic visualization.

successful intraoperative visualization of hepatoblastoma, rhabdomyosarcoma, and pulmonary metastases from Wilms tumor following intravenous ICG administration.[50]

- *Hepatoblastoma surgery:* ICG given 24 to 72 hours preoperatively enables clear delineation of tumor margins and intrahepatic satellite lesions, even in laparoscopic resections.[51] The dye accumulates in tumor tissue with impaired biliary excretion while being rapidly cleared from surrounding normal parenchyma, creating a favorable tumor-to-background ratio. FGS has been reported to identify otherwise occult nodules, altering the surgical plan in up to 20% to 30% of cases.[52]
- *Pulmonary metastasectomy:* In patients with metastatic Wilms tumor or osteosarcoma, ICG fluorescence can help localize small or deep-seated lung nodules not palpable through thoracoscopy or thoracotomy. Near-infrared thoracoscopy has detected additional metastases missed by preoperative imaging in several pediatric series. ICG is extremely valuable in resection of pulmonary metastases from hepatoblastoma and sarcoma.[53,54]
- *Lymphatic mapping and sentinel node identification:* When injected peritumorally or subdermally, ICG follows lymphatic drainage pathways, allowing visualization of sentinel lymph nodes.[55] This technique has been applied in pediatric melanoma and rhabdomyosarcoma to improve nodal staging.[55,56]

The safety profile of ICG in children is excellent, with anaphylactic reactions being exceedingly rare (<0.05%). However, its nonspecific uptake and relatively shallow tissue penetration remain limitations, particularly for deeply located or poorly vascularized tumors.

Targeted Fluorescent Agents

The next generation of FGS agents aims to improve specificity through molecular targeting, coupling a fluorescent dye to a ligand that binds a tumor-associated receptor or antigen. These agents can highlight tumor tissue with high sensitivity and contrast, potentially overcoming the limitations of nontargeted tracers.[10,57]

Folate receptor-targeted agents

The folate receptor (FR) is overexpressed in several pediatric tumors, including Wilms tumor, osteosarcoma, and some rhabdomyosarcomas.[57] Folate-conjugated fluorescent tracers, such as OTL38 (folate receptor-targeted NIR dye) have been used in adult ovarian and pulmonary cancers[58,59] and initial studies in pediatric oncology are being undertaken (NCT06235125).[8]

GD2-targeted fluorescence

Disialoganglioside GD2 is a well-established target in pediatric neuroblastoma and some sarcomas (ie, Ewing sarcoma and osteosarcoma).[60] Beyond neuroblastoma, GD2 is also an attractive target for fluorescence imaging in other small round blue cell tumors. GD2-targeted antibodies conjugated to NIR fluorophores (eg, IRDye800CW) have shown preclinical efficacy in identifying tumor foci in murine models.[61] Clinical translation in children is ongoing.

Other molecular targets

Additional molecular targets under investigation include vascular endothelial growth factor (VEGF), epidermal growth factor receptor (EGFR), and carbonic anhydrase IX (CAIX), among others.[62,63] The potential to combine these targeted fluorophores with therapeutic agents—yielding *theranostic* compounds—offers an exciting avenue for personalized pediatric oncology treatments.

However, regulatory approval for pediatric use poses significant hurdles. The small patient population, requirement for pediatric-specific toxicology, and ethical constraints on first-in-human studies make large-scale clinical trials difficult. Collaborative multicenter consortia and adaptive trial designs are essential to accelerate the evaluation of targeted tracers in children.

Integration of Fluorescence-Guided Surgery into Clinical Workflow

The integration of fluorescence imaging into routine pediatric oncologic surgery requires both technological and logistical considerations. Key steps include

- *Timing and dosing of tracer administration:* Optimal dosing protocols differ by agent and tumor type. For ICG, most studies recommend 0.5 to 1.0 mg/kg intravenously 24 to 72 hours before surgery for hepatoblastoma, whereas pulmonary metastasectomy often requires 24-hour preoperative administration
- *Imaging equipment:* Modern NIR-capable laparoscopes and open-field cameras allow seamless switching between white-light and fluorescence modes without disrupting surgical workflow
- *Quantitative imaging and calibration:* Efforts are underway to quantify fluorescence intensity for objective margin assessment, reducing operator dependency
- *Combination with other guidance modalities:* As described in Section 2, FGS can be integrated with image-guided navigation, intraoperative ultrasound, or RGS to create multimodal systems that combine anatomic and functional information. Such hybrid imaging may be particularly powerful in detecting satellite lesions or assessing resection margins in real time.

Limitations and Challenges

While FGS offers clear advantages, several limitations must be acknowledged before widespread adoption in pediatric oncology:

1. *Depth penetration*: Most NIR fluorophores penetrate only 5 to 10 mm below the tissue surface, limiting detection of deeper lesions.
2. *Specificity*: Nontargeted tracers may accumulate in inflammatory or necrotic tissue, producing false-positive signals.
3. *Standardization*: Variability in imaging systems and protocols complicates comparison between studies and hinders multicenter validation.
4. *Regulatory and ethical barriers*: Pediatric-specific approval processes for new tracers are lengthy, with limited commercial incentive for industry partners.
5. *Integration and cost*: Implementation requires dedicated imaging systems and training, which may be challenging in resource-limited pediatric centers.

Despite these barriers, the ongoing evolution of fluorescence imaging, particularly in combination with molecular targeting and artificial intelligence for automated detection, holds promise for transforming pediatric surgical oncology into a more precise, image-driven discipline.

FUTURE DIRECTIONS AND SUMMARY

The Convergence of Image-Guided and Fluorescence-Guided Surgery

The integration of image-guided and fluorescence-guided modalities represents a major step toward precision surgery in pediatric oncology. While IGS provides a *map*—a navigational framework derived from preoperative or intraoperative imaging—FGS supplies the *color*, offering real-time functional and molecular information. The convergence of these 2 technologies has the potential to redefine surgical practice by combining spatial accuracy with biological specificity.

Such multimodal integration can, for instance, allow simultaneous visualization of the resection plane, vascular structures, and residual fluorescent tumor deposits. As computing power and tracking algorithms improve, real-time multimodal fusion may become standard, enabling the surgeon to operate within a continuously updated, holographically enhanced digital twin of the patient.

Artificial Intelligence and Predictive Modeling

Artificial intelligence (AI) and machine learning are poised to play pivotal roles in the next phase of image-guided pediatric surgery. Deep-learning algorithms already assist in segmentation of CT and MRI scans, reducing manual workload and improving consistency.[17] Beyond segmentation, AI may enable predictive modeling—forecasting tumor growth, deformation under surgical manipulation, and likely resection margins.

For fluorescence imaging, machine-learning algorithms can analyze intensity patterns to distinguish true tumor signal from background autofluorescence, improving accuracy and enabling quantitative thresholding.[64,65]

Furthermore, the integration of intraoperative data into AI-driven registries may help establish large-scale, data-rich cohorts in pediatric surgical oncology—a crucial step toward evidence-based validation of new technologies. By combining preoperative imaging, intraoperative video, and histopathologic outcomes, such datasets could train algorithms to optimize future surgical planning and predict patient-specific risks.

Ethical and Safety Considerations

The adoption of advanced imaging and fluorescent tracers in children raises unique ethical considerations. Pediatric patients cannot provide informed consent in the same manner as adults, and parents must rely on the medical team's judgment regarding the risk–benefit balance of novel technologies.

Key ethical domains include

1. *Safety of novel agents*: Every fluorescent tracer requires rigorous toxicologic and pharmacokinetic evaluation in children, accounting for differences in metabolism, organ function, and developmental physiology.
2. *Radiation exposure*: Repeated imaging, particularly with CT-based navigation, should adhere to ALARA (as low as reasonably achievable) principles, and preference should be given to nonionizing modalities (MRI, ultrasound, NIR imaging) whenever possible.
3. *Data privacy and AI ethics*: The use of AI-assisted systems and digital data sharing demands robust safeguards for pediatric patient confidentiality and data security.
4. *Equity and accessibility*: The high cost of advanced navigation systems risks widening disparities between well-resourced and low-resource centers. Ensuring equitable access will require international collaboration and cost-effective adaptation of technologies.

Addressing these ethical challenges proactively is crucial to maintain public trust and ensure that innovation remains aligned with the principles of pediatric care: safety, compassion, and long-term well-being.

Vision for the Future

The ultimate goal of image- and fluorescence-guided surgery in pediatric oncology is complete, precise, and personalized resection with minimal collateral damage. In the envisioned operating room of the future, the pediatric surgeon will navigate within a digitally enhanced, multimodal environment:

- Preoperative MRI and CT scans are automatically segmented by AI and projected holographically onto the patient.
- Electromagnetic tracking aligns the virtual and real anatomy with submillimetric accuracy.
- Targeted fluorescent tracers highlight residual tumor tissue or sentinel nodes.
- Real-time feedback from RGS, optical sensors, and AI algorithms assists in defining safe dissection planes.

Such a *smart operating theater* would merge visualization, analytics, and human expertise into a unified system focused on curative and function-preserving surgery. Importantly, technological sophistication must never replace, but rather augment, surgical judgment and multidisciplinary collaboration.

SUMMARY

Pediatric surgical oncology is entering an era of technical transformation. Image-guided and fluorescence-guided technologies are no longer experimental curiosities but clinically relevant tools that enhance safety, accuracy, and understanding of complex anatomy. For children with solid tumors, where the margin between cure and long-term morbidity is narrow, such precision can profoundly influence both survival and quality of life.

The synergistic integration of 3D modeling, real-time navigation, and molecular fluorescence will continue to evolve, driven by technological innovation and multidisciplinary research. As these tools mature, they promise not only to improve surgical outcomes but also to reshape the philosophy of pediatric cancer surgery by transforming it from experience-based to data-driven, from intuitive to image-guided, and from purely anatomic to truly personalized.

CLINICS CARE POINTS

- IGS improves anatomic orientation.
- 3D modeling helps surgical preparation.
- FGS enables real-time visualization of tumors.
- Pitfall: specific correlation between pathology and non-targeted fluorescence is still lacking.

REFERENCES

1. Davidoff AM. Advocating for the surgical needs of children with cancer. J Pediatr Surg 2022;57(6):959–66. Epub 2022 Feb 23. PMID: 35331552.
2. von Allmen D. Pediatric surgical oncology: a brief overview of where we have been and the challenges we face. Semin Pediatr Surg 2019;28(6):150864. https://doi.org/10.1016/j.sempedsurg.2019.150864. Epub 2019 Nov 20. PMID: 31931962.
3. Kattner P, Strobel H, Khoshnevis N, et al. Compare and contrast: pediatric cancer versus adult malignancies. Cancer Metastasis Rev 2019;38(4):673–82.

4. Dasgupta R, Billmire D, Aldrink JH, et al. What is new in pediatric surgical oncology? Curr Opin Pediatr 2017;29(1):3–11.
5. Sanchez-Sanchez A, Giron-Vallejo O, Ruiz-Pruneda R, et al. Three-dimensional printed model and virtual reconstruction: an extra tool for pediatric solid tumor surgery. Eur J Pediatr Surg Rep 2019;6(1):e70–6.
6. Oeffinger KC, Mertens AC, Sklar CA, et al, Childhood Cancer Survivor Study. Chronic health conditions in adult survivors of childhood cancer. N Engl J Med 2006;355(15):1572–82.
7. Latoch E, Zubowska M, Młynarski W, et al. Late effects of childhood cancer treatment in long-term survivors diagnosed before the age of 3 years – a multicenter, nationwide study. Cancer Epidemiology 2022;80:102209.
8. Fusco JC, Abdelhafeez AH, Krauel L, et al. Imaging adjuvants in pediatric surgical oncology. Pediatr Blood Cancer 2025;72(Suppl 2):e31241. https://doi.org/10.1002/pbc.31241. Epub 2024 Aug 5. PMID: 39101518.
9. Simons DC, Dodd A, Tummers WSFJ, et al. Next-generation imaging techniques for surgical guidance in pediatric tumors. Ann Surg Oncol 2025;32(13):10057–65. Epub 2025 Sep 24. PMID: 40993464.
10. Goldstein SD, Heaton TE, Bondoc A, et al. Evolving applications of fluorescence guided surgery in pediatric surgical oncology: a practical guide for surgeons. J Pediatr Surg 2021;56(2):215–23. Epub 2020 Oct 19. PMID: 33189300.
11. van der Zee JM, Rahman AM, Klein Gunnewiek K, et al. Evaluation of UNeXt for automatic bone surface segmentation on ultrasound imaging in image-guided pediatric surgery. Bioengineering (Basel) 2025;12(10):1008. PMID: 41155007; PMCID: PMC12561024.
12. Fitski M, Meulstee JW, Littooij AS, et al. MRI-based 3-Dimensional visualization workflow for the pre-operative planning of nephron-sparing surgery in Wilms' tumor surgery: a pilot study. J Healthc Eng 2020;6:8899049.
13. Prasad K, Fassler C, Miller A, et al. More than meets the eye: augmented reality in surgical oncology. J Surg Oncol 2024;130(3):405–18. Epub 2024 Aug 19. PMID: 39155686.
14. Simons DC, Buser MAD, Fitski M, et al. Multi-modal 3-Dimensional visualization of pediatric neuroblastoma: aiding surgical planning beyond anatomical information. J Pediatr Surg 2024;59(8):1575–81. Epub 2024 Feb 24. PMID: 38461108.
15. Valls-Esteve A, Adell-Gomez N, Pasten A, et al. Exploring the potential of three-dimensional imaging, printing, and modeling in pediatric surgical oncology: a new era of precision surgery. Children 2023;10(5):832.
16. Wake N, Wysock JS, Bjurlin MA, et al. "Pin the Tumor on the Kidney:" an evaluation of how surgeons translate CT and MRI data to 3D models. Urology 2019;131:255–61. Epub 2019 Jun 22. PMID: 31233814; PMCID: PMC7036263.
17. Frush DP, Callahan MJ, Coley BD, et al. Comparison of the different imaging modalities used to image pediatric oncology patients: a COG diagnostic imaging committee/SPR oncology committee white paper. Pediatr Blood Cancer 2023;70-(Suppl 4):e30298. https://doi.org/10.1002/pbc.30298. Epub 2023 Apr 6. PMID: 37025033; PMCID: PMC10652359.
18. Buser MAD, van der Rest JK, Wijnen MHWA, et al. Deep learning and multidisciplinary imaging in pediatric surgical oncology: a scoping review. Cancer Med 2025;14(2):e70574. https://doi.org/10.1002/cam4.70574.
19. Wellens LM, Meulstee J, van de Ven CP, et al. Comparison of 3-Dimensional and augmented reality kidney models with conventional imaging data in the preoperative assessment of children with wilms tumors. JAMA Netw Open 2019;2(4):e192633.

https://doi.org/10.1001/jamanetworkopen.2019.2633. PMID: 31002326; PMCID: PMC6481457.

20. Shah NR, Weadock WJ, Williams KM, et al. Use of modern three-dimensional imaging models to guide surgical planning for local control of pediatric extracranial solid tumors. Pediatr Blood Cancer 2024;71(5):e30933. https://doi.org/10.1002/pbc.30933. Epub 2024 Mar 2. Erratum in: Pediatr Blood Cancer. 2024 Jul 12: e31168. doi: 10.1002/pbc.31168. PMID: 38430473.
21. van der Zee JM, Fitski M, Simonis FFJ, et al. Virtual resection: a new tool for preparing for nephron-sparing surgery in Wilms tumor patients. Curr Oncol 2022; 29(2):777–84. PMID: 35200565; PMCID: PMC8870999.
22. Valls-Esteve A, Tejo-Otero A, Lustig-Gainza P, et al. Patient-specific 3D printed soft models for liver surgical planning and Hands-On training. Gels 2023;9(4): 339. PMID: 37102951; PMCID: PMC10138006.
23. Hampshire J, Dicken BJ, Uruththirakodeeswaran T, et al. Pediatric patient-specific three-dimensional virtual models for surgical decision making in resection of hepatic and retroperitoneal tumors. Int J Comput Assist Radiol Surg 2023;18(10):1941–9. Epub 2023 Mar 11. PMID: 36905500.
24. de Groot NT, van der Zee JM, van Boheemen VJ, et al. Technical approach for infrared tracking for soft tissue navigation with a holographic head-mounted display and preclinical validation. J Vis Exp 2025;223. https://doi.org/10.3791/68607. PMID: 40982410.
25. Rohmer K, Becker M, Georgiades M, et al. Acceptance and feasibility of an augmented reality-based navigation system with optical tracking for percutaneous procedures in interventional radiology - a simulation-based phantom study. Röfo 2025;197(8):936–44. English, German.
26. van Doormaal TPC, van Doormaal JAM, Mensink T. Clinical accuracy of holographic navigation using point-based registration on augmented-reality glasses. Oper Neurosurg 2019;17(6):588–93. PMID: 31081883; PMCID: PMC6995446.
27. van Boheemen VJ, van der Zee JM, Kuipers M, et al. Phantom design for tracked ultrasound-based surgical navigation systems. MethodsX 2025;15:103697. https://doi.org/10.1016/j.mex.2025.103697. PMID: 41277992; PMCID: PMC 12637238.
28. Riva M, Hennersperger C, Milletari F, et al. 3D intra-operative ultrasound and MR image guidance: pursuing an ultrasound-based management of brainshift to enhance neuronavigation. Int J Comput Assist Radiol Surg 2017;12(10): 1711–25. Epub 2017 Apr 8. PMID: 28391583.
29. Hermann EJ, Krauss JK. Electromagnetic navigation in cranial neurosurgery. Adv Tech Stand Neurosurg 2025;55:181–95. PMID: 40608107.
30. Škapin AD, Brumat P, Vodičar M. Electromagnetic navigation guided tailored lamino-pedicular intralesional marginal resection of recurrent sacral osteoblastoma: a case report. J Spine Surg 2024;10(4):764–71. Epub 2024 Nov 5. PMID: 39816765; PMCID: PMC11732325.
31. Olthof KA, Fusaglia M, den Hartog AG, et al. The impact of 3-dimensional models and surgical navigation for open liver surgery. Int J Comput Assist Radiol Surg 2025;20(11):2213–8. Epub 2025 Jul 1. PMID: 40591242; PMCID: PMC12575497.
32. Bitterer F, Bauer A, Glehr G, et al. Intraoperative contrast-enhanced ultrasound has an outcome-relevant impact on surgery of primary and metastatic liver lesions. Ultraschall Med 2025;46(1):49–56. English.
33. Brouwer OR, Buckle T, Bunschoten A, et al. Image navigation as a means to expand the boundaries of fluorescence-guided surgery. Phys Med Biol 2012;57-(10):3123–36. Epub 2012 May 1. PMID: 22547491.

34. Klein Gunnewiek K, van Baarsen KM, Graus EHM, et al. Navigated intraoperative ultrasound in pediatric brain tumors. Childs Nerv Syst 2024;40(9):2697–705. Epub 2024 Jun 11. Erratum in: Childs Nerv Syst. 2025 Apr 14;41(1):156. doi: 10.1007/s00381-025-06824-2. PMID: 38862795; PMCID: PMC11322494.
35. Zhang P, Luo H, Zhu W, et al. Real-time navigation for laparoscopic hepatectomy using image fusion of preoperative 3D surgical plan and intraoperative indocyanine green fluorescence imaging. Surg Endosc 2020;34(8):3449–59. Epub 2019 Nov 8. PMID: 31705286.
36. Ma L, Huang T, Wang J, et al. Visualization, registration and tracking techniques for augmented reality guided surgery: a review. Phys Med Biol 2023;68(4). https://doi.org/10.1088/1361-6560/acaf23. PMID: 36580681.
37. van der Woude R, Fitski M, van der Zee JM, et al. Clinical application and further development of augmented reality guidance for the surgical localization of pediatric chest wall tumors. J Pediatr Surg 2024;59(8):1549–55. Epub 2024 Feb 24. PMID: 38472040.
38. Pelizzo G, Pierucci UM, Marinaro M, et al. Virtual reality for preoperative planning and education in pediatric surgery: preliminary results for the treatment of congenital malformations and tumors. World J Surg 2025;49(6):1497–507. Epub 2025 Apr 17. PMID: 40246557; PMCID: PMC12134200.
39. de Groot NT, van der Zee JM, Bökkerink GMJ, et al. Introducing holographic surgical navigation in pediatric wilms' tumor patients: a feasibility study during total nephrectomy. Bioengineering (Basel) 2025;12(8):896. PMID: 40868409; PMCID: PMC12383552.
40. Wang Z, Wu LC, Chen JQ. Sentinel lymph node biopsy compared with axillary lymph node dissection in early breast cancer: a meta-analysis. Breast Cancer Res Treat 2011;129(3):675–89. Epub 20110709.
41. Morton DL, Wen DR, Wong JH, et al. Technical details of intraoperative lymphatic mapping for early stage melanoma. Arch Surg 1992;127(4):392–9.
42. Sever RE, Rosenblum LT, Stanley KC, et al. Detection properties of indium-111 and IRDye800CW for intraoperative molecular imaging use across tissue phantom models. J Biomed Opt 2025;30(Suppl 1):S13705. https://doi.org/10.1117/1.JBO.30.S1.S13705. Epub 2024 Sep 20. PMID: 39310036; PMCID: PMC 11413652.
43. Predina JD, Newton AD, Keating J, et al. A phase I clinical trial of targeted intraoperative molecular imaging for pulmonary adenocarcinomas. Ann Thorac Surg 2018;105(3):901–8. Epub 2018 Feb 15. PMID: 29397932; PMCID: PMC10959252.
44. Gao RW, Teraphongphom NT, van den Berg NS, et al. Determination of tumor margins with surgical specimen mapping using near-infrared fluorescence. Cancer Res 2018;78(17):5144–54. Epub 2018 Jul 2. PMID: 29967260; PMCID: PMC6125224.
45. Keereweer S, Van Driel PB, Snoeks TJ, et al. Optical image-guided cancer surgery: challenges and limitations. Clin Cancer Res 2013;19(14):3745–54. Epub 2013 May 14. PMID: 23674494.
46. Esposito C, Settimi A, Del Conte F, et al. Image-guided pediatric surgery using indocyanine green (ICG) fluorescence in laparoscopic and robotic surgery. Front Pediatr 2020;8:314. PMID: 32626676; PMCID: PMC7311575.
47. Esposito C, Del Conte F, Cerulo M, et al. Clinical application and technical standardization of indocyanine green (ICG) fluorescence imaging in pediatric minimally invasive surgery. Pediatr Surg Int 2019;35(10):1043–50. Epub 2019 Jul 4. PMID: 31273452.

48. van Manen L, Handgraaf HJM, Diana M, et al. A practical guide for the use of indocyanine green and methylene blue in fluorescence-guided abdominal surgery. J Surg Oncol 2018;118(2):283–300. Epub 2018 Jun 24. PMID: 29938401; PMCID: PMC6175214.
49. Di Mitri M, Di Carmine A, Zen B, et al. Advancing pediatric surgery with indocyanine green (ICG) fluorescence imaging: a comprehensive review. Children 2025; 12(4):515. PMID: 40310106; PMCID: PMC12026291.
50. Szavay PO, Bondoc A, Esposito C, et al. Clinical consensus statement on the use of indocyanine green fluorescence-guided surgery in pediatric patients. J Pediatr Surg 2024;59(11):161657. https://doi.org/10.1016/j.jpedsurg.2024.07.042. Epub 2024 Jul 30. PMID: 39179501.
51. Lake CM, Bondoc AJ, Dasgupta R, et al. Indocyanine green is a sensitive adjunct in the identification and surgical management of local and metastatic hepatoblastoma. Cancer Med 2021;10(13):4322–43. Epub 2021 Jun 12. PMID: 34117727; PMCID: PMC8267136.
52. Yamada Y, Ohno M, Fujino A, et al. Fluorescence-guided surgery for hepatoblastoma with indocyanine green. Cancers (Basel) 2019;11(8):1215. PMID: 31434361; PMCID: PMC6721588.
53. Schermerhorn SMV, Vore E, Bondoc AJ, et al. Utilization of indocyanine green for augmentation of pulmonary metastases resection in pediatric, adolescent, and young adult sarcoma patients. Pediatr Blood Cancer 2026;73(3):e70096. https://doi.org/10.1002/1545-5017.70096. Epub 2026 Jan 8. PMID: 41502349.
54. Abdelhafeez AH, Mothi SS, Pio L, et al. Feasibility of indocyanine green-guided localization of pulmonary nodules in children with solid tumors. Pediatr Blood Cancer 2023;70(10):e30437. https://doi.org/10.1002/pbc.30437. Epub 2023 May 17. PMID: 37194488; PMCID: PMC10685698.
55. Jeremiasse B, van den Bosch CH, Wijnen MWHA, et al. Systematic review and meta-analysis concerning near-infrared imaging with fluorescent agents to identify the sentinel lymph node in oncology patients. Eur J Surg Oncol 2020;46(11): 2011–22. Epub 2020 Aug 3. PMID: 32826112.
56. Jeremiasse B, van Scheltinga CEJT, Smeele LE, et al. Sentinel lymph node procedure in pediatric patients with melanoma, squamous cell carcinoma, or sarcoma using near-infrared fluorescence imaging with indocyanine green: a feasibility trial. Ann Surg Oncol 2023;30(4):2391–8. Epub 2023 Jan 15. PMID: 36641516; PMCID: PMC10027760.
57. Paraboschi I, De Coppi P, Stoyanov D, et al. Fluorescence imaging in pediatric surgery: state-of-the-art and future perspectives. J Pediatr Surg 2021;56(4): 655–62. Epub 2020 Aug 15. PMID: 32900510.
58. Dodd AC, Wadhwani NR, Lehane A, et al. Widespread folate receptor expression in pediatric and adolescent solid tumors - opportunity for intraoperative visualization with the novel fluorescent agent pafolacianine. Oncotarget 2025;16:759–67. PMID: 41100709; PMCID: PMC12536893.
59. Tanyi JL, Randall LM, Chambers SK, et al. A phase III study of pafolacianine injection (OTL38) for intraoperative imaging of folate receptor-positive ovarian cancer (study 006). J Clin Oncol 2023;41(2):276–84. Epub 2022 Sep 7. PMID: 36070540.
60. Sarkaria IS, Martin LW, Rice DC, et al, ELUCIDATE Study Group. Pafolacianine for intraoperative molecular imaging of cancer in the lung: the ELUCIDATE trial. J Thorac Cardiovasc Surg 2023;166(6):e468–78. Epub 2023 Mar 3. PMID: 37019717; PMCID: PMC12507096.

61. Ustjanzwe A, Marini F, Wagner S, et al. Predicting GD2 expression across cancer types by the integration of pathway topology and transcriptome data. bioRxiv 2025;5:1705930.
62. Wellens LM, Deken MM, Sier CFM, et al. Anti-GD2-IRDye800CW as a targeted probe for fluorescence-guided surgery in neuroblastoma. Sci Rep 2020;10(1): 17667. https://doi.org/10.1038/s41598-020-74464-4. PMID: 33077751; PMCID: PMC7573590.
63. Hernot S, van Manen L, Debie P, et al. Latest developments in molecular tracers for fluorescence image-guided cancer surgery. Lancet Oncol 2019;20(7): e354–67. PMID: 31267970.
64. Steinkamp PJ, Pranger BK, Li MF, et al. Fluorescence-guided visualization of soft-tissue sarcomas by targeting vascular endothelial growth factor A: a phase 1 single-center clinical trial. J Nucl Med 2021;62(3):342–7. Epub 2020 Jul 17. PMID: 32680922.
65. Mao J, He H. Deep learning in fluorescence imaging and analysis. J Intell Med 2024;1:42–62.

Fertility Preservation for Children and Adolescents with Cancer

Kristine S. Corkum, MD[a,b,*], Amanda Buchanan, MD[c],
Erin E. Rowell, MD[d,e]

KEYWORDS

• Pediatric • Cancer • Survivorship • Infertility • Fertility preservation

KEY POINTS

- Pediatric oncofertility is a vital aspect of comprehensive oncology care, ensuring that future reproductive health is addressed for children and adolescents undergoing cancer treatment.
- Fertility preservation options for pre- and postpubertal patients include established methods (oocyte retrieval, ovarian tissue cryopreservation, sperm banking) and experimental approaches like testicular tissue cryopreservation.
- Autologous transplantation of cryopreserved postpubertal ovarian tissue reliably restores endocrine function and has achieved live births; prepubertal transplantation shows limited but promising outcomes.
- No human births have yet resulted from cryopreserved testicular tissue, though fertility restoration has been demonstrated in animal models.

BACKGROUND AND INFERTILITY RISK STRATIFICATION

As survival rates for childhood cancer continue to improve, there is a growing emphasis on enhancing the quality of life for survivors and their families. Many of the life-saving therapies that have been instrumental in improving overall survival can cause adverse effects that have a profound impact on survivors' quality of life posttreatment. In particular, the gonadotoxic effects of radiation and chemotherapy

[a] Department of Surgery, University of Colorado Anschutz Medical Campus, Aurora, CO, USA; [b] Fertility Preservation and Reproductive Late Effects Program, Children's Hospital Colorado, Aurora, CO, USA; [c] Golisano Children's Hospital, University of Kentucky, Lexington, KY, USA; [d] Department of Surgery, Northwestern Feinberg School of Medicine, Chicago, IL, USA; [e] Fertility & Hormone Preservation & Restoration Program, Ann & Robert H. Lurie Children's Hospital of Chicago, Chicago, IL, USA
* Corresponding author. Children's Hospital Colorado, 13123 E 16th Avenue, Aurora, CO 80045.
E-mail address: kristine.corkum@childrenscolorado.org

Surg Oncol Clin N Am 35 (2026) 885–897
https://doi.org/10.1016/j.soc.2026.04.011 surgonc.theclinics.com

Abbreviations	
ASRM	American Society for Reproductive Medicine
CED	cyclophosphamide equivalent dose
FP	fertility preservation
HSCT	hematopoietic stem cell transplantation
IVF	in vitro fertilization
OHS-ER	ovarian hormone stimulation with egg retrieval
OTC	ovarian tissue cryopreservation
OTT	ovarian tissue transplantation
TESE	testicular sperm extraction
TTC	testicular tissue cryopreservation

have been identified as one of the most distressing concerns for survivors and their families, making fertility preservation (FP) counseling and interventions an essential component of comprehensive survivorship care.[1]

The field of pediatric oncofertility has become an integral component of comprehensive pediatric oncology care by addressing the reproductive health needs of children and adolescents undergoing cancer treatment. It is a multidisciplinary specialty aimed at mitigating the gonadotoxic effects of chemotherapy and radiation by implementing FP techniques before, during, or after cancer treatment.[2–4] Immediate oncofertility care begins with gonadotoxicity risk stratification followed by counseling, and potential FP interventions such as egg freezing, sperm banking, or surgery to remove ovarian or testicular tissue for cryopreservation to provide patients with the possibility of biological parenthood in the future. Long-term oncofertility care includes ongoing reproductive late effect care with potential restoration of reproductive hormone function and fertility potential. This review will discuss FP risk stratification, counseling, options, and outcomes for both male and female patients at risk for treatment-related fertility loss. It will also cover the current outcomes for fertility and hormone restoration efforts as well as research advances for ovarian and testicular tissue cryopreservation (TTC). In addition, it will address current oncofertility ethical, legal, and financial controversies and access to care concerns.

Oncofertility Counseling

FP counseling is a critical component of comprehensive cancer care. Leading medical organizations, including the Children's Oncology Group, American Academy of Pediatrics, the American Society for Reproductive Medicine (ASRM), and the American Society of Clinical Oncology, underscore the importance of FP counseling for patients who receive a cancer diagnosis. Current clinical guidelines recommend that all pediatric and adolescent patients diagnosed with cancer receive timely and individualized counseling (**Fig. 1**). This counseling includes a thorough risk assessment based on the patient's diagnosis, pubertal status, and proposed treatment regimen, as well as anticipatory guidance regarding potential impacts on future reproductive potential.[5] Providers are strongly encouraged to review both standard and investigational FP options and to discuss the potential future use of preserved reproductive tissue. These conversations should occur as soon as possible after diagnosis and ideally before treatment begins given that gonadotoxic effects from chemotherapy and radiation may occur as soon as the first treatment.[4]

Counseling should be carried out by a provider with a foundational knowledge of reproductive biology, gonadotoxic therapies, infertility risk stratification, and the available nonexperimental and experimental FP options for children. In settings where local providers lack this expertise, referral to specialized oncofertility centers or utilization of

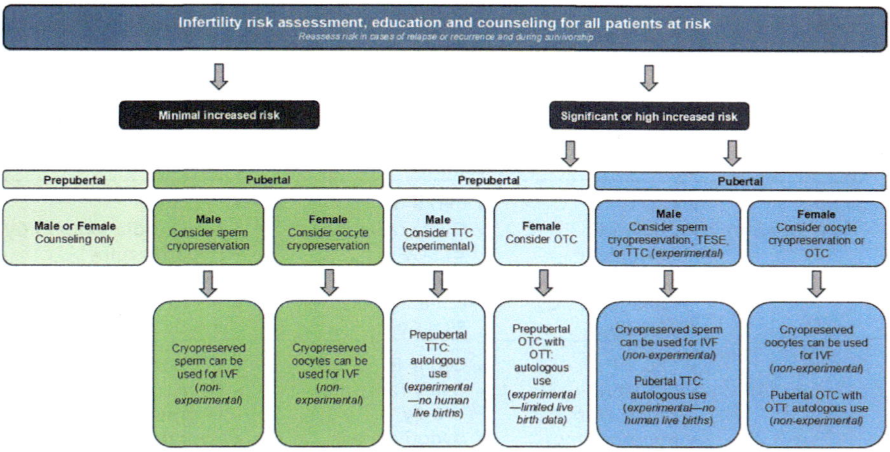

Fig. 1. Pediatric oncofertility counseling workflow for infertility risk assessment, education, and counseling. IVF, in vitro fertilization; OTC, ovarian tissue cryopreservation; OTT, ovarian tissue transplantation; TTC, testicular tissue cryopreservation.

established online resources is recommended to ensure high-quality, evidence-based care coordination.[6]

Importantly, oncofertility counseling should be viewed as an ongoing process rather than a single encounter. Treatment plans may evolve over time, and any escalation in therapy or change in diagnosis may necessitate re-evaluation of fertility risk and re-engagement of the FP team. At every stage, these discussions are essential to support informed, value-aligned decision-making by patients and their families regarding future reproductive health. It is equally important to communicate that FP interventions do not guarantee future fertility, and that assisted reproductive technologies, such as in vitro fertilization, may be required to achieve biological parenthood. Counseling should also encompass alternative family-building options, including adoption, surrogacy, and the use of donor gametes or embryos, to provide patients and families with a comprehensive understanding of potential reproductive pathways.[4]

The Best Practice Committee of the Pediatric Initiative Network of the Oncofertility Consortium has developed a standardized framework for oncofertility risk stratification based on patient sex, pubertal status (for female individuals), and planned treatment regimen[5] (**Table 1**). This system categorizes patients into 3 risk levels (minimally increased, significantly increased, and high level of increased risk) to guide clinical discussions regarding future infertility risk and appropriate FP strategies.

Infertility Risks to Ovaries

In female patients, the gonadotoxic effects of chemotherapy and radiation therapy can result in infertility and premature ovarian insufficiency or failure. Female individuals are born with a finite number of primordial follicles that constitute the ovarian reserve. These follicles may remain quiescent, undergo maturation and ovulation during and after puberty, or be activated and undergo atresia.[7] Gonadotoxic therapies can disrupt the ovarian reserve through multiple mechanisms: inducing granulosa cell apoptosis and reducing estrogen production, accelerating follicular depletion, and causing microvascular damage to the ovarian cortex.[4] Collectively, these effects contribute to diminished ovarian function and increased risk of premature ovarian insufficiency or failure.

Table 1
Infertility risk stratification system

Gonad (Pubertal Status)	Level of Increased Risk: Minimal	Significant	High
Ovaries (*Prepubertal*)	• CED <8[a] • Cisplatin/ carboplatin • Hypothalamus radiation 22 Gy–29.9 Gy	• CED 8–12[a] • Ovary radiation <15 Gy • Hypothalamus radiation >30 Gy–39.9 Gy	• CED >12[a] • Ovary radiation ≥15 Gy • Hypothalamus radiation >40 Gy • Alkylator ± total body irradiation in HSCT
Ovaries (*Pubertal*)	• CED <4[a] • Cisplatin/ carboplatin • Hypothalamus radiation 22 Gy–29.9 Gy	• CED 4–8[a] • Ovary radiation <10 Gy • Hypothalamus radiation > 30 Gy–39.9 Gy	• CED >8[a] • Ovary radiation 10 Gy or greater • Hypothalamus radiation >40 Gy • Alkylator ± total body irradiation in HSCT
Testes (*Prepubertal and Pubertal*)	• CED <4[a] • Cisplatin/ carboplatin • Testicular radiation 0.2 Gy–0.6 Gy • Hypothalamus radiation 26 Gy–29.99 Gy	• Cisplatin >500 mg/m^2 • Testicular radiation 0.7 Gy–3.9 Gy • Hypothalamus radiation >30 Gy–39.9 Gy • RPLND	• CED ≥4[a] • Alkylator ± total body irradiation, myeloablative and reduced intensity regimens • Testicular radiation ≥4 Gy • Hypothalamus radiation >40 Gy

[a] CED units are g/m^2 (or 1000 mg/m^2).

Modified from Meacham LR, Burns K, Orwig KE, et al. Standardizing Risk Assessment for Treatment-Related Gonadal Insufficiency and Infertility in Childhood Adolescent and Young Adult Cancer: The Pediatric Initiative Network Risk Stratification System. J Adolesc Young Adul 2020;9:662–666.

Prepubertal female individuals exhibit a relative resistance to gonadotoxic injury due to the quiescent state of their follicles, larger number of primordial follicles, and the absence of active folliculogenesis. As a result, higher thresholds of chemotherapy and radiation exposure are required to induce comparable ovarian damage; therefore, pubertal status is a critical component of female-specific risk stratification. Notably, female individuals exposed to pelvic irradiation are also at an increased risk for adverse pregnancy outcomes, including spontaneous abortion, low birth weight, and preterm labor.[8]

Infertility Risks to Testes

The testis is composed of 2 main cell types—Sertoli cells which make sperm and Leydig cells which make testosterone. Unlike female individuals, male individuals continue to produce sperm throughout their lifetime and thus have potential for more reserve. In general, the risk of infertility to male individuals is independent of age and can occur immediately upon receiving radiation therapy (XRT) or chemotherapy.[9] Sertoli cells are supremely sensitive to gonadotoxicity, even at a young age. Damage will usually result in temporary azoospermia (absence of sperm in the ejaculate), with eventual recovery over time (usually within 5 years). However, it may be permanent if Sertoli cell damage is too significant, as may be seen with more intensive therapy.[10] Leydig cells, on the other hand, are more resistant to damage from XRT and chemotherapy, so it is much more common to have normal testosterone levels and progression through puberty while receiving or after receiving gonadotoxic therapy.[11]

Chemotherapy-related Risk Factors

Chemotherapy is the major backbone of childhood cancer treatment, and many agents carry significant risks of gonadotoxicity. Alkylating agents, such as cyclophosphamide, ifosfamide, procarbazine, and busulfan, are non–cell cycle–specific and induce apoptosis in both quiescent and proliferating cells making them highly gonadotoxic and the most studied in this realm.[12] To standardize exposure across regimens, cumulative doses are calculated using the cyclophosphamide equivalent dose (CED) in gram per square meter.[5,13] Current guidelines define high-risk thresholds as a CED greater than 4 g/m^2 in male individuals, greater than 12 g/m^2 in prepubertal female individuals, and greater than 8 g/m^2 in postpubertal female individuals.[5] Platinum-based chemotherapeutic agents, particularly cisplatin, are associated with male infertility risk, with cumulative doses exceeding 500 mg/m^2 linked to abnormal sperm motility and reduced sperm counts.[9] Unlike male patients, female patients exposed to platinum-based therapies do not experience long-term adverse effects on fertility or reproductive endocrine function. As patients receive combination therapy or additional therapy with relapsed disease, the risks of gonadotoxicity are additive.[13] There is currently limited evidence regarding the long-term reproductive effects of biologic agents and immunotherapies for pediatric-aged patients.[4]

Radiation-related Risk Factors

Radiation exposure to the gonads may be direct or result from scatter during treatment of intra-abdominal, pelvic, or lower extremity malignancies. Collaboration with radiation oncology is essential to estimate gonadal dose and inform risk stratification. In male individuals, direct testicular radiation 4 Gy or greater is associated with a high risk of infertility, with no protective effect of prepubertal status due to ongoing spermatogenesis.[5,14] Even radiation doses as low as 2 Gy, may result in oligospermia or azoospermia (low to no sperm in ejaculate), or abnormal spermatic function that may not recover.[10] In female individuals, high-risk thresholds are defined as 15 Gy or greater for prepubertal ovaries and 10 Gy or greater for postpubertal ovaries, reflecting the greater resilience of quiescent primordial follicles in younger patients (see **Table 1**).

Hematopoietic Stem Cell Transplantation

The myeloablative conditioning regimens used prior to hematopoietic stem cell transplantation (HSCT) pose a substantial risk to fertility due to the combined effects of high-dose alkylating agents and total body irradiation. All patients undergoing HSCT, including those receiving reduced-intensity conditioning regimens, are classified as high-risk for treatment-related infertility.[5]

Surgical Interventions

Surgical interventions may contribute to overall fertility risk and should be integrated into comprehensive oncofertility assessment. For male patient, rarely is bilateral orchiectomy performed, but unilateral orchiectomy is common. While this removes 50% of the testicular tissue, fertility is rarely affected.[15] Retroperitoneal surgery, such as retroperitoneal lymph node dissection, carries a risk of sympathetic nerve damage, which does not impair the testis directly, but may impair ejaculation and thus contribute to difficulties with conception.[16] Since the testicles themselves are normal, sperm can usually be obtained from the testicles themselves or through postejaculatory bladder washing.

In female individuals, unilateral oophorectomy alone does not appear to significantly impair reproductive hormonal function, yet it may hasten the onset of menopause by 1 year.[17] The effects of unilateral oophorectomy should be considered alongside chemotherapeutic and radiologic exposures when counseling patients and families about fertility risks and preservation strategies.

FERTILITY PRESERVATION PROCEDURES AND OPTIONS

Female Individuals

Since the 2019 publication of ASRM practice committee opinion, ovarian tissue cryopreservation (OTC) has been considered non-experimental for both prepubertal and postpubertal female individuals. For prepubertal girls, OTC remains the only pretreatment option for FP for those at a high level of increased risk because they are hormonally immature and cannot undergo ovarian stimulation for egg retrieval. Postpubertal girls may be a candidate for ovarian hormone stimulation with egg retrieval (OHS-ER) if the treatment timeline allows for 2 to 3 weeks for hormone stimulation and ultrasound-guided retrieval procedure. Postpubertal girls are also candidates for OTC.

For all patients undergoing OTC, laparoscopic unilateral oophorectomy, without salpingectomy, is the preferred surgery to obtain healthy ovarian tissue for cryopreservation and to allow enough tissue for future fertility and/or hormone restoration. Surgery ought to be done using a no-touch technique and maintaining dissection at least 1 cm away from the ovarian cortex for optimal tissue health.[18] The laparoscopic oophorectomy can be performed under one anesthetic exposure at the time of another necessary procedure such as bone marrow biopsy or central venous access surgery. Recent data found that laparoscopic oophorectomy for OTC is successful even following open abdominopelvic surgery for tumor biopsy or excision.[2,19] In this situation, patients are counseled that a small open Pfannenstiel incision could be needed if the laparoscopic approach were unsuccessful.

Several patients who had planned HSCT underwent both OHS-ER and OTC. After infertility risk assessment and counseling, these patients desired egg freezing and also the option for ovarian tissue transplantation (OTT) for fertility and hormone restoration in the future. The timeline for these patients is typically about 4 to 6 weeks since patients need 2 to 3 weeks for OHS-ER, then approximately 2 weeks for the ovaries to recover from stimulation and return to normal size prior to laparoscopic oophorectomy. This also allows the option for a second round of hormone stimulation if the first yield from egg retrieval is lower than expected.[20] Cryopreservation of both eggs and ovarian tissue costs slightly more per year than freezing eggs or ovarian tissue alone with average cost for ovarian tissue cryostorage of approximately US$400 per year with need-based cost adjustment available through contract with the storage company (https://reprotech.com/for-customers/storage-fees/).

Once the ovarian tissue has been removed for OTC, it needs to be processed by a specialized laboratory with appropriate Food and Drug Administration certification. This involves thinning the ovarian cortex and then slicing it into cortical strips that are individually placed in vials for slow rate freezing, then transferred into liquid nitrogen tanks for long-term cryostorage. Recent research has determined the ovary size and density of follicles through the pubertal transition and has established best practice guidelines for pediatric ovarian tissue processing.[21] Surgical programs need to have a relationship with a tissue processing laboratory to facilitate the cryopreservation process. Many hospitals can perform the oophorectomy locally, then ship tissue to a specialized laboratory.

Egg freezing is a well-established option for FP, and cryopreserved eggs can be thawed to create an embryo, which can then be implanted in the same patient or used by a surrogate through in vitro fertilization (IVF). In adult women of reproductive age, ovarian tissue can be thawed and currently used for autologous reimplantation of cortical strips on the exposed medulla of the remaining ovary to allow natural conception. Ovarian cortical strips can also be implanted in subcutaneous tissue or in a peritoneal bursa to allow hormone stimulation for egg retrieval for IVF. For women who were postpubertal at the time of OTC, the transplantation of tissue (OTT) is considered a standard of care option, with over 300 live births worldwide. For women who were prepubertal at the time of OTC, the OTT procedure is considered experimental with only 2 reported cases of live birth in this group.[22]

Male Individuals

Tissue or sperm preservation, regardless of patient age, is of highest quality when done prior to receiving any oncologic therapy. However, even after therapy has begun, there may be identifiable germ cells present. At a CED greater than 7 g/m^2, there are few germ cells identified, so this is used as a general threshold after which FP is not performed.[23] TTC can be pursued without a delay in subsequent therapy.[3] Sertoli cells do not produce mature sperm until puberty, thus puberty is the timepoint distinction for male preservation options.

Prior to puberty, the only option for preservation is TTC. This is essentially a testicular biopsy where spermatogonial cells are identified and preserved, with the hopes of future maturation and reimplantation to achieve pregnancy. While there are reports of achieving pregnancy with this technology in primates, human pregnancies have not been achieved, and it is thus considered experimental.[23,24] The procedure can be done through a small scrotal incision at the time of another procedure. It has a low complication rate and removal of such a small volume of tissue typically results in acceptable cosmetic appearance of the scrotum and future growth of the testis.[3]

After puberty, mature sperm is produced and can be seen in the ejaculate. As such, sperm cryopreservation through sperm banking is the preferred method for retrieval. Multiple human pregnancies have been achieved with this method. Because sperm are mature, they are immediately sensitive to potential DNA damage and it is critical that preservation be done prior to initiation of therapy. For boys in the process of pubertal transformation, it can be difficult to know who can and cannot produce an ejaculate sample for cryopreservation. In general, boys who are Tanner 3 or who experience nocturnal emissions should be offered cryopreservation.[25] Adding another level of complexity is determining a patient and family's comfort with discussion of and around manual stimulation. Practice navigating this discussion is important, often with a dedicated fertility specialist guiding this. Overall, about 93% of Tanner 3 boys who report nocturnal emissions are able to produce sperm by manual stimulation, and 68% are successful with sperm cryopreservation.[26]

For postpubertal male individuals who cannot produce a sample for cryopreservation or for peripubertal boys, TTC, electroejaculation, and mature testicular sperm extraction (TESE) are additional options. An initial attempt at sperm cryopreservation should be made, but these samples may be oligospermatic. As such, TTC can be offered and combined with TESE, if available. This allows the preservation of both stem cells and any available mature germ cells, to maximize options for the patient in the future. While rare, postpubertal patients who are unwilling or otherwise unable to produce an ejaculated specimen, TESE or electroejaculation can be used to cryopreserve mature sperm.

Meeting with a dedicated fertility specialist, recommendations from provider/parents to bank and a greater ability to provide a sample to bank are all associated with a higher likelihood of successful sperm banking.[25] Yet sperm banking tends to be underutilized in teenage boys, with a 2025 study reporting less than 25% of male individuals completing sperm cryopreservation, and most being those with testicular cancer presumably treated by urologists familiar with fertility.[27] Reasons are likely multifactorial and include comfort of usually oncologists with discussions related to fertility, availability of counseling services, availability of laboratories/facilities to provide these services, and concerns surrounding costs and future use. The improved education surrounding fertility counseling facilitated by large consortiums and national society guideline statements, development of dedicated oncofertility teams and easier access to has increased significantly over time.

Use of cryopreserved sperm is a well-established option for FP for creating an embryo for IVF. Testicular tissue reimplantation and spermatogonial stem cell injection remain experimental, and there have been no human live births from TTC to date.

CHALLENGES TO FERTILITY PRESERVATION ACCESS

Access to FP counseling and services remains challenging for children with cancer, with barriers including institutional resources, geography, local laws/politics, and financial costs.

Knowledge Gaps and Institutional Variation

Evidence still suggests gaps in access to infertility risk assessment and to FP procedures for pediatric patients.[28] Recent study by Corona and colleagues[29] found that the presence of a formal FP program, defined by a multidisciplinary team who can provide infertility risk assessment and FP procedures when indicated, identifies patients at the highest level of infertility risk 100% of the time and that FP procedures are offered in an equitable way. Another recent study by McElhinney and colleagues[30] demonstrates with a formal program in place, FP procedures can be offered in a coordinated and short time frame to fulfill FP goals and not cause delay in the patient's start of definitive medical therapy.

Access to pediatric oncofertility care varies significantly depending on the resources and infrastructure available at the treating institution. FP programs are generally categorized into 3 models. Full-service programs provide comprehensive care, including patient and family education, individualized counseling, access to both standard-of-care and experimental FP procedures, in-house tissue processing, and active research participation. Limited-service programs offer counseling and facilitate FP procedures but rely on external centers for tissue processing and storage. Education-only and counseling-only programs focus on risk assessment and consultation, referring patients to other institutions for procedural interventions. Some centers caring for children and adolescents with cancer lack any formal FP capabilities, resulting in missed opportunities for timely counseling and intervention.[31] Specialty counseling has been offered through telemedicine although this is not available in every state and often not available across state lines. This variability underscores the need for standardized, equitable access to oncofertility services across pediatric cancer care settings.

Financial

Costs associated with FP interventions vary widely, often depending on insurance coverage (public or private) and whether procedures are considered standard of care or experimental. Expenses may include operative fees, tissue processing and handling, and long-term storage. Families can incur total costs ranging from several hundred to several thousand dollars, representing a substantial barrier for those with limited financial resources. Obtaining specific costs regarding FP procedures from hospitals is generally difficult, even for a quote for families to consider. Philanthropic support can be leveraged to cover FP services but may be limited based on the values of the sponsoring organization (eg, covering male but not female cryopreservation due to perceived religious concerns). In some cases, institutional or third-party financial assistance is available to help cover FP services, but most costs are covered directly by the patients and families. These financial challenges further complicate an already difficult situation and contribute to inequities in access to FP services for children with cancer. Moreover, institutional costs associated with establishing and maintaining FP programs can be prohibitive, limiting program development and availability across centers.

Ethical Issues

Offering FP for children at risk for infertility from their medical diagnosis or treatment is now viewed by most medical providers as a crucial component of their care, yet for some patients, the lack of access to FP counseling and procedures, financial considerations, social and political forces create inequality in care which is ethically problematic. Additional ethical complexities arise regarding posthumous disposition of cryopreserved tissue. Some programs mandate that the tissue be destroyed in the event of the child's death, while other programs have policies to allow donation of the tissue for research purposes, and the disposition of tissue is addressed as part of the informed consent process for the OTC/TTC itself.[32] Situations requiring heightened ethical consideration include diagnoses necessitating complete gonadal removal, where time for FP counseling and procedures is warranted even if treatment timelines must adjust, and cases of a cancer diagnosis with a very poor prognosis, where beneficence and nonmaleficence must be balanced to avoid causing additional suffering while ensuring parents understand fertility risks.[33] These scenarios ought to involve multidisciplinary team discussion between the child, when applicable, parents, the child's oncologist, and the fertility specialist team for individualized care. Thorough and timely documentation in the medical record regarding discussions and decisions related to infertility and FP is paramount to avoid miscommunication and possibly traumatizing, repetitive discussions.

RESEARCH: CURRENT STATE AND FUTURE DIRECTIONS

Use of Ovarian Tissue

For postpubertal patients, OTC with subsequent OTT is considered a standard of care option for FP, and hundreds of women worldwide have now achieved pregnancy and live birth using cryopreserved ovarian tissue with autologous transplantation. The most recent fertility restoration data from a systematic review by Erden and colleagues[34] evaluated pregnancy outcomes using autologous transplantation of cryopreserved ovarian tissue, finding that of 162 deliveries of 170 newborns (8 sets of twins), 67% of the pregnancies were conceived naturally while 33% were achieved using assistive reproductive technology. In this review, perinatal complication rates did not differ from that of the general pregnancy population, except for the incidence of pre-eclampsia, which was suspected to be related to chemotherapy exposure, underlying medical condition, and use of assisted reproductive techniques. The study also found that not receiving chemotherapy prior to OTC and natural conception were associated with a lower perinatal complication rate.[34] Recent outcomes data from Europe show that current best estimates for success of OTT in adult women include restoration of endocrine function in over 80% of patients with hormone effects for at least 5 years, pregnancy and live birth rate of approximately 40% and 30%, respectively, with natural conception, and pregnancy and live birth rate of approximately 36% and 21%, respectively, with IVF.[35] Another large cohort study of adult women in Australia who had OTC and subsequent OTT reported a live birth rate of 25%.[36] For prepubertal patients who underwent OTC, only 1 case report exists documenting pregnancy and live birth in adulthood, with a second report of pregnancy and livebirth after prepubertal OTC and subsequent OTT.[22] Laparoscopic oophorectomy for OTC is considered a standard FP option in prepubertal patients while OTT remains experimental in this group due to the small numbers of patients who have had OTT and live birth from prepubertal OTC.[37]

Future research focusing on the use of ovarian tissue for surrogacy and to mature follicles from prepubertal tissue in vitro, known as in vitro follicle maturation is critical since this will allow fertility options beyond autologous tissue transplant, particularly important for patients with leukemia or Ewing's sarcoma who may have a risk of retransfer of malignancy in cryopreserved ovarian tissue. Current ongoing research is also evaluating ovarian tissue for possible presence of malignant cells prior to OTT.[35]

Use of Testicular Tissue

There have been no documented live births from cryopreserved testicular tissue. Restoration of male fertility in a murine model from injection/transplantation of spermatogonial stem cells has been described.[38] More recently, sperm cells were found in the ejaculate of a previously sterile Rhesus monkey after injection of spermatogonial stem cells into the rete testis. The sperm produced were able to successfully fertilize an oocyte using intracytoplasmic sperm injection (ICSI), resulting in the birth of the first graph drive baby primate.[24] Fertility restoration in nonhuman primates has allowed practitioners to more confidently and positively offer TTC to patients.[39] Additional research has focused on the isolation of spermatogonia for autologous sperm cell transplantation, autologous testicular tissue grafting, and in vitro spermatogenesis.[40]

SUMMARY

Pediatric oncofertility is a vital aspect of comprehensive oncology care, ensuring that future reproductive health is addressed for children and adolescents undergoing cancer treatment. FP options exist for both prepubertal and postpubertal patients, ranging from established approaches such as oocyte retrieval, OTC, and sperm banking to experimental strategies like TTC. Autologous transplantation of cryopreserved postpubertal ovarian tissue has demonstrated consistent success in restoring endocrine function and achieving live births, with limited but promising reports following transplantation of prepubertal ovarian tissue. No human births have yet resulted from cryopreserved testicular tissue, though fertility restoration has been demonstrated in animal models. Oncofertility counseling is essential to support informed, values-based decision-making, yet universal access remains challenging due to institutional resources, geography, legal constraints, and financial barriers. Ongoing efforts to standardize care, expand institutional capabilities, and promote access are critical to ensuring equitable opportunities for FP among pediatric patients.

CLINICS CARE POINTS

- Infertility risk assessment and counseling should be offered to the families of all children receiving therapies that place them at an increased risk for infertility or premature hormonal failure, and standardized risk assessment tools exist to help quantify this risk.
- FP options exist for both prepubertal and postpubertal patients, including both nonexperimental (oocyte harvest, OTC, and sperm cryopreservation) and experimental (TTC) options for FP depending on the patient's gender and pubertal status.
- Sperm banking in postpubertal male individuals is often underutilized and should occur prior to any chemotherapy.

DISCLOSURE

The authors have no commercial or financial conflicts of interest to disclose. The authors have no sources of funding to report.

REFERENCES

1. Ellis SJ, Wakefield CE, McLoone JK, et al. Fertility concerns among child and adolescent cancer survivors and their parents: a qualitative analysis. J Psychosoc Oncol 2016;34(5):347–62.
2. Rowell EE, Corkum KS, Lautz TB, et al. Laparoscopic unilateral oophorectomy for ovarian tissue cryopreservation in children. J Pediatr Surg 2019;54(3):543–9.
3. Corkum KS, Lautz TB, Johnson EK, et al. Testicular wedge biopsy for fertility preservation in children at significant risk for azoospermia after gonadotoxic therapy. J Pediatr Surg 2019;54(9):1901–5.
4. Talbot L, Corkum KS, McCracken K, et al. Oncofertility care for children, adolescents, and young adults at risk for treatment-related fertility loss. Pediatr Blood Cancer 2025;72(Suppl 2):e31277.
5. Meacham LR, Burns K, Orwig KE, et al. Standardizing risk assessment for treatment-related gonadal insufficiency and infertility in childhood adolescent and young adult cancer: the pediatric initiative network risk stratification system. J Adolesc Young Adult Oncol 2020;9(6):662–6.
6. Quinn GP, Bowman Curci M, Reich RR, et al. Impact of a web-based reproductive health training program: ENRICH (educating nurses about reproductive issues in cancer healthcare). Psychooncology 2019;28(5):1096–101.
7. Wallace WH, Kelsey TW. Human ovarian reserve from conception to the menopause. PLoS One 2010;5(1):e8772.
8. Metzger ML, Meacham LR, Patterson B, et al. Female reproductive health after childhood, adolescent, and young adult cancers: guidelines for the assessment and management of female reproductive complications. J Clin Oncol 2013;31(9):1239–47.
9. Green DM, Liu W, Kutteh WH, et al. Cumulative alkylating agent exposure and semen parameters in adult survivors of childhood cancer: a report from the St jude lifetime cohort study. Lancet Oncol 2014;15(11):1215–23.
10. Kenney LB, Antal Z, Ginsberg JP, et al. Improving Male reproductive health after childhood, adolescent, and young adult cancer: progress and future directions for survivorship research. J Clin Oncol 2018;36(21):2160–8.

11. Chemaitilly W, Liu Q, van Iersel L, et al. Leydig cell function in Male survivors of childhood cancer: a report from the St jude lifetime cohort study. J Clin Oncol 2019;37(32):3018–31.
12. Skinner R, Mulder RL, Kremer LC, et al. Recommendations for gonadotoxicity surveillance in male childhood, adolescent, and young adult cancer survivors: a report from the International Late Effects of Childhood Cancer Guideline Harmonization Group in collaboration with the PanCareSurFup Consortium. Lancet Oncol 2017;18(2):e75–90.
13. Green DM, Nolan VG, Goodman PJ, et al. The cyclophosphamide equivalent dose as an approach for quantifying alkylating agent exposure: a report from the childhood cancer survivor study. Pediatr Blood Cancer 2014;61(1):53–67.
14. Green DM, Kawashima T, Stovall M, et al. Fertility of Male survivors of childhood cancer: a report from the childhood cancer survivor study. J Clin Oncol 2010; 28(2):332–9.
15. Ferreira U, Netto Junior NR, Esteves SC, et al. Comparative study of the fertility potential of men with only one testis. Scand J Urol Nephrol 1991;25(4):255–9.
16. Hudson MM. Reproductive outcomes for survivors of childhood cancer. Obstet Gynecol 2010;116(5):1171–83.
17. Bjelland EK, Wilkosz P, Tanbo TG, et al. Is unilateral oophorectomy associated with age at menopause? A population study (the HUNT2 survey). Hum Reprod 2014;29(4):835–41.
18. Rowell EE, Corkum KS, Even KA, et al. Ovarian tissue health after laparoscopic unilateral oophorectomy: a porcine model for establishing optimized fertility preservation techniques in children. J Pediatr Surg 2020;55(8):1631–8.
19. Harris CJ, Lautz TB, Rowell EE. Feasibility of laparoscopic ovarian tissue cryopreservation after open abdominopelvic tumor surgery. Am J Surg 2020;220(5): 1249–52.
20. Harris CJ, Rowell EE, Corkum KS. Special considerations in pediatric female fertility preservation. Semin Pediatr Surg 2025;37:151545.
21. Tsui EL, Harris CJ, Rowell EE, et al. Human ovarian gross morphology and subanatomy across puberty: insights from tissue donated during fertility preservation. F S Rep 2023;4(2):196–205.
22. Corkum KS, Rhee DS, Wafford QE, et al. Fertility and hormone preservation and restoration for female children and adolescents receiving gonadotoxic cancer treatments: a systematic review. J Pediatr Surg 2019;54(11):2200–9.
23. Valli-Pulaski H, Peters KA, Gassei K, et al. Testicular tissue cryopreservation: 8 years of experience from a coordinated network of academic centers. Hum Reprod 2019;34(6):966–77.
24. Fayomi AP, Peters K, Sukhwani M, et al. Autologous grafting of cryopreserved prepubertal rhesus testis produces sperm and offspring. Science 2019;363-(6433):1314–9.
25. Klosky JL, Lehmann V, Flynn JS, et al. Patient factors associated with sperm cryopreservation among at-risk adolescents newly diagnosed with cancer. Cancer 2018;124(17):3567–75.
26. Adank MC, van Dorp W, Smit M, et al. Electroejaculation as a method of fertility preservation in boys diagnosed with cancer: a single-center experience and review of the literature. Fertil Steril 2014;102(1):199–205.e1.
27. Lehmann V, Vlooswijk C, van der Graaf WTA, et al. Pre-treatment fertility preservation and post-treatment reproduction in long-term survivors of adolescent and young adult (AYA) cancer. J Cancer Surviv 2025;19(4):1143–54.

28. Nelson M, Levine J. Current issues in fertility preservation among pediatric and adolescent cancer patients. Curr Oncol Rep 2023;25(7):793–802.
29. Corona LE, Bak M, Farje D, et al. Formal fertility preservation program facilitates equitable fertility care among pediatric oncology and stem cell transplant patients. J Pediatr Surg 2025;60(9):162400.
30. McElhinney KL, McLean SK, Zarnegar-Lumley S, et al. Comprehensive fertility preservation can be offered in a timely manner around gonadotoxic therapy in children and adolescents. Pediatr Blood Cancer 2024;71(10):e31232.
31. Lautz TB, Harris CJ, Laronda MM, et al. A fertility preservation toolkit for pediatric surgeons caring for children with cancer. Semin Pediatr Surg 2019;28(6):150861.
32. Schmidt KT, Larsen EC, Andersen CY, et al. Risk of ovarian failure and fertility preserving methods in girls and adolescents with a malignant disease. BJOG 2010; 117(2):163–74.
33. McDougall RJ, Gillam L, Delany C, et al. Ethics of fertility preservation for prepubertal children: should clinicians offer procedures where efficacy is largely unproven? J Med Ethics 2018;44(1):27–31.
34. Erden M, Uyanik E, Demeestere I, et al. Perinatal outcomes of pregnancies following autologous cryopreserved ovarian tissue transplantation: a systematic review with pooled analysis. Am J Obstet Gynecol 2024;231(5):480–9.
35. Dolmans MM, Demeestere I, Anckaert E, et al. Proceedings of the oncofertility congress of the "Freezing Ovarian Tissue and Oocytes" (FOTO) consortium brussels. J Assist Reprod Genet 2022;39(8):1715–25.
36. Finkelstein T, Rolnik DL, Agresta F, et al. Pregnancy outcomes following ovarian tissue cryopreservation: an Australian cohort study. Am J Obstet Gynecol 2025;233(2):108.e1-e11.
37. Mulder RL, Font-Gonzalez A, Hudson MM, et al. Fertility preservation for female patients with childhood, adolescent, and young adult cancer: recommendations from the PanCareLIFE Consortium and the International Late Effects of Childhood Cancer Guideline Harmonization Group. Lancet Oncol 2021;22(2):e45–56.
38. Goossens E, De Rycke M, Haentjens P, et al. DNA methylation patterns of spermatozoa and two generations of offspring obtained after murine spermatogonial stem cell transplantation. Hum Reprod 2009;24(9):2255–63.
39. Barraud-Lange V, Boissel N, Gille AS, et al. A 10-year experience in testicular tissue cryopreservation for boys under 18 years of age: what can be learned from 350 cases? Andrology 2024;12(2):385–95.
40. Younis N, Caldeira-Brant AL, Chu T, et al. Human immature testicular tissue organ culture: a step towards fertility preservation and restoration. Front Endocrinol 2023;14:1242263.

Pediatric Palliative Surgical Oncology

Principles, Practice, and Evolving Roles

Nelson Piché, MD, MSc[a], Hau D. Le, MD[b,*]

KEYWORDS

• Pediatric palliative care • Pediatric surgical oncology • Holistic care • Cancer

KEY POINTS

- Pediatric palliative surgical oncology lies at a vital intersection of surgery, oncology, and palliative care.
- Pediatric surgeons can play a central role in this journey, not only as technical experts but as communicators, partners, advocates, and witnesses.
- Intergrating palliative principles from diagnosis through end-of-life ensures surgical recommendations align with patient and family priorities, the child's developmental needs and lived experience.
- Evidence increasingly demonstrates that palliative surgery can offer substantial benefits when guided by thoughtful communication, interdisciplinary collaboration, and clear goals of care.

INTRODUCTION

A diagnosis of cancer in childhood introduces profound uncertainty and distress into the lives of affected children and their families. Although significant therapeutic advances have improved survival for many pediatric cancers, the illness and its treatment still pose substantial physical, emotional, and psychological challenges. Cancer remains the leading nontraumatic cause of death among children in the United States. Every year, approximately 10,000 children (birth to 14 years) and 5000 adolescents (aged 15–19 years) will be diagnosed with cancer, and 1000 and 500, respectively, will die from the disease.[1] Despite advances in multimodal therapies that

[a] Division of Pediatric Surgery, Centre Hospitalier Universitaire Sainte-Justine, Université de Montréal, Montréal, Québec, Canada; [b] Division of Pediatric Surgery, American Family Children's Hospital, University of Wisconsin School of Medicine and Public Health, Madison, WI, USA

* Corresponding author. Department of Surgery, University of Wisconsin School of Medicine and Public Health, 600 Highland Avenue CSC H4, Madison, WI 53792-0466.
E-mail address: leh@surgery.wisc.edu

Surg Oncol Clin N Am 35 (2026) 899–912
https://doi.org/10.1016/j.soc.2026.04.009 **surgonc.theclinics.com**
1055-3207/26/

Abbreviations	
BC/WC	best case/worst case
EOL	end-of-life
EPEC	Education in Palliative and End-of-Life Care–Pediatrics
PPC	pediatric palliative care

have increased survival across many childhood malignancies, the diagnosis of pediatric cancer introduces significant ambiguity and hardship for children and families.

Pediatric surgical oncologists play an important role in diagnosis, staging, definitive treatment, symptom management, and end-of-life (EOL) care.[2] Historically regarded primarily as technical specialists, surgeons today navigate a clinical landscape that requires sophisticated communication, prognostic awareness, and the capacity to integrate primary palliative care principles into practice.[3] Surgical decisions often occur under conditions of emotional stress and time pressure, requiring clinicians to balance procedural benefits with overall patient-centered goals and quality-of-life considerations.

The purpose of this article is to present a comprehensive, evidence-informed framework for pediatric palliative surgical oncology. Drawing upon emerging literature, multidisciplinary practice models, and the evolving needs of children with serious illness, this work aims to guide pediatric surgeons in delivering holistic, developmentally appropriate, and goal-concordant care throughout the continuum of pediatric cancer treatment.

BACKGROUND AND EVOLUTION OF PEDIATRIC PALLIATIVE CARE

Modern pediatric palliative care emerged in the late 20th century as clinicians recognized the need to address suffering and improve the quality of life for seriously ill children, as a large majority of children with cancer suffered a great deal in their last month of life.[4] Disparities exist between parents' perceptions of their child's suffering and those of their physicians. The World Health Organization defines pediatric palliative care (PPC) as the prevention and relief of physical, psychological, social, and spiritual suffering from the time of diagnosis onward, regardless of prognosis.[5] Unlike adult palliative care, which often centers on advanced chronic illness and occurs later in the course of the disease, PPC spans diverse conditions, including malignancies, congenital anomalies, neuromuscular disorders, and genetic syndromes, and is encouraged to be involved early in the disease course.[6,7]

Over recent years, research has demonstrated the value of early integration of palliative care for children with life-threatening illnesses. The American Academy of Pediatrics has recommended that PPC be offered *at diagnosis and continued throughout the course of illness, whether the outcome ends in cure or death*.[8] Benefits include improved symptom management, reduced health care utilization, enhanced family satisfaction, and, in some cases, improved survival.[9–12] However, access remains variable, and many pediatric patients still receive palliative care only late in the course of illness.[13,14]

Pediatric surgery has been slow to integrate palliative care principles, due partially to limited training, a curative surgical culture, parental and physician misperception of PPC involvement, and discomfort with EOL realities. These issues lead to palliative care consultation only when illness acuity and severity are high, the possibility of curability is low, and death seems imminent.[15] Yet, many children receiving palliative care undergo at least one surgical procedure following program enrollment, reflecting the reality that surgical interventions represent a major component of care in serious pediatric illness.[16–20] As a result, pediatric surgeons can elevate the care they provide by adopting palliative care frameworks and collaborating with interdisciplinary teams to ensure that interventions align with family priorities, minimize suffering, and meaningfully contribute to the child's remaining life.

DIFFERENT LEVELS OF PALLIATIVE CARE

Palliative care can be considered as a 3-level care.[21,22] The first level of palliative care is called Palliative Care Approach, which is geared for students, generalists, nurses, and hospital staff to integrate palliative care methods in settings where PPC is not available.

The second level of palliative care is Primary Palliative Care, which all clinicians, including surgeons, should be prepared to provide.[23,24] Primary Palliative Care encompasses foundational competencies such as basic symptom management, developmentally appropriate communication, routine elicitation of family values, and ongoing goals-of-care discussions across the trajectory of serious illness. Although there is usually no formal Primary Palliative Care education during surgical training, pediatric surgeons learn these skills informally from observation and from mentorship.[3,25]

Specialized Palliative Care, the third level of palliative care, is delivered by a multidisciplinary team to provide expert support for refractory symptom management, high-stakes decision-making, anticipatory grief, psychosocial and spiritual needs, and coordination across inpatient, outpatient, and home settings. In general, Specialized Palliative Care was associated with the most optimal child quality of life, but it requires more resources that smaller hospitals might not be able to afford.[26,27]

Drawing on all the experiences from the disciplines of surgery, pediatrics and palliative care, the American Pediatric Surgery Association's cancer committee recently recommended the following 7 principles of Pediatric Palliative Surgical Oncology: (1) respecting values, (2) effective communication, (3) expert symptom management, (4) commitment to longitudinal care, (5) collaborative practice, (6) access to subspecialty palliative care, and (7) enhanced provider resilience. These principles provide the framework for educational and training initiatives, research, and support for resources at the health care system level.[28]

THE EXPANDING ROLE OF PEDIATRIC SURGICAL ONCOLOGISTS IN PALLIATIVE CARE

Pediatric surgical oncologists are involved at almost every phase of the cancer care continuum, from diagnosis and staging to the management of complications, symptom relief, and, not infrequently, EOL support.[3,19] Historically, surgeons were viewed primarily as technical experts; however, modern pediatric oncology requires surgeons to participate in shared decision-making, prognostication, and longitudinal care planning.[29] Surgical consultations often occur under emotionally charged conditions and within compressed timelines, making communication skills and the ability to elicit family values essential competencies.

GOALS OF SURGICAL TREATMENTS AND THEIR PALLIATIVE PURPOSES

Surgical interventions in pediatric oncology span a continuum from diagnosis and cure to symptom relief and facilitation of meaningful experiences near the end of life. Understanding the range of surgical goals and clarifying the intention behind each intervention is essential to ensure that treatments remain aligned with patient and family priorities.[2,25]

Diagnosis and Staging

Biopsies and staging procedures are critical to defining disease biology and planning therapy. Even at this early stage, surgeons lay the groundwork for rapport-building and values-based discussions.[16,29,30]

Curative or Palliative Resection

For many solid tumors, surgical resection remains a cornerstone of curative therapy. Although framed as curative, such surgeries may also provide palliative benefits by reducing tumor burden and improving function. The distinction between curative and palliative intent is therefore often fluid and should be explored explicitly with families.[3,31]

Management of Complications

Complications of cancer or its treatment, including intestinal obstruction or perforation, infection, hemorrhage, and device-related problems, may require operative or procedural intervention. These procedures frequently improve comfort and quality of life, even when they do not alter the disease trajectory.[20]

Symptom Relief

Procedures such as gastrostomy or gastrojejunostomy tube placement, diverting stomas, pleural or peritoneal drainage, tumor debulking, central venous access, or tracheostomy may directly target symptom relief. Evidence demonstrates that palliative surgical interventions can reduce pain, improve feeding and breathing, facilitate home care, and enable participation in age-appropriate activities.[29,32,33]

Facilitating Emotional, Functional, or Practical Goals

Some surgical interventions are performed to enable children and families to accomplish personal goals near the end of life, such as spending time at home, participating in meaningful activities, or enhancing interaction with loved ones.[34,35] For example, tracheostomy may allow a child to communicate more effectively, and gastrostomy may reduce the burden of repeated hospitalizations.[20]

Supporting Nonoperative Management

Even when surgery is not feasible or recommended, a surgical consultation may still provide value.[36] Families often wish to hear directly from surgeons about why an operation would not be beneficial, which may provide a sense of closure and confirm that *everything possible* was considered.[29,30]

PROGNOSTICATION, UNCERTAINTY, AND DECISION-MAKING IN PEDIATRIC SURGICAL ONCOLOGY

Prognostication in pediatric oncology is inherently challenging. Childhood cancers encompass a diverse group of diseases with variable trajectories, evolving therapies, and heterogeneous responses to treatment. Prognostic uncertainty complicates decision-making for families and clinicians, particularly when evaluating the potential benefits and burdens of surgical intervention. Prognostication in pediatric oncology involves assessing and predicting the future clinical course and outcomes for children diagnosed with cancer, using a range of clinical, pathologic, and increasingly sophisticated molecular and computational approaches.[37]

Surgeons contribute uniquely to prognostic discussions by integrating clinical data with firsthand knowledge of operative risks, recovery trajectories, and likely postoperative outcomes. Families frequently rely on surgeons to help them visualize what recovery may entail, whether an intervention could meaningfully change quality of life, and what outcomes might be unacceptable or overly burdensome.[29] Importantly, uncertainty should not be minimized. Explicit acknowledgment of what is known, what remains uncertain, and how decisions can be revisited over time supports trust and shared decision-making.

Communication frameworks such as the best case/worst case (BC/WC) model can help structure conversations around prognosis and potential surgical outcomes.[38] Originally developed in adult surgery, BC/WC has been effectively adapted for pediatrics and promotes presenting a *best possible*, *worst possible*, and *most likely* scenario to help families understand a range of outcomes without feeling coerced. This method also encourages surgeons to articulate the anticipated functional and emotional impacts of surgery, which are factors that matter deeply to children and caregivers.

In pediatric contexts, prognostic communication is iterative rather than a single event. As conditions evolve, surgeons and interdisciplinary teams must revisit goals of care and adjust recommendations accordingly. This approach honors family preferences, reduces decisional conflict, and ensures that interventions remain aligned with the child's and family's values.[6]

COMMUNICATION FRAMEWORKS FOR PEDIATRIC SURGEONS

High-quality communication is essential for effective pediatric surgical oncology care. Decisions about surgery often occur during periods of acute stress, heightened emotion, and evolving prognostic understanding. Despite this, communication skills have historically received limited emphasis in surgical training. Pediatric surgeons routinely deliver life-altering information, making structured, evidence-informed communication approaches indispensable.

Using Structured Serious-Illness Communication Models

Educational initiatives such as the Education in Palliative and End-of-Life Care–Pediatrics (EPEC-Pediatrics) curriculum demonstrate improved clinician knowledge, attitudes, and skills following structured PPC training. Participants consistently report greater confidence in communication, enhanced capacity for difficult conversations, and perceived improvements in institutional quality of care.[39] These findings reinforce the need to integrate PPC education into pediatric surgical training, as children receiving PPC frequently undergo one or more surgical procedures during their illness.[20]

These approaches support surgeons in: (1) Assessing family understanding, (2) Eliciting hopes and worries, (3) Responding empathetically to emotion, (4) Presenting information in digestible segments, and (5) Aligning treatment recommendations with family values.

The EPEC–Pediatrics (SICG) also offers validated prompts, for example, *"If your child's illness was to get worse, how much would s/he and you be willing to go through for the possibility of more time?*, to elicit values that can guide surgical decision-making and improve clinician's confidence in conducting difficult conversation with families of children living will serious illness.[40,41]

Five Cardinal Questions for Perioperative Assessment

Building on Joanne Wolfe's 5 cardinal questions,[42] pediatric surgical teams can use the following perioperative adaptations to understand family priorities quickly: (1) *What was your child like before s/he got sick*? (2) *What is your understanding of your child's illness and the role of this surgery*? (3) *What is most important to you and your child*? (4) *What are you hoping for from this surgery? What are your worries about this surgery*? (5) *Where is your source of strength in this situation*?

These questions deepen understanding of family motivations, clarify expectations, and support the identification of goal-concordant recommendations.

Responding to Emotion

Surgeons may hesitate to discuss patients' and families' emotions for fear that it may cause distress. Yet studies demonstrate that even brief empathic statements, such as *can see how much you care about your child* or *This sounds incredibly difficult*, significantly improve trust, reduce conflict, and strengthen therapeutic alliance.[6,20] Naming emotions directly (eg, *You seem worried*) validates families' experiences and builds rapport.

Incorporating these techniques requires practice. Simulation, role-play, and interdisciplinary teaching with PPC teams can reduce surgeon anxiety about difficult conversations and increase communication proficiency.

SPIRITUALITY, HOPE, AND MEANING IN SURGICAL ENCOUNTERS

Severe illness in a child often prompts profound existential, emotional, and spiritual questions for families and clinicians alike. Spirituality in pediatric palliative care is broad, encompassing sources of meaning, connection, purpose, and hope, and is not limited to religious belief. Families may simultaneously hope for a cure while preparing for possible decline, a duality that clinicians must recognize and support.[43]

Surgeons frequently encounter moments when families express fear, despair, or yearning for miracles. Rather than viewing these expressions as obstacles to decision-making, they can be understood as natural coping strategies. Acknowledging these emotional and spiritual dimensions, for example, *It sounds like your hope for more time is very strong, and I also hear how much you want your child to be comfortable,* helps families feel seen and supported.[6]

Balancing Hope and Realism

Pediatric oncology families often hold multiple simultaneous hopes: for a cure, for more time, for comfort, and for dignity.[44] Hope is not monolithic; adolescents, younger children, and parents may hold different hopes at different times. Surgeons can honor this complexity by exploring what families hope for *today*, in the context of updated prognostic information.[45]

Honest communication about prognosis is critical. Delaying discussions of likely outcomes can inadvertently increase invasive, nonbeneficial interventions near the end of life and limit opportunities for home time, memory-making, and symptom-focused care.[20] Providing compassionate realism, grounded in both medical facts and empathy, allows families to align their decisions with their deepest values.

Addressing Unfixable Suffering

Many stressors affect families (eg, financial hardship, caregiving strain, and housing insecurity) and fall outside the surgeon's direct control. Yet acknowledging these burdens and inviting interdisciplinary support (social work, psychology, spiritual care, and palliative care) reinforces that the family is not alone. Surgeons do not need to solve every problem; they need to recognize suffering, connect families to resources, and remain present.

END-OF-LIFE DISCUSSIONS

EOL discussions in pediatric surgical oncology require a balance of honesty, compassion, clinical expertise, and emotional attunement as families facing the imminent death of a child experience intense fear, anticipatory grief, and uncertainty. Surgeons, often viewed as authorities in cure-focused care, may struggle to shift toward conversations centered on comfort, dignity, and quality of life.[43]

Core Principles of Effective End-of-Life Communication

Successful EOL discussions share several components:

- Acknowledging emotions. Naming feelings, such as *I can see how heartbreaking this is,* helps families feel validated. Evidence shows that empathic statements decrease distress and increase trust.[6]
- Listening to family values and priorities. Asking families what they hope for and what they fear most provides critical insight into decision-making.
- Providing clear, compassionate medical information. EOL decision-making requires families to understand prognosis and realistic outcomes. Clarity prevents false hope and allows families to make informed choices aligned with their values.[46]
- Offering recommendations when appropriate. Families often feel overwhelmed and look to surgeons for guidance. Providing a recommendation, which can be framed as supportive rather than directive, can reduce decisional burden.
- Avoiding harmful or ambiguous language. Phrases like *withdraw care* or *nothing more we can do* can be interpreted as abandonment. Instead, clinicians can say, *We will always care for your child, and at this point, the focus is on comfort and being together.*

Timing of End-of-Life Discussions

EOL conversations should occur early enough to allow families time to process, plan, and engage meaningfully.[47] Early EOL discussions are associated with better goal-concordant care and improved preparedness.[26,48] Surgeons play a role in initiating or revisiting these conversations, especially when surgical options no longer offer meaningful benefit.

Interdisciplinary Support

EOL care is inherently multidisciplinary. Pediatric palliative care, social work, chaplaincy, child life, psychology, and ethics teams provide essential support. Therefore, pediatric surgeons need not carry the entire burden; instead, they can anchor communication within the broader care team to ensure consistent, coordinated messaging.

WHEN DOES IT END?

The relationships formed between pediatric surgeons, their patients, and families are unique, often intense, emotionally charged, and forged under extraordinary circumstances. Unlike many adult specialties, pediatric surgical oncology involves caring for children and families through prolonged diagnostic uncertainty, complex operations, recurrent hospitalizations, and, in some cases, the dying process. These relationships do not automatically end when surgical intervention ceases or when cure is no longer possible.[29]

Continuity, Closure, and the Surgeon–Family Relationship

When a child dies, families frequently look to the surgeon, who may have performed biopsies, resections, or palliative procedures, as an important part of the child's care. Many parents express appreciation when surgeons attend memorials, reach out with condolence messages, or acknowledge the child's life and the family's loss. Such gestures can facilitate healthy bereavement and reinforce that their child was known, valued, and remembered.[6]

For surgeons, staying connected with families after a child's death can also serve as a source of meaning and closure. Although these interactions can be emotionally challenging, they may protect against burnout and compassion fatigue by helping surgeons process grief, reflect on the care they provided, and reaffirm their purpose within pediatric medicine.[8]

Boundaries and Professionalism

Maintaining professional boundaries remains important. Surgeons differ in how they navigate postbereavement contact, and practices vary across institutions. However, families consistently report that follow-up and continued connection with their physicians and health care providers are important for their bereavement experience.[49,50] They want acknowledgment that their child mattered, that their suffering was witnessed, and that their health care team remembers them.

Team-Based Reflection

After a patient's death, interdisciplinary debriefings can help identify successes, missed opportunities, and opportunities for system-level improvement. These reflective practices also support clinicians' well-being and contribute to continuous quality improvement in palliative surgical care.[51]

OUTCOMES OF PALLIATIVE SURGERY IN CHILDREN WITH CANCER

Evidence increasingly demonstrates that palliative surgical interventions can offer meaningful benefits to children with serious illness. Contrary to long-held assumptions, palliative surgery does not inherently shorten survival, nor does it necessarily increase suffering. Instead, when aligned with family goals and integrated within interdisciplinary care, surgery may improve symptom control, enhance functional status, support home-based care, and even correlate with improved survival in some cohorts.[16,20]

Symptom Relief and Functional Improvement

Common palliative procedures, including gastrostomy or gastrojejunostomy tube placement, tumor debulking, pleural or peritoneal drainage, tracheostomy, and central venous catheter placement, can substantially improve quality of life. Benefits may include reduced pain, improved breathing or feeding, decreased hospitalization frequency, and increased ability to participate in developmentally meaningful activities.[29]

Facilitation of Home Time and Preferred Location of Care

For many families, particularly near the end of life, goals of care prioritize time at home. Procedures such as tracheostomy, gastrostomy, and tunneled drain placement can enable symptom management in home or hospice settings, reduce crisis-driven admissions, and facilitate memory-making.[43]

Survival Outcomes

A common misconception is that palliative surgery merely prolongs the dying process or adds burdens without benefits. Recent data counter this view. Ellis and colleagues reported that among pediatric patients receiving palliative care, those who underwent surgical interventions had longer survival than those who did not, even after adjusting for disease severity.[20] Although this does not imply that surgery directly increases survival, it highlights that palliative procedures often occur within broader care plans that support stability, symptom management, and improved caregiving capacity.

Alignment with Goals of Care

Outcomes of palliative surgery must be assessed not only through clinical metrics but also through family-centered measures such as comfort, communication, participation in milestones, and achievement of specific family goals. Even when life-prolongation is not possible, procedures can meaningfully enhance a child's final weeks or months.

COMPARISONS TO ADULT PALLIATIVE SURGERY

Palliative surgery in pediatrics differs fundamentally from adult practice due to developmental, prognostic, ethical, and psychosocial factors. Although both fields aim to relieve suffering and support quality of life, the guiding principles and clinical contexts diverge significantly.

Prognostic Complexity

Adult patients referred for palliative surgery often have advanced malignancies with relatively predictable trajectories. In contrast, children with life-limiting illnesses, whether oncologic, genetic, or congenital, may live for extended periods despite significant disease burden. Prognostication is therefore more uncertain, complicating decisions about when and whether to perform surgical intervention that aligns with long-term goals.[43]

Family-Centered Decision-Making

Whereas adult patients typically make autonomous decisions, pediatric decisions rely on parents or guardians acting as surrogate decision-makers within the *best interest* standard. This requires clinicians to support families as they balance hopes for a cure, desire to relieve suffering, and concerns about the long-term implications of procedures. Family management style, coping strategies, and cultural values play an important role in outcomes and decisional conflict, including discussion regarding EOL.[52]

Developmental Considerations

Children's developmental stages influence symptom expression, understanding of illness, and goals of care.[53] Child life specialists, psychologists, and educational supports are therefore integral to PPC, a model rarely mirrored in adult palliative surgery.[54] Many pediatric procedures aim not only to reduce symptoms but to preserve developmentally important activities such as play, communication, school engagement, and independence.[55]

Different Definitions of Benefit

In adult practice, palliative surgery is often considered when expected to prolong life or meaningfully improve function. In pediatrics, benefit may be defined more broadly: enabling a child to attend school, celebrate milestones, reduce caregiver burden, or spend time at home. These goals reflect the lived realities and family-centered priorities inherent to pediatric care.[6]

FUTURE DIRECTIONS

Integrating Palliative Care into Surgical Training

Formal palliative care competencies must be embedded into pediatric surgical residency and fellowship programs.[56] Communication skills, prognostication, symptom management, and shared decision-making are not optional. They are essential components of high-quality surgical care for children with serious illness. Curricula such as EPEC-Pediatrics, VitalTalk, and simulation-based training offer proven frameworks that should be adapted and adopted across surgical education.[39]

Enhancing Early and Longitudinal Pediatric Palliative Care Integration

PPC should be introduced at diagnosis for all children with cancer, regardless of prognosis.[57] Early involvement supports goal formation, reduces crisis-driven decision-making, and improves continuity. Standardizing referral pathways and embedding palliative clinicians within oncology and surgical teams can reduce variability and ensure consistent access.[6]

Developing Pediatric-Specific Decision Aids

Tools such as the BC/WC model require pediatric-specific adaptations that reflect developmental needs, surrogate decision-making, and the nuanced goals of childhood and adolescence. Visual aids, stories, and developmentally informed examples can help families better understand the likely impacts of surgical interventions.[38]

Advancing Multicenter Research

Large, prospective, multicenter studies are needed to define surgical outcomes, identify patient-centered metrics, and clarify which interventions provide meaningful benefit across disease trajectories. Standardized quality-of-life measures, including child-reported outcomes when feasible, are essential for building a robust evidence base.[16]

Promoting Global Equity in Pediatric Palliative Care Access

Efforts must address global disparities in palliative care availability, opioid access, and trained interdisciplinary teams, as countries with lower income also have poorer access to PPC.[58] Programs should support capacity building in low-resource settings and advocate for policy changes that ensure children receive equitable, compassionate care regardless of geography.[43,59]

Addressing Social Determinants and Ensuring Inclusive Care

Future work must prioritize equity, diversity, and inclusion across PPC and surgical oncology. Studies show that socioeconomic stressors profoundly shape outcomes and care experiences. Tailored supports such as family navigation, financial assistance, and culturally sensitive communication are critical for overcoming structural barriers.[60]

Supporting Clinician Well-being

Pediatric palliative surgical oncology can be emotionally taxing. Institutions should provide structured debriefings, access to mental health resources, mentorship, and protected time for reflection, all of which support resilience and reduce burnout.

Healthy clinicians are better positioned to deliver compassionate, high-quality care.[28,39]

SUMMARY

Pediatric palliative surgical oncology lies at a vital intersection of surgery, oncology, and palliative care. Children with cancer and their families navigate a landscape marked by uncertainty, intensive treatments, and profound emotional challenges. Pediatric surgeons can play a central role in this journey, not only as technical experts but as communicators, partners, advocates, and witnesses.

Integrating palliative principles throughout the continuum of care, which begins at diagnosis and extends beyond the end of life, ensures that surgical recommendations remain aligned with family priorities, developmental needs, and the child's lived experience. Evidence increasingly demonstrates that palliative surgery can offer substantial benefits when guided by thoughtful communication, interdisciplinary collaboration, and clear goals of care.

As research grows, training evolves, and systems strengthen globally, pediatric surgical oncologists are uniquely positioned to advance a model of care that both alleviates suffering and honors the humanity of every child and family they serve. The future of the field rests in our collective commitment to compassionate, goal-concordant, and scientifically grounded care.

CLINICS CARE POINTS

- Introduce pediatric palliative care early, ideally at diagnosis, not at end-of-life; early integration improves symptom control, family satisfaction, and survival in some cohorts.
- Clarify and revisit the intent of every surgical intervention with the family; palliative procedures can improve comfort and enable home-based care without shortening lives.
- Use structured frameworks like Best Case/Worse Case to elicit values and align recommendations; avoid phrases such as "withdraw care" that families may interpret as abandonment.
- The surgeon-family relationship continues beyond the child's death; condolence outreach, funeral or memorial attendance, and team debriefing support bereavement and clinician resilience.

DECLARATION OF AI AND AI-ASSISTED TECHNOLOGIES IN THE WRITING PROCESS

During the preparation of this work the authors used Gen AI. After using this tool/service, the authors reviewed and edited the content as needed and takes full responsibility for the content of the publication.

REFERENCES

1. Siegel RL, Miller KD, Fuchs HE, et al. Cancer statistics, 2022. CA Cancer J Clin 2022;72:7–33.
2. Inserra A, Narciso A, Paolantonio G, et al. Palliative care and pediatric surgical oncology. Semin Pediatr Surg 2016;25:323–32.
3. Le HD, Braungart S, Shalkow-Klincovstein J, et al. Roles of pediatric surgeons in palliative pediatric oncology. Pediatr Blood Cancer 2025;72(Suppl 2):e31354.
4. Wolfe J, Grier HE, Klar N, et al. Symptoms and suffering at the end of life in children with cancer. N Engl J Med 2000;342:326–33.

5. Organization WH. In: Organization WH, editor. Integrating palliative care and symptom relief into paediatrics: a WHO guide for health care planners, implementers and managers. Geneva: Licence: CC BY-NC-SA 3.0 IGO; 2018.
6. Widger K, Medeiros C, Trenholm M, et al. Indicators used to assess the impact of specialized pediatric palliative care: a scoping review. J Palliat Med 2019;22:199–219.
7. Chelazzi C, Villa G, Lanini I, et al. The adult and pediatric palliative care: differences and shared issues. J Anesth Analg Crit Care 2023;3(1).
8. Section on Hospice and Palliative Medicine and Committee on Hospital Care. Pediatric palliative care and hospice care commitments, guidelines, and recommendations. Pediatrics 2013;132:966–72.
9. Kaye EC, Weaver MS, DeWitt LH, et al. The impact of specialty palliative care in pediatric oncology: a systematic review. J Pain Symptom Manage 2021;61:1060–79.e2.
10. Wolfe J, Hammel JF, Edwards KE, et al. Easing of suffering in children with cancer at the end of life: is care changing? J Clin Oncol 2008;26:1717–23.
11. Schmidt P, Otto M, Hechler T, et al. Did increased availability of pediatric palliative care lead to improved palliative care outcomes in children with cancer? J Palliat Med 2013;16:1034–9.
12. Green DJ, Bennett E, Olson LM, et al. Timing of pediatric palliative care consults in hospitalized patients with heart disease. J Pediatr Intensive Care 2023;12:63–70.
13. Massie AM, Ebelhar J, Allen KE, et al. Defining and timing of palliative opportunities in children with central nervous system tumors. Neurooncol Pract 2021;8:451–9.
14. Rossfeld ZM, Miller R, Fosselman DD, et al. Timing of palliative consultation for children during a fatal illness. Hosp Pediatr 2019;9:373–8.
15. Ellis D, Mazzola E, Wolfe J, et al. Comparing pediatric surgeons' and palliative care pediatricians' palliative care practices and perspectives in pediatric surgical patients. J Pediatr Surg 2024;59:37–44.
16. Ellis DI, Chen L, Gordon Wexler S, et al. Goals of surgical interventions in youths receiving palliative care. JAMA Netw Open 2024;7:e2444072.
17. Goudreault M, Humbert N, Gauvin F, et al. Interventions in the operating room for children near end of life: a multidisciplinary approach. J Pediatr Surg 2018;53:1065–8.
18. Corkum KS, Lautz TB, Hebal FN, et al. Procedural burden experienced by children with cancer during their terminal hospital admission. J Pediatr Surg 2019;54:133–9.
19. Ellis DI, Chen L, Wexler SG, et al. Mapping surgical intervention trajectories in seriously ill children receiving palliative care. J Pediatr Surg 2025;60:161905.
20. Ellis DI, Nye RT, Wolfe J, et al. Surgical intervention in patients receiving pediatric palliative care services. Pediatrics 2023;151.
21. Downing J, Ling J, Benini F, et al. A summary of the EAPC white paper on core competencies for education in paediatric palliative care. European Journal of Palliative Care 2014;21:245–9.
22. Benini F, Papadatou D, Bernada M, et al. International standards for pediatric palliative care: from IMPaCCT to GO-PPaCS. J Pain Symptom Manage 2022;63:e529–43.
23. Marterre B, Kopecky K, Miller P. Primary palliative care for surgeons: a narrative review and synthesis of core competencies. Ann Palliat Med 2022;11:885–906.
24. Navaneethan H. Pediatric palliative care. Pediatric Care Online; 2024.

25. Shelton J, Jackson GP. Palliative care and pediatric surgery. Surg Clin North Am 2011;91:419–28.ix.
26. Marcus KL, Santos G, Ciapponi A, et al. Impact of specialized pediatric palliative care: a systematic review. J Pain Symptom Manage 2020;59:339–64.e10.
27. Halix SJ, Porter AS, Robbins AJ, et al. What pediatric palliative care offers to pediatric surgeons. J Pediatr Surg 2025;60:162127.
28. Halix SJ, Robbins AJ, Cameron DB, et al. Principles of pediatric palliative surgical oncology: a guide to palliative care for pediatric surgeons. Ann Surg 2024;281(2): 215–8.
29. Ott KC, Vente TM, Lautz TB, et al. Pediatric palliative care and surgery. Ann Palliat Med 2022;11:918–26.
30. Carlisle EM, Shinkunas LA, Lieberman MT, et al. Empowering parents of pediatric surgical oncology patients through collaborative engagement with surgeons. J Pediatr Surg 2023;58:1736–43.
31. Snaman J, McCarthy S, Wiener L, et al. Pediatric palliative care in oncology. J Clin Oncol 2020;38:954–62.
32. Hawkins CM, Gill AE. Introduction to interventional radiology's role in palliative care for children with cancer: a COG Diagnostic Imaging Committee/SPR Oncology Committee White Paper. Pediatr Blood Cancer 2023;70(Suppl 4): e30238.
33. Burlo F, Bortolin I, Grasso DL, et al. Safety and feasibility of tracheostomy and gastrostomy home replacement: a five-year experience from a palliative care center. Front Pediatr 2025;13:1644830.
34. Adams J, Auger J, Schiff D. Outcome of indwelling tunneled PleurX(R) catheter placement in pediatric and young adult patients with malignant effusions. Pediatr Blood Cancer 2014;61:1118–20.
35. den Hollander BS, Connolly BL, Sung L, et al. Successful use of indwelling tunneled catheters for the management of effusions in children with advanced cancer. Pediatr Blood Cancer 2014;61:1007–12.
36. Louie AD, Miner TJ. Palliative surgery and the surgeon's role in the palliative care team: a review. Ann Palliat Med 2022;11:907–17.
37. Varga P, Obeidat M, Mate V, et al. From simple factors to artificial intelligence: evolution of prognosis prediction in childhood cancer: a systematic review and meta-analysis. EClinicalMedicine 2024;78:102902.
38. Taylor LJ, Nabozny MJ, Steffens NM, et al. A framework to improve surgeon communication in high-stakes surgical decisions: best case/worst case. JAMA Surg 2017;152:531–8.
39. Postier AC, Wolfe J, Hauser J, et al. Education in palliative and end-of-life care-pediatrics: curriculum use and dissemination. J Pain Symptom Manage 2022; 63:349–58.
40. Ardiadne Labs. Serious illness conversation guide. 2023. Available at: https://www.ariadnelabs.org/wp-content/uploads/2023/05/Serious-Illness-Conversation-Guide.2023-05-18.pdf.
41. van Breemen C, Lusney N, Doherty M, et al. Education initiative for essential conversations with parents-serious illness guide for pediatrics (SICG-Peds(c)-Peds). J Med Educ Curric Dev 2024;11:23821205241298590.
42. Wolfe J. Pediatric palliative care is a social issue. Courageous Parents Network; 2015.
43. Salins N, Hughes S, Preston N. Palliative care in paediatric oncology: an update. Curr Oncol Rep 2022;24:175–86.

44. Sisk BA, Kang TI, Mack JW. Sources of parental hope in pediatric oncology. Pediatr Blood Cancer 2018;65:e26981.
45. Feudtner C. The breadth of hopes. N Engl J Med 2009;361(2).
46. van Breemen C, Johnston J, Carwana M, et al. Serious illness conversations in pediatrics: a case review. Children (Basel) 2020;7.
47. Marsac ML, Kindler C, Weiss D, et al. Let's talk about it: supporting family communication during end-of-life care of pediatric patients. J Palliat Med 2018; 21:862–78.
48. Ullrich CK, Lehmann L, London WB, et al. End-of-Life care patterns associated with pediatric palliative care among children who underwent hematopoietic stem cell transplant. Biol Blood Marrow Transplant 2016;22:1049–55.
49. Lichtenthal WG, Sweeney CR, Roberts KE, et al. Bereavement follow-up after the death of a child as a standard of care in pediatric oncology. Pediatr Blood Cancer 2015;62(Suppl 5):S834–69.
50. Snaman JM, Kaye EC, Torres C, et al. Helping parents live with the hole in their heart: the role of health care providers and institutions in the bereaved parents' grief journeys. Cancer 2016;122:2757–65.
51. Friedrichsdorf SJ, Remke S, Hauser J, et al. Development of a pediatric palliative care curriculum and dissemination model: education in palliative and end-of-life care (EPEC) pediatrics. J Pain Symptom Manage 2019;58:707–20.e3.
52. Kenney AE, Bedoya SZ, Gerhardt CA, et al. End of life communication among caregivers of children with cancer: a qualitative approach to understanding support desired by families. Palliat Support Care 2021;19:715–22.
53. Michelson KN, Steinhorn DM. Pediatric end-of-life issues and palliative care. Clin Pediatr Emerg Med 2007;8:212–9.
54. Thompson AL, Kentor RA, Schaefer MR, et al. Psychologists as pivotal members of the pediatric palliative care team. J Pain Symptom Manage 2024;67:e907–13.
55. Boucher S, Downing J, Shemilt R. The role of play in children's palliative care. Children (Basel) 2014;1:302–17.
56. Istl AC, Johnston FM. Role of palliative medicine training in surgical oncology. Surg Oncol Clin N Am 2021;30:591–608.
57. Levine DR, Mandrell BN, Sykes A, et al. Patients' and parents' needs, attitudes, and perceptions about early palliative care integration in pediatric oncology. JAMA Oncol 2017;3:1214–20.
58. McNeil MJ, Ehrlich B, Wang H, et al. Ideal vs actual timing of palliative care integration for children with cancer in Latin America. JAMA Netw Open 2023;6: e2251496.
59. Siddiqui MF, Nohra L, Saleh M, et al. Pediatric oncology, palliative care and low- or middle- income countries: a call for action. Glob Pediatr Health 2023;10: 2333794X231188591.
60. Boyden JY, Umaretiya PJ, D'Souza L, et al. Disparities in pediatric palliative care: where are we and where do we go from here? J Pediatr 2024;275:114194.

United States Postal Service

Statement of Ownership, Management and Circulation
(All Periodicals Publications Except Requester Publications)

1. Publication Title: SURGICAL ONCOLOGY CLINICS OF NORTH AMERICA	2. Publication Number: 0 1 2 - 5 6 5	3. Filing Date: 08/24/2026
4. Issue Frequency: JAN, APR, JUL, OCT	5. Number of Issues Published Annually: 4	6. Annual Subscription Price: $351.00

7. Complete Mailing Address of Known Office of Publication (Not printer) (Street, city, county, state, and ZIP+4)
Addr 1: Elsevier INC
Addr 2: 230 Park Ave Ste 800
City, State ZIP: New York NY 10169
Contact Person: Mohana Priya Damodharan
Telephone: 91-44-4299-4077

8. Complete Mailing Address of Headquarters or General Business Office of Publisher (Not Printer)
Addr 1: Elsevier INC
Addr 2: 230 Park Ave Ste 800
City, State ZIP: New York NY 10169

9. Full Names and Complete Mailing Addresses of Publisher, Editor and Managing Editor (do not leave blank)
Publisher (Name and complete mailing address)
Name: Dolores Meloni, ELSEVIER INC.
Addr 1: 1600 JOHN F KENNEDY BLVD. SUITE 1600
Addr 2:
City, State ZIP: PHILADELPHIA, PA 19103-2899

Editor (Name and complete mailing address)
Name: ASHLIE JACKMAN, ELSEVIER INC.
Addr 1: 1ST FLOOR, NIELSEN HOUSE, JOHN SMITH DRIVE, OXFORD, OX4 2WB, UK
Addr 2:
City, State ZIP: PHILADELPHIA, PA 19103-2899

Managing Editor (Name and complete mailing address)
Name: PATRICK MANLEY, ELSEVIER INC.
Addr 1: 1600 JOHN F KENNEDY BLVD. SUITE 1600
Addr 2:
City, State ZIP: PHILADELPHIA, PA 19103-2899

10. Owner (Do not leave blank. If the publication is owned by a corporation, give the name and address of the corporation immediately followed by the names and addresses of all stockholders owning or holding 1 percent or more of the total amount of stock. If not owned by a corporation, give the names and addresses of all the individual owners. If owned by a partnership or other unincorporated firm, give its name and address as well as those of each individual owner. If the publication is published by a nonprofit organization, give its name and address.)

Full Name	Complete Mailing Address
WHOLLY OWNED SUBSIDIARY OF REED/ELSEVIER,	1600 JOHN F KENNEDY BLVD. SUITE 1600
US HOLDINGS	PHILADELPHIA, PA 19103-2899

11. Known Bondholders, Mortgagees, and Other Security Holders Owning or Holding 1 Percent or more of Total Amount of Bonds, Mortgages, or Other Securities. If none, check box → None

Full Name	Complete Mailing Address
NA	

12. Tax Status (For completion by nonprofit organizations authorized to mail at nonprofit rates) (Check one)
The purpose, function, and nonprofit status of this organization and the exempt status for federal income tax purposes:
[X] Has Not changed During Preceding 12 Months
[ ] Has Changed During Preceding 12 Months (Publisher must submit explanation of change with this statement below)

PS Form 3526, July 2014

13. Publication Title: SURGICAL ONCOLOGY CLINICS OF NORTH AMERICA
14. Issue Date for Circulation Data Below: October 2026

15. Extent and Nature of Circulation		Average No. Copies Each Issue During Preceding 12 Months	No. Copies of Single Issue Published Nearest to filing Date
a. Total Number of Copies (Net press run)		72	71
b. Paid and/or Requested Circulation	(1) Mailed Outside-County Paid Subscriptions Stated on PS Form 3541 (Include paid distribution above nominal rate, advertiser's proof copies, and exchange copies)	43	44
	(2) Mailed In-County Paid Subscriptions Stated on PS Form 3541 (Include paid distribution above nominal rate, advertiser's proof copies, and exchange copies)	0	0
	(3) Paid Distribution Outside the Mails Including Sales Through Dealers and Carriers, Street Vendors, Counter Sales, and Other Paid Distribution Ouside USPS	18	16
	(4) Paid Distribution by Other Classes of Mail Through the USPS (e.g. First-Class Mail)	11	11
c. Total Paid Distribution [Sum of 15b. (1), (2), (3), and (4)] ▶		72	71
d. Free or Nominal Rate Distribution (By Mail and Outside the Mail)	(1) Free or Nominal Rate Outside-County Copies Included on PS Form 3541	0	0
	(2) Free or Nominal In-County Copies Included on PS Form 3541	0	0
	(3) Free or Nominal Rate Copies Mailed at Other Classes Through the USPS (e.g. First-Class Mail)	0	0
	(4) Free or Nominal Rate Distribution Outside the Mail (Carriers or other means)	0	0
e. Total Free or Nominal Rate Distribution (Sum of 15d. (1), (2), (3) and (4)) ▶		0	0
f. Total Distribution (Sum of 15c. and 15e.) ▶		72	71
g. Copies not Distributed (See Instructions to Publishers #4 (page #3))		0	0
h. Total (Sum of 15f. and g.) ▶		72	71
i. Percent Paid (15c. Divided by 15f. Times 100) ▶		100.00%	100.00%

* if you are claiming electronic copies, go to line 16 on page 3. If you are not claiming electronic copies, skip to line 17 on page 3.

16. Electronic copy Circulation		
If present, check box →		
a. Paid Electronic Copies		
b. Total Paid Print Copies (Line 15c) + Paid Electronic Copies (Line 16a) ▶	72	71
c. Total Print Distribution (Line 15F) + Paid Electronic Copies (Line 16a) ▶	72	71
d. Percentage Paid (Both Print & Electronic Copies (16b divided bt 16c x 100) ▶	100.00%	100.00%

[X] I certify that 50% of all my distribution copies (electronic and Print) are paid above a nominal price

17. Publication of Statement of Ownership
[X] Publication required. Will be printed in the **October 2026** issue of this publication. [ ] Publication not required

18. Signature and Title of Editor, Publisher, Business Manager, or Owner: **Mohana Priya Damodharan** Title: **Distribution Controller** Date: 8/24/2026

I certify that all information furnished on this form is true and complete. I understand that anyone who furnishes false or misleading information on this form or who omits material or information requested on the form may be subject to criminal sanctions (including fines and imprisonment) and/or civil sanctions (including civil penalties)

PS Form 3526, July 2014

9780443432286